*Running as Therapy: An Integrated Approach* examines both the psychology of running and the use of running as a mode of psychotherapy. Sixteen authors, including psychologists, psychiatrists, and professors of physical education, provide the most recent findings in research and clinical practice about what can and cannot be expected of running as therapy. This is the first book to address directly running as therapy in an organized, systematic, and thorough fashion.

After explaining the rationale for the use of running as therapy, the authors outline specific programs that can be prescribed and discuss how different approaches can be applied to different groups (such as women or children) and different problems (depression, anxiety). The book is directed to practitioners who want to know why, how, and when to use this therapeutic technique and to researchers who want to know how the effectiveness of the therapy has been measured and what results have been obtained. It is written to be accessible to the many men and women who run for health or pleasure.

The authors also explore important topics in the psychology of running, of interest to runners and therapists alike: addiction to running, the personality of the runner, the ''runner's high,'' and cognitive strategies used during running. They critically review the research literature on the psychology and therapeutics of running, and a selected bibliography of major books and articles gives access to a body of research that is widely dispersed across many scientific disciplines. The book is a state-of-the-art presentation of what running can do to solve certain kinds of psychological problems (stress, anxiety) or remove their troublesome symptoms (headaches, fatigue). It presents a form of therapy which, if guided by professional help, can be an effective and inexpensive alternative to analysis or drugs.

Michael L. Sachs is a research project coordinator at the University of Maryland School of Medicine. From 1979 to 1983 he was editor of *The Running Psychologist*. Gary W. Buffone is a psychologist in private practice in Jacksonville, Florida.

EDITED BY
MICHAEL L. SACHS AND GARY W. BUFFONE

# Running as Therapy

## An Integrated Approach

UNIVERSITY OF NEBRASKA PRESS
LINCOLN AND LONDON

Copyright 1984 by
the University of Nebraska Press
All rights reserved
Manufactured in the United States
of America

The paper in this book meets the
guidelines for permanence
and durability of the Committee on
Production Guidelines for
Book Longevity of the Council on
Library Resources.

Library of Congress Cataloging
in Publication Data

Main entry under title:

Running as therapy.

Includes bibliographical
references and index.
1. Running – Therapeutic use.
2. Psychotherapy.
I. Sachs, Michael L.
II. Buffone, Gary W., 1951-
[DNLM: 1. Running.
2. Psychotherapy. 3. Psychology.
QT 260 R943]
RC489.R86R86 1984
616.89'1653    83-10342
ISBN 0-8032-4139-9

# Contents

By chase our long-liv'd fathers earn'd their food;
Toil strung the nerves and purified the blood;
But we, their sons, a pamper'd race of men,
Are dwindled down to threescore years and ten.
Better to hunt in fields for health unbought
Than fee the doctor for a nauseous draught.
The wise for cure on exercise depend;
God never made his work for man to mend.

JOHN DRYDEN

# Introduction

# Running Therapy and Psychology

The therapeutic effects of physical activity have been recognized for centuries, and the use of exercise—particularly running—in psychotherapy has been drawing great interest over the past five years. According to various accounts (see Eischens and Greist, chap. 3, and Kostrubala, chap. 7) the roots of this approach are only ten to fifteen years old, but as early as 1905 Franz and Hamilton published a paper dealing with the effects of exercise in "retarding" depression. This paper is rarely cited, however, and does not appear to have influenced recent developments in the therapeutic use of exercise. The attention currently given to exercise and running as therapy in the popular, research, and applied literatures suggests that its relative newness is matched by great interest and excitement.

Running is virtually the only exercise discussed in this book and in the literature on exercise therapy. Generally, aerobic (meaning "with oxygen," so that oxygen uptake balances need for oxygen), rhythmic, continuous activities such as running, swimming, bicycling, and walking are most effective as therapy. Anaerobic ("without oxygen") activities, which usually involve discontinuous action (as in tennis and basketball), are considered less effective. In this book the term *running therapy,* rather than *exercise therapy,* will be used most of the time, though other forms of exercise, particularly other aerobic activities, may prove effective in therapeutic situations. Let us emphasize that running is not for everyone, for physical or psychological reasons. For example, brisk walking—another aerobic activity—may be better suited for many individuals. Running, of course, can be done at various speeds, and we do not distinguish here between jogging and running.

### What is Running Therapy?

*Running therapy* is the use of running as a mode of psychotherapy, alone or more frequently as an adjunct to other modes of therapy, by a trained mental health professional to promote physical or psychological adjustment (or both). This supervision by a professional, with specific therapeutic goals in mind, distinguishes running therapy from simpler forms of running.

### When is Running Therapy Used?

Aerobic running as therapy has a wide range of applications, from specific clinical uses in treating phobias to the general treatment of depression and anxiety. This work is reviewed in several chapters in this book, particularly Buffone (chap. 1) and Berger (chap. 9).

### What is the History of Running Therapy?

Although Franz and Hamilton reported using exercise as therapy almost eighty years ago, the use of running is more recent. Greist has used running in therapy for more than fifteen years (see Eischens and Greist, chap. 3). The work of Orwin dates to the early 1970s, and Kostrubala presented one of the first written expositions on the subject in his 1976 book *The Joy of Running* (see also Kostrubala, chap. 7). Kostrubala assembled his first running therapy group in March 1973.

Since the mid-1970s interest in running as therapy has increased exponentially. The references listed in part 1 and in the selected bibliography (part 3) illustrate this growth, and a considerable number of doctoral dissertations have also been conducted in this area (Sachs and Buffone 1982). The existence of this book reflects the interest in and need for knowledge about this rapidly growing area of therapy.

### How Many Therapists Use Running in Their Practice?

Although the organization called Running Psychologists (see the introduction to part 3 for more on this group) has many names on its mailing list, not all are running therapists. It is likely that many therapists incorporate some form of physical activity (most likely walking) in their practice, but the number who would say that running forms an integral component of their therapeutic approach is impossible to estimate accurately. There probably are more therapists who run than who use running to treat patients (they may be using running as "self-therapy").

### Need One Be Certified to Practice Running Therapy?

No particular certification is required to use running in therapy. It is at the disposal of any therapist. There may be a need to establish a governing body to develop and implement ethical and professional guidelines for this approach, as has happened with many other therapeutic techniques.

In 1979/80 the International Association of Running Therapists (IART) was founded. IART trained health professionals (psychiatrists, psychologists, teachers, nurses, etc.) for certification as running therapists and promoted noncompetitive running as a means of improving mental and physical health. The group is no longer in existence, but similar associations may develop again in the future.

### What is the State of the Art of Running Therapy?

Running therapy has many proponents, and several approaches to incorporating running in therapy have been presented (see part 1). Although it may seem relatively simple, using running in therapy is fairly complicated. Running therapy incorporates the basic prescription of exercise for a given individual with a particular clinical problem. A patient must gradually develop a capacity for running if therapeutic effects are to result, but running may be contraindicated for some, perhaps because of physical problems or medication. Furthermore, running, like any other therapeutic approach, has not been demonstrated to be effective with all mental illnesses—for example, depression (see Eischens and Greist, chap. 3, for more on this subject).

The therapist must decide whether running therapy is likely to be effective with a given individual and problem, see that the client obtains medical clearance, and decide whether to use running alone or in combination with other therapies. Although we have case studies and reports on running therapy, with numerous examples in part 1, no guidelines for using running in specific therapeutic situations are yet available.

### What Is the State of the Need in Running Therapy?

More high-quality research and practice is needed to clarify the particular parameters within which running can be effective therapy. Three areas must be emphasized.

First, for which emotional problems will running therapy be effective? Preliminary research has shown running to be effective with such common clinical problems as anxiety and depression, specifically state anxiety and mild to moderate depression. But there is little evidence that running significantly alters trait anxiety levels, more severe chronic depression, or affective disorders such as bipolar illness.

Although anecdotal reports and exploratory studies have indicated that running therapy may also be effective in treating substance abuse (alcoholism and drug addiction) and phobic conditions, some questions remain. Would running therapy be effective with such problems as obsessive-compulsive neurosis and specific phobic disorders, schizophrenia and other psychoses, psychosexual problems, and the prevalent personality disturbances? Although exercise may in some way ameliorate these conditions, there is at present little evidence for such effectiveness, and a running treatment may even exacerbate certain clinical problems if poorly managed (e.g., severe depression, schizoid or obsessive-compulsive personality disorder).

Second, given individual differences in therapeutic approaches, what basic guidelines can be offered concerning use of running as therapy? Very few guidelines are available other than those presented in part 1 (see in particular chaps. 2, 3, and 4). We do seem to know the correct prescription for exercise in terms of what intensity, duration, and frequency produce a therapeutic effect, but that is where our knowledge ends. Considering the intrapersonal factors (cognitions, affects, biochemical changes) and interpersonal factors (therapist, therapeutic relationship) inherent in running therapy, it is difficult to determine exactly what produces the desired outcomes, especially when a running program is combined with other therapies.

The final question concerns whether running is more effective when it is the sole therapeutic mode or when it is combined with other therapies in a comprehensive treatment program. But can a running treatment be "purely" administered? The available information suggests that, even when running therapy is used alone, nonspecific treatment factors come into play. Much of the work conducted thus far has combined running with other methods of therapy (e.g., cognitive-behavioral, psychodynamic). Assuming that most clinical problems do not manifest themselves in a single part of a patient's system (e.g., cognitively, affectively, or behaviorally), multiple interventions directed at more than one area of the patient's functioning are likely to be more effective than a single intervention. This is discussed further by Buffone in chapters 1 and 12.

## What Is the Role of the Psychology of Running in This Book?

It is important to be aware of psychological aspects of the running experience—in particular, addiction to running, the effect of exercise on personality, the "runner's high," the mind of the runner (cognitive strategies used during running), and research in the psychology and therapeutics of running. At present, running therapy is in its infancy, and only through careful scientific nurturing can we hope to assist in its development into a respected and mature approach.

We would like to acknowledge the encouragement and support of several people, particularly Dr. Bonnie G. Berger of Brooklyn College. M. Paul Laurin and the University of Quebec at Trois-Rivières were generous in providing financial support for work related to the book. In addition, the evaluations by two anonymous reviewers aided greatly in the refinement of the final work. It would have been impossible, as well, to complete this book without the continued loving support of our wives, Fay Sachs and Norma Buffone, who helped so very much.

MICHAEL L. SACHS

GARY W. BUFFONE

## References

Franz, S. I., and Hamilton, G. V. 1905. The effects of exercise upon the retardation in conditions of depression. *American Journal of Insanity* 62: 239–56.

Kostrubala, T. 1976. *The joy of running*. Philadelphia: J. B. Lippincott.

Orwin, A. 1973. "The running treatment": A preliminary communication on a new use for an old treatment (physical activity) in the agoraphobic syndrome. *British Journal of Psychiatry* 122: 175–79.

———. 1974. Treatment of a situational phobia: A case for running. *British Journal of Psychiatry* 125: 95–98.

Sachs, M. L., and Buffone, G. W. 1982. Bibliography: Psychological considerations in exercise, including exercise as psychotherapy, exercise dependence (exercise addiction), and the psychology of running. Unpublished manuscript, Université du Québec à Trois-Rivières.

# Part 1

---

# Running as Therapy

# Introduction

There is increasing public concern with the cost and quality of mental health care in the United States, and attention is being given to methods of treatment that are proving cost-effective. Running provides therapists with a natural form of psychotherapy that is practical, time-efficient, and inexpensive, since it requires less professional participation. This becomes more and more important as the spiraling cost of health care reinforces the current trend toward cost-effectiveness and accountability in therapy.

The purpose of part 1 is to encourage dialogue among researchers and clinicians who are using running therapy to treat mental health problems by having a number of such workers share their ideas and experiences. We hope to offer a better understanding and appreciation of a diverse and sometimes controversial field.

Considering the prevalence of clinical depression and its apparent amenability to exercise treatments, we have devoted several chapters to this topic. The first chapter, by Gary W. Buffone, addresses some commonly asked questions concerning the use of running in the treatment of depression. Buffone includes such issues as the advantages of a running treatment, methodological problems, possible causes of improvement, factors common to running and to "pure" forms of psychotherapy, the use of running as adjunct or primary treatment, running therapy with or without a therapist's direct involvement, contraindications, and the rates of depression for runners versus nonrunners.

The second chapter, by Bonnie G. Berger, presents running strategies for women and men interested in running or for therapists considering running as a therapeutic tool. Berger discusses intensity, duration, frequency, developing endurance, keeping a running log, making running enjoyable, and contraindications to running as well as providing material on the therapist as runner. This chapter provides a base for using running as therapy and for understanding the programs employed in subsequent chapters.

Roger R. Eischens and John H. Greist combine their experience and knowledge in chapter 3, on beginning and continuing running, further developing and expanding upon the base presented in chapter 2. They furnish a comprehensive guide to developing and maintaining a running therapy program, a guide that can be used by either the therapist or the client. This program, written for beginners, has been used over the past fifteen years with only an 11 percent attrition rate in recent years. Eischens and Greist follow this introduction by sharing the basis of their success in using running to treat depression. They present several guiding principles for using running therapy with depressed patients and offer two alternative treatment plans for different types of depressed individuals that can be used with minimal professional supervision.

Frederick D. Harper, in chapter 4, offers a form of running therapy he calls "jogotherapy." He stresses the need for delineating specific, measurable treatment goals. Some of the clinical problems he suggests are amenable to jogotherapy include alcoholism, anxiety, depression, and obesity. Harper also discusses the role of the psychotherapist in jogotherapy.

In chapter 5 Jaylene Summers and Henry Wolstat discuss their program of "creative running." They relate this approach to the blossoming holistic health model and note a number of psychological techniques they have found useful in training runners in therapy. They also discuss the clinical application of running in psychotherapy and provide a number of case examples.

In chapter 6 Michael H. Sacks presents a psychoanalytic perspective on running that attempts to understand motivation by exploring the runner's unconscious. He explores in detail the antidepressant effects of running, including a number of case examples. In some people running may serve as a creative means of dealing with conflict and learning about the self.

In chapter 7 Thaddeus Kostrubala presents a synthesis of his experiences with running as therapy. Kostrubala was one of the first to effectively use running in this way, and he includes a number of case reports. His coverage ranges from anthropology to neurochemistry.

A population rarely addressed in the running therapy literature, yet of considerable interest and importance, is children. W. Mark Shipman, in chapter 8, discusses the emotional and behavioral effects that long-distance running has on children. He suggests that over time long-distance running generates changes within the runner that overflow into the surrounding community. Running programs appear to be accompanied by increasing enthusiasm, a sense of creativity, and optimism.

In chapters 9 and 10 Bonnie G. Berger addresses special concerns in running and running therapy, particularly directed toward women but relevant to men as well. These chapters are written for psychologists, psychiatrists, and other practitioners of behavioral medicine. In chapter 9 Berger evaluates experimental literature dealing with the value of running for treating anxiety and depression. Chapter 10 discusses the use of running to enhance psychological well-being, particularly self-esteem and self-concept. Chapter 9 focuses on correcting psychological deficits; chapter 10, on attaining optimal psychological health.

As many clinicians have realized, exercise therapy may produce improvement, but *adherence* to the exercise program is crucial if improvement is to continue beyond formal treatment. Gary W. Buffone, Michael L. Sachs, and E. Thomas Dowd, in chapter 11, present cognitive-behavioral strategies for maintaining exercise behavior. They review recent advances in behavioral maintenance strategies and discuss their applicability to exercise, and they present specific cognitive, behavioral, and social techniques that can be used to modify and sustain exercise participation.

To complete part 1, Gary W. Buffone presents his observations on the state of running or exercise therapy and proposes possible future directions. He discusses the current state of research and theory, the limitations of this approach, assessment and treatment, implications for practitioners, and the application of running therapy to special populations.

GARY W. BUFFONE

# 1

# Running and Depression

Depression has been referred to as the "common cold" of emotional disorders because it is so frequent in clients presenting themselves for psychotherapy. Depression ranks second only to schizophrenia as the reason for first and second admissions to state mental hospitals in the United States, and it has been estimated that its prevalence outside psychiatric hospitals is five times greater than that of schizophrenia (Dunlop 1965). Not only is depression a primary cause of human misery, but its by-product, suicide, is a leading cause of death in certain age groups.

While tricyclic medications, electroconvulsive therapy, and long-term psychotherapy have been mainstays in the treatment of depressive disorders, there appears to be no clearly superior method for dealing with the more prevalent neurotic or reactive depressions. There is certainly a need to develop a treatment more efficient and readily available than those currently in use. At present a few approaches such as cognitive-behavior therapy (Foreyt and Rathjen 1978) and aerobic running seem to offer promise. This chapter will focus on the latter method.

A number of preliminary studies (Blue 1979; Brown, Ramirez, and Taub 1978; Buffone 1980b; Greist et al. 1978; Kavanaugh et al. 1977) have shown that aerobic running produces significant improvement in the condition of moderately depressed clients. Berger presents an excellent discussion and review of the literature in chapter 9. The results of one study (Greist et al. 1978) suggest that aerobic running is as effective as two forms of verbal psychotherapy, and four times as cost-effective. Although these and other preliminary results appear promising, there is still much to learn before running can be reliably prescribed for depressed clients. In some ways, perhaps fortunately so, this early research has generated more questions than it has answered. This is at best a time for cautious optimism.

This chapter will offer some thoughts and cite research results in response to questions that have arisen from this early research on running and depression. More carefully controlled research is needed to assess the potential of such an approach in actual clinical practice.

## How Has Research into the Use of Exercise as Therapy Come About?

Although considerable attention has been directed toward cognitive methods (Beck 1976; Foreyt and Rathjen 1978; Meichenbaum 1974) and behavioral approaches in psychotherapy (Bandura 1969; Lazarus 1968), the use of physical interventions such as exercise has generally been neglected in the professional literature until recently (Dickerson 1978; Greist et al. 1978). Two separate but related events in recent years appear to have set the stage for physical exercise as a form of psychotherapy.

First, the "aerobics explosion" has prompted increasing numbers of Americans to take to the streets and courts to improve their general health and physical fitness. Of the aerobic exercises available (Cooper 1968), running seems to offer several advantages and has received much attention in the popular literature (Fixx 1977, 1980; Sheehan 1975, 1978). A 1977 Gallup poll estimated that 25 million persons run or jog regularly. Concurrently, numerous studies have investigated the physiological effects of exercise (Bonanno and Lies 1974; Buccola and Stone 1975; Cooper 1968). These studies have produced evidence that exercise reduces the risk of coronary attacks and arterial disease, obesity, hypertension, and the associated elevated blood lipids. It appears even more certain that regular exercise can reduce the risk of certain life-threatening physical diseases and thereby increase longevity. Regular jogging programs undertaken by sedentary middle-aged males have consistently produced decreases in resting heart rate and increases in maximum oxygen consumption, which normally declines with age (Kasch 1976; Paolone et al. 1976). Other studies have shown that running can improve the functioning of the cardiovascular and respiratory systems and retard disease and deterioration of the body. Now that the physiological benefits of exercise have become widely accepted, researchers have begun to focus on the associated psychic consequences (Sacks and Sachs 1981).

Second, in the past two decades there has been a resurgence of professional interest in a psychobiological or mind-body perspective (Bakal 1979; Morgan 1973). Health practitioners have begun to recognize that the complex functions of the human system are interrelated and interdependent. Researchers in psychosomatic and behavioral medicine have firmly established that the mind can affect the body (Brown 1974; Pelletier 1977), as in such disorders as migraine headaches, peptic ulcers, hypertension, arthritis, bronchial asthma, and sexual impotence. It is now becoming apparent that the reverse also holds true. The body, appropriately used, can affect the mind in constructive ways.

These two influences—popular interest in exercise and research on the subject and the resurgence of the psychobiological perspective in the health professions—seem to have contributed heavily to the application of exercise as a form of psychotherapy. Although research in this area is in its infancy, exercise undertaken solely for physical benefits has been shown to have a positive effect on psychological state. Such results have been demonstrated with a variety of individuals in diverse settings (Greist et al. 1978).

## What Advantages Does a Running Approach Offer in the Treatment of Depression?

Running as a somatic intervention for the depressed client seems to offer several advantages not typically available through more traditional means of treatment (Buffone 1980a). One advantage is its cost-effectiveness (Greist et al. 1978) in view of the rising cost of health care and the trend toward accountability in psychotherapy. This method is also easily learned by the patient and requires no special skill or coordination.

A second advantage is that running provides additional health benefits by increasing cardiovascular endurance and respiratory efficiency, by improving muscle tone, digestion, and blood volume, and by promoting fat loss. Running also seems to have positive psychological effects, including increased energy, decreased anxiety, improved sleep, greater sense of well-being, and enhanced body awareness and image (Collingwood 1972; Driscoll 1976; Kuntzleman 1977; Mitchum 1976; Morgan 1979a). Strenuous exercise such as running may also encourage a more positive, health-promoting approach, as opposed to the remediation model so often encountered in psychotherapy. Patients are required to accept more responsibility in therapy and to take an active role in their own improvement.

Of particular importance is that, once learned, running can be used by patients as a self-regulatory tool to control depression, helping them generalize the effect of treatment beyond the counseling situation, which is often a problem (Stokes and Baer 1977). Getting patients to continue the prescribed exercise regimen after the formal termination of treatment is vital, for if they discontinue exercise the therapeutic effects will soon subside. As with other somatic therapies, such as medication, continued regular dosage is necessary. Clients should be taught compliance strategies during treatment so that regular exercise can be established as a habit that helps them cope with the stresses of daily life.

Another advantage of this approach is that clinicians who participate in running, either alone or with their clients, may also experience the positive benefits of relaxation, time-outs, and a change in what can become a routine and hectic schedule. This may aid the helping professions in reducing their high rate of burnout and job-related psychopathology, which affect the quality of service provided (Freudenberger and Richelson 1980; Maslach 1976).

## What Methodological Problems Are Inherent in the Research Supporting This Approach?

Although preliminary results on the use of running to treat depression are generally positive, there appear to be several methodological limitations that make their interpretation difficult. These limitations appear in six major areas: sample size, subject characteristics, evaluation methods, the effect of non-specific treatment variables, vague treatment guidelines, and follow-up. These problems are discussed more fully by Silva and Shultz in chapter 17, and Dienstbier (chap. 14) also presents a number of points related to research.

SAMPLE SIZE

Most of the studies conducted to date have used small samples (Blue 1979; Buffone 1980b; Greist et al. 1978), which has severely restricted any broad generalizations from their results. In the future it would be advisable to increase sample size to avoid the idiosyncratic conclusions often drawn from small-$N$ research (Hersen and Barlow 1976).

SUBJECT CHARACTERISTICS

A second major limitation has been the subjects themselves, since those willing to participate in research of this kind may be different in some ways from the depressed population in general. Subjects in these studies were willing to participate in a strenuous physical exercise program, and this selection process, coupled with subject attrition during the study, would render the final population highly select and probably atypical.

In one study (Buffone 1980b) where subject attrition was approximately 50 percent, certain self-report measures showed that the final sample was different from those who dropped out of treatment. Those who completed the study reported themselves to be both more motivated and more depressed, and historically they appeared to demonstrate more chronic patterns of depression. Though this information is retrospective, it points out the need to examine more closely those subjects who complete these vigorous therapy programs. Are they truly representative of the general depressed population? Probably not. Measures therefore must be taken to determine what differences exist between participants and nonparticipants in this area of research and what types of subjects tend to complete these rather demanding treatment programs.

### EVALUATION

A third problem inherent in preliminary research is the method of evaluating subject change. Thus far, the intensity of depression has been measured by self-report instruments such as the Beck Depression Inventory (Beck et al. 1978) and the Zung Depression Scale (Zung 1965). The problem with using only self-report inventories to measure subject change is that these instruments are highly vulnerable to experimenter bias and demand characteristics (Hersen and Barlow 1976). Multifaceted measures of change are needed so that the degree of depression can be assessed on several different levels, including not only intrasubject perception of change (i.e., cognitions, belief systems, affective areas), but also assessment by outside observers. One such scale, the Hamilton Rating Scale, is a simple, reliable means of rating degree of depression through a brief interview (Hamilton 1960). More objective assessment might compensate for the obvious shortcomings so often found in studies employing only self-report methods.

### NONSPECIFIC TREATMENT VARIABLES

A fourth problem that traditional research models (prepost comparative group) neglect is the many nonspecific treatment variables that may contribute to reported outcomes. It appears that prior studies of running as a treatment for depression have assumed that the observed improvement was specifically attributable to the aerobic running. Buffone (1980b) questioned this assumption, reporting that the improvement observed was the result of the specific treatment *plus* a number of nonspecific treatment variables, including the physical condition of the subjects at the initiation of the study, the experience level of the therapist, social and group interaction effects, subjects' expectations regarding treatment, and lifestyle changes during the course of the study. For example, significant life events dramatically altered the intensity of depression despite experimentally controlled conditions. Such variables must be measured or controlled for in future studies if we are to accurately determine the effect of the treatment intervention. It was also apparent in this study (Buffone 1980b) that individuals responded differently to the therapy methods used (i.e., running versus cognitive-behavioral therapy). These results suggest that research designs that control for these nonspecific treatment variables are needed to clarify the specific effect of the running method.

## VAGUE TREATMENT PACKAGES

A fifth problem is the vagueness of the treatment methods used in the preliminary research. What kinds of exercise prescriptions (intensity, duration, frequency) are being used? Quantification of running programs is seriously lacking and has created problems for experimenters who wish to replicate these studies, as though a drug study failed to monitor or report dosages. A well-outlined, detailed treatment manual should be made available to others conducting research on aerobic running.

## FOLLOW-UP

A final difficulty in the early research is the lack of follow-up. A most important, but often neglected, aspect of behavior change programs is determining whether reported improvements are maintained after the original controlling conditions have been discontinued. Buffone (1980b) conducted a two-month follow-up that indicated there was little maintenance of initial improvement, primarily because the subjects stopped running. How permanent are treatment-related improvements? And are the skills learned in therapy continued after treatment ends? Perhaps periodic booster sessions might help patients maintain the improvements and skills acquired in treatment. This should be investigated in future research.

## Why Does Aerobic Running Cause Improvement in Depressed Individuals?

A number of theories attempt to explain this. They can be divided into physiological and psychological theories. It has been suggested that a change mechanism associated with running works through the increase in blood flow and oxygenation, which affect the central nervous system (Kostrubala 1977). A second, somewhat more complex explanation is that a specific central nervous system chemical substance is released during running. Riggs (1981) presents an excellent discussion of the biochemical factors related to strenuous physical exercise. Howley (1976) demonstrated that the norepinephrine urinary excretion level of healthy young males was four and a half times the preexercise value thirty minutes after exercising on a treadmill at 80 percent of maximum aerobic power. Norepinephrine is known to be low in many depressed persons. The catecholamine theory of affective disorders posits that the level of brain norepinephrine may be related to chronic emotional illness (Schildkraut 1965). As has been reported, norepinephrine production (as measured by urinary excretion) increases dramatically during exercise. As a depressed patient's workload increases, as in running programs, norepinephrine output rises to maintain biological functions. The positive psychological changes reported in the literature are attributed to this specific chemical increase. Research conducted thus far (Glasser 1978, 1979) has failed to confirm this or other intriguing biochemical hypotheses. (See Sachs, chap. 15, for more on this.)

The psychological models appear more subject to scientific scrutiny and may be more easily substantiated. The meditation model, for example, proposes that regular exercise is an active form of meditation (Kostrubala 1977). The repetitive, rhythmic motions of aerobic activity may trigger mechanisms similar to centering devices in sedentary forms of meditation. This model has received some support in explaining the effects of running in the treatment of anxiety. Bahrke and Morgan (1978) compared the effectiveness of meditation and of strenuous physical activity in reducing state anxiety. Their results tend to support the hypothesis that running may relieve anxiety through a "time-out" from anxious cognitions, as occurs in meditation. This same explanation may hold for depression. Running, which requires a close monitoring of bodily functions such as foot strike and breathing, may distract an individual from negative thoughts and depressive symptoms (Greist et al. 1978).

A second psychological explanation for the improvement accompanying a running treatment for depression relates to the mastery experienced as one gradually increases distance and endurance. Solomon and Bumpus (1978, 588) commented: "Running, by giving a patient a feeling of being in charge over functions such as heart rate, breathing, and muscles, automatically gives him a sense of mastery. This is a therapeutic maneuver frequently employed in behavior therapy, and in the course of biofeedback treatment." This mastery explanation is supported by research (Seligman 1974) showing that depressed patients improve when they realize they can control themselves or their environment through their actions. The awareness that behavior and subsequent reinforcement are related, not independent of each other, may be curative in itself.

A third psychological hypothesis is related to changing self-perception as patients begin to run regularly. Running improves physical health, appearance, and body image, which may cause corresponding changes in self-acceptance and self-esteem (Collingwood 1972; Collingwood and Willet 1971). Clients may generalize this more positive self-image from the exercise experience to other areas of their lives. Also, people who exercise tend to view this activity as positive and may begin to substitute it for negative habits and defenses. Sacks (chap. 6) presents a psychoanalytic explanation of why running seems to reduce subjective rates of depression, discussing the discharge of repressed aggression into physical activity as a possible factor.

### Are the Factors That Cause Improvement Also Found in Other Forms of Psychotherapy?

Yes. Mastery, for example, is very closely linked to the behavioral theory of depression and its treatment. In the cognitive-behavioral treatment of depression (Beck et al. 1978) the patient is encouraged to engage in activities that produce feelings of pleasure or of mastery, defined as a sense of accomplishment. The patient is assigned the task of engaging in a certain number of mastery experiences each day and then rating the sense of mastery (0–5) and accompanying feelings. Typically the patient feels less depressed after engaging in activities that produce a sense of mastery. This can easily be linked to the sense of accomplishment people experience after running their first hundred yards or their first mile.

A second behavioral technique, graded task assignment, is also similar to the experience of running patients. This approach assumes that depressed patients perceive themselves as unable to control the environment. Patients are assigned specific tasks that show they can do so. Like running, a graduated task program is designed to demonstrate to patients that they do have some control over their lives.

Distraction, which is sometimes a product of running, can also result from the cognitive-behavioral approach. It is taught by the therapist as an active treatment ingredient so that patients can temporarily reduce painful affect through a skill that can be used outside the office. Such distraction is also produced by the sedentary recreational activities typically assigned to hospitalized patients, but aerobic activities may prove more effective because they are more intrusive and physically demanding, requiring patients to concentrate on the activity rather than on their depressive affects and cognitions.

Recent research into treatments for depression has also revealed broader commonalities, suggesting that the specific components of the running therapy for depression may be less important than certain essential ingredients. Zeiss, Lewinsohn, and Munoz (1979) compared training in interpersonal skills, pleasant activities, and cognitive training in the treatment of depressed outpatients and found that the outcome of treatment was not related to the specific interventions used. They suggest that treatment should include several basic components: (1) an elaborate, well-planned structure that helps patients believe they can control their behaviors and thereby their depression; (2) training in skills that make patients feel more effective in handling their daily lives; (3) emphasis on the use of these skills outside therapy; and (4) encouragement to attribute improvement to the patient, not the therapist.

Buffone's program (1980b) included these ingredients, as should any running program for treating depression. Initial structuring was aimed at convincing subjects that they could overcome their depression by acquiring certain skills (cognitive-behavioral and running). Subjects were then trained in these skills and encouraged to employ them outside the weekly therapy sessions. Finally, improvement was attributed to the subjects themselves rather than to the therapy or therapist.

This theory of why subjects improve is also supported by Bandura's (1977) work on self-efficacy. Bandura has suggested that "psychological procedures, whatever the form, alter the level and strength of self-efficacy" (p. 191). He further states that "self-directed mastery experiences are then arranged to reinforce a sense of personal efficacy. Through this form of treatment incapacitated people rapidly lose their fears" (p. 196–97). In this case "depression" might be substituted for "fears."

In running programs that contain these essential ingredients, patients learn they can control their behaviors and thereby their depression, a conclusion supported by Seligman's theory (1974) of learned helplessness. The purpose of therapy, running or other forms, is thus to restore the patient's efficacy.

## What about Combining Running with Other Forms of Therapy? Would Exercise Serve Best as a Primary or an Adjunct Treatment?

Ideally, running would be prescribed for the right patients, (motivated to exercise), at the right time (when they are receptive to such an approach), to deal with the right problems (those that appear amenable to this method). Since one can rarely make such exact and appropriate treatment prescriptions, therapists should be flexible in their use of this approach. It is unwise to attempt to fit the patient to the treatment; for optimal results, the opposite must occur. In prescribing running, the therapist must realize that any presenting problem, especially depression, is a multifaceted syndrome consisting of clusters of specific problems that will require multiple interventions.

Thus there should be comprehensive and thorough assessment of the presenting complaint. Lazarus (1976) outlines a number of areas that should be covered in the initial history and assessment. Because depression often includes affective, motivational, cognitive, behavorial, and physiological components, the therapist may concentrate on any combination of these to produce change in the depressive syndrome. Each has a reciprocal relation to other components, so improvement in one area generally affects other areas, and it thus seems likely that running therapy would be most effective in conjunction with other forms of therapy (Driscoll 1976; Rueter and Harris 1980).

The effects of an aerobic running treatment may be enhanced by other methods designed to affect other areas of functioning. It has already been suggested (Lazarus 1976) that a multimodal approach is more effective than a single intervention. For example, one might expect that aerobic running could ameliorate the physiological symptoms of depression (e.g., sleep and appetite disturbance, diminished libido) while leaving other problem areas unchanged (e.g., affects, long-standing dysfunctional thinking or belief systems).

## Would a Running or Exercise Regimen Alone Be Sufficient to Reduce Depression, without a Therapist's Direct Involvement?

This is doubtful. Certainly, for well-functioning individuals in a nonclinical population, aerobic exercise may prove helpful in controlling depression (Colt et al. 1981). But for mild to moderate clinical depression a therapist's assistance is necessary. Two factors that Buffone's subjects (1980a) all noted as crucial to their improvement were relationship variables: the concern and interest of the therapist, and interaction with the other group members.

The characteristics of the therapist (e.g., style, competence, enthusiasm) affect patients' response to therapy (Bergin and Strupp 1972). Therapists using the aerobic running method with depressed clients must be aware of how their own attitudes and behaviors influence their patients.

Improvement also may be promoted by the social contact and support of a group setting. Group sessions can provide patients with regular peer contact and reviews of their progress, so group treatment not only may enhance a successful outcome, but can be used after treatment to prolong the treatment effect, through regular "booster sessions" or alumni meetings. These interpersonal factors should not be overlooked in considering a running treatment for clinically depressed individuals.

### If Regular Running or Aerobic Exercise Does Reduce Depression, Do Regular Runners Experience Less Depression Than Nonrunners?

If running does affect depression levels, it seems to follow that there should be a lower rate of depression among runners than among nonrunners. Unfortunately, this hypothesis has little empirical support. An informal survey conducted by Lilliefors (1978) with an unspecified number of runners reported that 56 percent of those questioned felt they were less depressed since they began running. Although this anecdotal information lends some credence to the hypothesis that runners have lower rates of depression, it raises more questions than it answers. For example, what of the runners who responded otherwise — the large group of 44 percent? Had running little or no effect on their depression? Do some people who run (and become injured or quit) experience an increase in the intensity and frequency of their depressive episodes? What about runners who are negatively addicted (Morgan 1979b) and become depressed when they must discontinue running? (See Sachs and Pargman, chap. 13, for more on running addiction.) An interesting study by Colt et al. (1981) suggests that long-distance runners, particularly women, manifest a high level of affective disorders. Colt et al. hypothesize that these runners are motivated to continue by the mood-improving action (reduction of depression?) of running.

In contrast, there are studies that suggest that regular exercisers experience less depression than nonexercisers. Only a few of the studies that compared the psychological characteristics of athletes and nonathletes have measured level of depression.

Tharp and Schlegelmilch (1977) compared habitual exercisers from a YMCA and the University of Nebraska with a group of nontrained subjects on several psychological indexes. The trained subjects scored significantly lower in anxiety and depression as measured by the Multiple Affect Adjective

Checklist (Zuckerman and Lubin 1965). Their scores suggested that they were more self-assured, relaxed, and emotionally stable than their nontrained counterparts.

A second, more comprehensive study of depression in athletes (Morgan and Pollock 1977) suggested that highly trained rowers, wrestlers, and runners possessed similar psychological characteristics as measured by the Profile of Mood States (POMS) (McNair, Lorr, and Droppleman 1971). The trained athletes scored below the mean reported for college students in depression, fatigue, confusion, and anxiety. Morgan (1980), in a more recent report, has stated that successful athletes in all sports "consistently show fewer signs of psychopathology and lower levels of anxiety, neuroticism, and depression than less successful athletes and the general population" (p. 93).

Wilson, Morley, and Bird (1980) compared the depression levels of "marathoners" who ran between six and twenty miles six or seven days a week ($N = 10$) to those of "joggers" who averaged one to two miles three to five days a week ($N = 10$) and of nonexercisers who had not participated in any regular physical activity during the year before the study ($N = 10$). Marathoners and joggers were significantly less depressed than nonexercisers as measured by the POMS (McNair, Lorr, and Droppleman 1971), and marathoners had significantly lower rates of depression than joggers.

The design and nature of studies of depression among exercisers and nonexercisers make it difficult to determine whether the observed differences in depression levels were caused by exercise or by other factors. The subjects' expectation of positive results, the types of people attracted to strenuous exercise, or a number of other variables may have contaminated these outcomes. Although anecdotal evidence and research conducted thus far do suggest that runners are less depressed than nonrunners, present evidence does not support a causal relation.

## When Is Running Contraindicated for the Depressed Patient?

Aerobic running is certainly not appropriate for every depressed patient. Although some evidence supports the therapeutic use of running to reduce moderate levels of depression, Greist and his colleagues (1978) sound a note of caution: "In our opinion, running as treatment for depression remains experimental, in need of replication by additional controlled studies and potentially dangerous to depressed individuals" (p. 287).

Running therapy is probably appropriate for only a small proportion of the patients seen in clinical practice. The therapist should consider several factors before assigning such treatment. One factor is values. Does the patient value physical exercise? This type of treatment is not likely to be accepted by some less well educated, indigent patients, though they might benefit from the method because of their lower capacity for verbal, insight-oriented psychotherapies. The approach will not work if the patient does not value physical exercise and will not comply with the exercise prescription. Running as a treatment would probably be most easily accepted by those who both value physical exercise and respond well to other therapeutic interventions, such as educated middle-class patients.

Running therapy certainly should not be prescribed for patients who are at risk of a cardiovascular accident. These patients may suffer a number of physical complications, such as gross obesity (40 percent over ideal body weight), severe heart disease, enlarged heart, or high blood pressure. Patients who present any physical abnormality or who are more than thirty years old should be evaluated by a physician before starting such a program.

Running is obviously contraindicated for patients who lack the interest or motivation to initiate physical activity or exercise. In my own experience, this seems more the rule than the exception. Although a clever, enthusiastic therapist might provide the encouragement and technology necessary to start such a patient on an exercise program, it is doomed to failure unless the patient becomes addicted (Sachs and Pargman 1979; see also Sachs and Pargman, chap. 13).

Running should be prescribed only with caution for obsessive-compulsives or for type-A individuals (Friedman and Rosenman 1974), who fight time because they want to accomplish too much in too little time. These competitive, hard-driving persons may take to jogging because they feel they can intensify their exercise by compressing it into less time, but they are likely to become obsessed with running and may turn it into a physically or emotionally destructive experience.

Running therapy is also contraindicated for patients with severe depression or suicidal inclinations (Kostrubala 1976). If a patient's ego is extremely fragile, one more failure might precipitate an intensive depressive episode or a suicidal gesture. DeFries (1981) reported that running appeared to have contributed to psychotic breaks in two young, "psychologically" vulnerable women. There is also no evidence that aerobic running is helpful for severe forms of depressive illness or for bipolar affective disorders. It is certainly important to constantly monitor clients' progress, and if running is not effective, the treatment strategy should be changed.

## What Does the Future Hold for Running as a Treatment for Depression?

Obviously, much more research is needed to achieve understanding of the potential effect of running on depression. The results of preliminary research call for more carefully designed studies that better define the roles and limitations of such an approach. Additionally, the role of follow-up and continued evaluation after formal treatment has ended should be stressed.

## References

Bahrke, M. S., and Morgan, W. P. 1978. Anxiety reduction following exercise and meditation. *Cognitive Therapy and Research* 2:323–33.

Bakal, D. A. 1979. *Psychology and medicine: Psychological dimensions of health and illness*. New York: Springer.

Bandura, A. 1969. *Principles of behavior modification*. New York: Holt, Rinehart and Winston.

———. 1977. Self-efficacy: Toward a unifying theory of behavioral change. *Psychological Review*, 191–215.

Beck, A. T. 1976. *Cognitive therapy and the emotional disorders*. New York: International Universities Press.

Beck, A. T.; Rush, A. J.; Emery, G.; and Shaw, B. F. 1978. *Cognitive therapy of depression*. New York: Guilford Press.

Bergin, A. E., and Strupp, H. H. 1972. *Changing frontiers in the science of psychotherapy*. Chicago: Aldine.

Blue, R. F. 1979. Aerobic running as a treatment for moderate depression. *Perceptual and Motor Skills* 48:228.

Bonanno, J. A., and Lies, J. E. 1974. Effects of physical training on coronary risk factors. *American Journal of Cardiology* 33:760–64.

Brown, B. 1974. *New mind, new body, bio-feedback: New directions for the mind*. New York: Bantam Books.

Brown, R. S.; Ramirez, D.; and Taub, J. 1978. The prescription of exercise for depression. *Physician and Sportsmedicine* (12):34–45.

Buccola, V., and Stone, W. J. 1975. Effects of jogging and cycling programs on physiological and personality variables in aged men. *Research Quarterly* 46:134–39.

Buffone, G. W. 1980a. Exercise as therapy: A closer look. *Journal of Counseling and Psychotherapy* 3(2):101–15.

———. 1980b. Psychological changes associated with the use of cognitive-behavior therapy and an aerobic running program in the treatment of depression. Ph.D. diss., Florida State University.

Collingwood, R. 1972. The effects of physical training upon behavior and self-attitudes. *Journal of Clinical Psychology* 28:583–85.

Collingwood, R., and Willet, L. 1971. Effects of physical training upon self-concept and body attitude. *Journal of Clinical Psychology* 27:411–12.

Colt, E. W. D.; Dunner, D. L.; Hall, K.; and Fieve, R. R. 1981. A high prevalence of affective disorder in runners. In *Psychology of running,* ed. M. H. Sacks and M. L. Sachs. Champaign, Ill.: Human Kinetics Publishers.

Cooper, K. H. 1968. *Aerobics.* New York: Bantam Books.

DeFries, Z. 1981. "Running madness": A prelude to real madness. In *Psychology of running,* ed. M. H. Sacks and M. L. Sachs. Champaign, Ill.: Human Kinetics Publishers.

Dickerson, D. D. 1978. Mind body unity: An interactional study of the psychological effects of physiological change. Ph.D. diss., California School of Professional Psychology.

Driscoll, R. 1976. Anxiety reduction using physical exertion and positive images. *Psychological Record* 26:87–94.

Dunlop, E. 1965. Use of antidepressants and stimulants. *Modern Treatment* 2:543–68.

Fixx, J. F. 1977. *The complete book of running.* New York: Random House.

———. 1980. *The second complete book of running.* New York: Random House.

Foreyt, J. P., and Rathjen, D. P. 1978. *Cognitive behavior therapy: Research and application.* New York: Plenum Press.

Freudenberger, H. H., and Richelson, G. 1980. *Burn out: The high cost of high achievement.* New York: Anchor Press.

Friedman, M., and Rosenman, R. H. 1974. *Type A behavior and your heart.* Greenwich, Conn.: Fawcett.

Glasser, W. 1978. The positive addiction experiment. *Starting Line* 2:2.

———. 1979. Glasser experiment: Results. *Arc* 4:7.

Greist, J. H.; Klein, M. H.; Eischens, R. R.; Faris, J.; Gurman, A. S.; and Morgan, W. P. 1978. Running through your mind. *Journal of Psychosomatic Research* 22:259–94.

Hamilton, M. 1960. A rating scale for depression. *Journal of Neurology, Neurosurgery and Psychiatry* 23:56–62.

Hersen, M., and Barlow, D. H. 1976. *Single case experimental designs: Strategies for studying behavior change.* New York: Pergamon Press.

Howley, E. T. 1976. The effect of different intensities of exercise on the excretion of epinephrine and norepinephrine. *Medicine and Science in Sports* 8:219–22.

Kasch, F. 1976. The effects of exercise on the aging process. *Physician and Sportsmedicine* 4:64–68.

Kavanaugh, T.; Shephard, R. J.; Tuck, J. A.; and Qureshi, S. 1977. Depression following myocardial infarction: The effects of distance running. *Annals of the New York Academy of Sciences* 301:1029–38.

Kostrubala, T. 1976. *The joy of running.* Philadelphia: J. B. Lippincott.

———. 1977. Jogging and personality change. *Today's Jogger* 1 (2):14–15, 56.

Kuntzleman, C. T. 1977. Jog to improve your productivity. *Today's Jogger* 1 (2):13, 29–31, 45, 56.

Lazarus, A. A. 1968. Learning theory and the treatment of depression. *Behavior Research and Therapy* 6:83–89.

————. 1976. *Multimodal behavior therapy*. New York: Springer.

Lilliefors, J. 1978. *The running mind*. Mountain View, Calif.: World Publications.

McNair, D. M.; Lorr, M.; and Droppleman, L. F. 1971. *The profile of mood states manual*. San Diego: Educational and Industrial Testing.

Maslach, C. 1976. Burned out. *Human Behavior* 5:16–23.

Meichenbaum, D. 1974. *Cognitive behavior modification*. Morristown, N.J.: General Learning Press.

Mitchum, M. L. 1976. The effect of physically exerting leisure activity on state anxiety level. M.S. thesis, Florida State University.

Morgan, W. P. 1973. Efficacy of psychobiologic inquiry in the exercise and sports sciences. *Quest* 20:39–47.

————. 1979a. Anxiety reduction following acute physical activity. *Psychiatric Annals* 9(3):36–45.

————. 1979b. Negative addiction in runners. *Physician and Sportsmedicine* 7(2): 56–63, 67–70.

————. 1980. Test of champions: The iceberg profile. *Psychology Today* 14, 2:92–99, 101–8.

Morgan, W. P., and Pollock, M. L. 1977. Psychologic characterization of the elite distance runner. *Annals of the New York Academy of Sciences* 301:382–403.

Paolone, A. M.; Lewis, R. R.; Lanigan, W. T.; and Goldstein, W. J. 1976. Results of two years of exercise training in middle aged men. *Physician and Sportsmedicine* 4:72–77.

Pelletier, K. R. 1977. *Mind as healer, mind as slayer: A holistic approach to preventing stress disorders*. New York: Dell.

Riggs, C. E. 1981. Endorphins, neurotransmitters, and/or neuromodulators and exercise. In *Psychology of running*, ed. M. H. Sacks and M. L. Sachs. Champaign, Ill.: Human Kinetics Publishers.

Rueter, M. A., and Harris, D. V. 1980. The effects of running on individuals who are clinically depressed. Paper presented at the American Psychological Association Convention, Montreal, Canada, September 1980.

Sachs, M. L., and Pargman, D. 1979. Running addiction: A depth interview examination. *Journal of Sport Behavior* 2:143–55.

Sacks, M. H., and Sachs, M. L., eds. 1981. *Psychology of running*. Champaign, Ill.: Human Kinetics Publishers.

Schildkraut, J. J. 1965. The catecholamine hypothesis of affective disorders: A review of supporting evidence. *American Journal of Psychiatry* 122:509–22.

Seligman, M. E. 1974. *Helplessness*. San Francisco: Freeman.

Sheehan, G. 1975. *Dr. Sheehan on running*. Mountain View, Calif.: World Publications.

————. 1978. *Running and being: The total experience*. New York: Simon and Schuster.

Solomon, E. G., and Bumpus, A. K. 1978. The running meditation response: An adjunct to psychotherapy. *American Journal of Psychotherapy* 32:583–92.

Stokes, T. F., and Baer, D. M. 1977. An implicit technology for generalization. *Journal of Applied Behavior Analysis* 10:349–67.

Tharp, G. D., and Schlegelmilch, R. P. 1977. Personality characteristics of trained versus non-trained individuals. *Medicine and Science in Sports* 9:55.

Wilson, V. E.; Morley, M. C.; and Bird, E. I. 1980. Mood profiles of marathon runners, joggers, and non-exercisers. *Perceptual and Motor Skills* 50:117–18.

Zeiss, A. M.; Lewinsohn, P. M.; and Munoz, R. F. 1979. Nonspecific improvement effects in depression using interpersonal skills training, pleasant activity schedules or cognitive training. Unpublished manuscript, Arizona State University.

Zuckerman, M., and Lubin, B. 1965. *Manual for the Multiple Affect Adjective Checklist.* San Diego: Educational and Industrial Testing.

Zung, W. K. 1965. A self-rating depression scale. *Archives of General Psychiatry* 12:63–70.

BONNIE G. BERGER

# 2

# Running Strategies
# for Women and Men

Although the psychological benefits of running and other forms of aerobic exercise have not been completely substantiated (Folkins and Sime 1981), the converging lines of evidence (see my chap. 9, "Running away from Anxiety and Depression" and chap. 10, "Running toward Psychological Well-being" argue strongly for its application. In addition to the psychological effects of running, desirable physical effects such as increased cardiovascular fitness, muscular strength, and muscular endurance, the absence of undesirable side effects, and cost-effectiveness support the use of running as a therapeutic strategy.

Because of the newness of running as a therapeutic technique, I will focus on practical guidelines critical to the therapist's success and the client's continuation of running after therapy is over. A major purpose of this chapter is to enable the therapist to approach this new form of treatment confidently. After considering the important issues in exercise prescription, I will review the question whether the therapist need be a runner, the advantages of running therapy over other forms of therapy, and practical methods of encouraging running adherence. Finally, I will consider the physiological and social concerns of women runners to illustrate the importance of developing a flexible, personalized running program that can be continually adapted to fit each client's needs.

## Exercise Prescription: How Fast, How Far, How Often?

Like any drug or treatment strenuous exercise should be prescribed with care to maximize its benefits, minimize the possibilities of harmful side effects

(Lamb 1974a, b, 1976a, b, 1979; Noakes and Opie 1979) and allow for any diseases and ailments that may already have developed (Lamb 1974c, 1975, 1976c, 1977, 1978). A comprehensive, concise, and clearly written guide to exercise by Sharkey (1979) is highly recommended as background reading for therapists who plan to employ running as a form of therapy. In the following discussion of running intensity, duration, and frequency I shall briefly define each parameter and then discuss the essential characteristics of running programs that have been therapeutically effective.

Of primary importance in exercise prescription is determining the appropriate *intensity, duration,* and *frequency* for clients of different fitness levels and ages. As I indicate in chapter 9, it seems likely that strenuous aerobic exercise is more likely to have therapeutic effects than is light exercise (Brown, Ramirez, and Taub 1978; Buffone 1980a; Morgan 1979). But strenuous exercise for one person may be light for another. Brown, Ramirez and Taub (1978) have aptly noted that individualized "dosage," as with any other prescription, should be established on the basis of a client's life circumstances and level of fitness. Refer to Sharkey (1979), appendix B, for an example of a graded walk-run fitness program designed for people of various fitness levels.

Exercise that most reliably results in decreased ongoing levels of anxiety and depression, enhanced self-esteem, and increased self-knowledge (1) is performed three times a week (*frequency*); (2) is conducted for at least twenty minutes without stopping (*duration*),[1] and (3) is characterized by sustained heavy breathing or is performed at between 70 percent and 85 percent of the client's maximum heart rate (intensity).

FREQUENCY

An exercise frequency of *three times a week* with one day off between exercise sessions provides a training effect that noticeably increases the physiological ease of running and serves as an intrinsic reward as clients observe their increasing ability to run. Running five days a week has been observed to result in even greater reductions of depression (Brown, Ramirez, and Taub 1978) and to be significantly related to lower prerunning anxiety levels (Wilson, Berger, and Bird 1981).

*Limit the Schedule*

Even though running five days a week might be more effective than running three days a week, it is important to limit the running schedule until the novice runner is able to run continuously for twenty minutes with relative ease. Limiting a running program to three or four days a week has several advantages. It reduces the likelihood of injury by allowing the body to recover. Pollock et al. 1977 reported that the percentage of injuries tripled when clients ran five days a week compared with three days a week. The lighter program presents less of a time problem for the client and tends to reduce monotony, and it can be incorporated rather easily into a variety of lifestyles. For example, a client who protects weekends from all infringements would prefer a Monday, Wednesday, Friday running schedule. Another who is busy during the week may prefer to run Friday, Sunday, and Tuesday.

### Follow a Set Routine

An advantage of running on specific days and even at a specific time of day is that running becomes an integral component of a person's schedule. With a set running routine it is clear when the runner misses a day. If the schedule is not preset as to the days of the week, the likelihood of missing a day is substantially increased.

Related to frequency is the time of day a client runs. Dienstbier (1977) recommended that running be scheduled at a time that does not interfere with one's lifestyle and said that running should enhance other activities. A "morning" person may prefer to rise early to include a run before daily activities begin and to reap the benefits of increased energy, relaxation, and feelings of accomplishment for the entire day. An "afternoon" person, however, may choose to substitute a run for a martini after a stressful day.

Regardless of the time of day selected, a regular running period three to four days a week is important for the novice runner who has yet to become committed or "addicted" to exercise (see Sachs and Pargman, chap. 13, for more on this topic).

INTENSITY

Of the three components of exercise strenuousness, intensity is the most important for developing a training effect (Katch and McArdle 1977) and is the best single indicator of strenuousness. It is most accurately measured by the amount of oxygen consumed during one minute of exercise, expressed in relation to weight, but since this method requires sophisticated laboratory equipment, a convenient way to assess intensity is to estimate one's *maximum heart rate* and *aerobic training zone*. When running intensity is over the aerobic threshold, the running becomes anaerobic and produces no additional improvement in aerobic fitness. Though cardiovascular fitness is not a goal of running therapy, the client may welcome this secondary benefit because the training effect makes running easier. Running at the lower end of the zone produces primarily muscular training effects; running at the upper end produces central circulatory benefits (Sharkey 1979). Detailed procedures for calculating one's aerobic training zone are presented clearly by Katch and McArdle (1977, 304–5) and by Sharkey (1979, 36–41).

An easy and fairly accurate way to estimate running intensity is to measure one's heart rate for ten seconds, during or immediately after exercise, then multiply the figure by six for the rate per minute. Measuring heart rate for a longer period tends to be inaccurate because the trained person's heart rate quickly returns to normal when exercise stops. A client's maximum exercise heart rate can be calculated by subtracting age in years from 220. A moderately intense running program would result in a heart rate between 70 percent and 85 percent of one's maximum heart rate (Burke 1979). Thus a forty-year-old client would plan to run at a heart rate between 126 and 153 beats per minute ($220 - 40 = 180; 180 \times .70 = 126; 180 \times .85 = 153$). For a thirty-year-old client of average fitness, heart rates between 133 (70 percent maximum heart rate) and 162 beats per minute (85 percent maximum heart rate) indicate that moderately intense effort is recommended. Unless a client has an exceedingly low fitness level, a heart rate below 130 beats per minute does not have much of a training effect (Sharkey 1979, 37), and thus running does not become pro-gressively easier in ensuing weeks. In general heart rates between 160 and 180 beats per minute are considered to be high-intensity aerobic effort (Sharkey 1979) and cannot be maintained for twenty to sixty minutes unless the client is highly fit. Although no studies have compared the psychological effects of running at different intensity levels, running at between 130 and 160 beats per minute has been observed to reduce anxiety and depression.

DURATION

Although the duration of the run can be expressed in terms of time, distance run, or calories burned, time is the measure suggested for initial use in running therapy. Both time and distance are more easily measured than calories. Time-based measures of running duration are employed more often than mileage in the experimentally based running literature, so clients can relate their own running to the literature. As clients become physiologically conditioned, they can still maintain the recommended twenty to thirty minute exercise schedule. Clearly, the speed of running and thus the distance must increase for the client to maintain a heart rate within the target zone. Conversely, the client may choose to maintain the same speed and increase the duration to thirty or forty minutes. If a client is habitually conserving energy so as to run for twenty to thirty minutes and thus is not running fast enough to maintain the target heart rate, it may be preferable to run a specific distance[2] regardless of the amount of time spent.

The suggested exercise duration of twenty to thirty minutes is based more on the body's physiological response to exercise and on the incidence of injury than on research indicating that psychological changes are more pronounced in this amount of running. In fact, forty to sixty minutes of running seems to result in positive feelings more often than do briefer runs (Carmack and Martens 1979; Glasser 1976; Kostrubala 1976; Mandell 1979).

The suggested twenty to thirty minutes of continuous running improves cardiovascular health (Kirby 1980; Squires 1980), reduces the risk of heart disease (Foster 1980; Paffenbarger, Wing, and Hyde 1979), and has desirable effects on blood lipids (Hartung and Squires 1980; Kirby 1980; Squires 1980). Twenty to thirty minutes can feasibly be garnered from a busy day, and it results in less than half as many injuries as occur in forty-five-minute running programs: "Although the results showed a greater increase in cardiorespiratory fitness for the 45-minute duration and 5-day/week groups, these programs are not recommended for beginning joggers because of the significantly greater percentage of injuries" (Pollock et al. 1977, 31).

If the diversionary aspect of exercise is one of the factors that promotes changes in psychological well-being (Bahrke and Morgan 1978; Dienstbier et al. 1981; Wilson, Berger, and Bird 1981), twenty minutes seems to be the "minimum" time that would decrease feelings of anxiety and depression. The total length of time spent exercising, like exercise frequency, should be limited if the client is running for therapeutic reasons rather than for performance. Six-mile runs have resulted in *larger decreases* of depression as measured before and after the runs than a marathon distance run (Dienstbier et al. 1981). A six-mile run obviously requires more than twenty minutes, but it was probably run in less than sixty minutes, since the runners were of marathon caliber. This particular study indicates that running longer than an hour may be less effective therapeutically than running between twenty and sixty minutes. A client who runs to the point of exhaustion may be literally running away from problems rather than examining and resolving them.

## How Do I Get There from Here?

For the client who has never participated in strenuous physical activity (more women than men will probably be in this category), running continuously for twenty minutes three times a week may seem impossible. Rather than immediately running for the entire twenty minutes, courting physiological disaster, and vowing never to run again, such clients should begin with a *brisk walking* program. A week or two of brisk walking will help novices develop stronger leg muscles, become familiar with the sensations of an elevated heart rate, establish some confidence in their physical abilities, and become familiar with the area where they plan to run. They can intersperse walking with a little jogging when they think they are able. When they are tired, gasping for breath, or frightened by their bodies' response to exercise, they can walk until their hearts return to a more normal rate, then do a little more jogging. With this procedure, novice runners can immediately fulfill the *duration, frequency,* and *intensity* components of the suggested running program.

The following information, well known to the habitual runner, is of particular importance in helping novice runners tailor the running program to their own fitness level.

1. *Keep moving*. A suggestion for novice runners that I once read has been particularly helpful to me in my own running—to just "keep moving" for a predetermined time, either by walking or by running, regardless of how tired one might be. This approach has helped me complete a run many times when I have wanted to stop, to my surprise and pleasure. To keep moving is particularly important for novice exercisers who wish to become runners. As fitness level and understanding of the body's response to exercise improve, one can increase the distance while keeping constant the frequency, duration, and intensity of the run.

2. *Talk test*. The runner should be able to converse with a companion, real or imaginary, while running. If not, the runner should reduce speed until this is possible. The "talk test" protects the novice from overextension.

3. *Keep running frequency, duration, and intensity constant*. Until the client can run consistently for the entire twenty-minute period without walking and is not fatigued for more than an hour after exercising, frequency, duration, and intensity should not be increased. By keeping running parameters constant, one can see progress—the distance covered in twenty minutes, the lesser effort required—and thus feel accomplishment, pride, and self-satisfaction. Maintaining rather than increasing running goals discourages the tendency to compete with oneself and lets one experience the joy of running.

4. *An hour to recover.* When the body recovers quickly after exercise, preferably within an hour, the person has adapted to that particular level of exercise and can increase one of the exercise parameters. Duration is frequently recommended for lengthening by psychologists and physiologists. Running between forty and sixty minutes enhances the likelihood of euphoric states while running, tends to clear the mind, and encourages exercise commitment or addiction (Carmack and Martens 1979; Glasser 1976; Kostrubala 1976, 1981; Mandell 1979; see also Sachs and Pargman, chap. 13, on running addiction).

5. *More is not always better.* Novice runners tend to think that if a little running is good for their minds and bodies, a lot must be even better. They require guidance in learning "to listen to their bodies" to determine the extent of their running at any particular time. Sore muscles the day after a run mean the client should temporarily reduce running intensity or duration.

6. *The therapist's support.* Heaps (1978) has provided experimental evidence that the therapist's support and belief in novice runners' abilities is important to their perception of their physical capabilities. College men (who were neither physically inactive nor highly trained runners) were significantly influenced in their perceptions of their personal fitness levels by the predetermined evaluative comments of a peer who ran with them as they completed Cooper's (1977) twelve-minute running test for fitness. In the two experimental conditions of positive or negative social comparison, the peer—who was actually Heap's confederate—either ran more slowly than the subject and said, "I sure had trouble keeping up with you; you must be in good shape" or ran faster than the subject and said, "You sure had trouble keeping up with me; you must be out of shape" (Heaps 1978, 401). The men's *perceptions* of their fitness (1) were significantly influenced by these brief comments, (2) were significantly and positively related to feelings of self-acceptance, and (3) were negatively related to concern for bodily functioning. Interestingly, the men's *actual* fitness was not related to any self-attitudes and was only minimally ($r = .27$) related to their estimates of their fitness levels. Thus a therapist's positive evaluation seems to directly influence clients' perception of their running capabilities, like or dislike of the running itself, and the success of running therapy.

RUNNING LOG

As Brown, Ramirez, and Taub (1978) noted, exercise novices often feel discouraged until their bodies adjust to the stress of running. Within these first weeks or months it is crucial that the therapist support the client's efforts and help resolve running problems before they become major obstacles. It may take six to twelve weeks for the running to become its own reward. For those who find running unpleasant this may never happen, and alternate forms of therapy should be chosen.

Maintaining a running log during the early exercise period is helpful for both client and therapist. One of the several diary versions available in bookstores (Editors of Consumer Guide 1978; Glover and Shepherd 1978) can be used, or client and therapist can design their own. A possible format is presented in table 1. Data that might affect the quality of the run, such as time of day, weather conditions, running alone or with a companion, and location can be recorded in the first column. The client also may wish to record mood (happy, relaxed, tense, angry, energetic, etc.). This qualitative information allows the client to note positive or negative characteristics of the running with the objective of reducing the number of unpleasant runs.

A systematic log serves several key functions:

1. *a source of motivation* (when contemplating whether to run on a particular day, a client might decide to run so as to record a more systematic running pattern in the diary)

2. *immediate and positive reinforcement* for completing a run

3. *a chronicle of progress* over time

4. *an opportunity to note and then solve problems* before they become of major importance

5. *an indication of compliance* with the program

Another function of diary maintenance was noted by Brown, Ramirez, and Taub (1978), who conducted extensive running therapy programs for depressed individuals: "We required daily records of exercise, mood change, and pulse rates from subjects who were not patients because it tended to ensure adherence to the exercise schedule. Many people who consider themselves staunch adherents of the old goals of *mens sana in corpore sano* delude themselves about the actual amount of time and care they give their bodies" (p. 41).

## Sources of Additional Information

### FOR CLIENTS

Most clients benefit by reading books by runners who address the common problems and concerns of novices. Such books provide additional motivation to run and eliminate the need to discuss the mechanics of running during therapy sessions. Most such books cover the need for stretching exercises, warmup and cool-down periods, running shoes and other apparel, and dietary changes.

Table 1. Weekly Jogging Log

| Frequency | Intensity | | Duration | |
|---|---|---|---|---|
| Date _____ | My run today felt | | Today's run was | |
| | easy | ____ | 1–20 minutes | ____ |
| Comments [a] _____ | average | ____ | 21–30 minutes | ____ |
| _____ | difficult | ____ | 31–40 minutes | ____ |
| _____ | | | 41–60 minutes | ____ |
| | My breathing | | 61 + minutes | ____ |
| Mood _____ | came easily | ____ | | |
| _____ | was labored | ____ | Distance run | ____ |
| _____ | was labored | | | |
| _____ | throughout | ____ | | |
| | | | | |
| | Heart rate | ____ | | |
| Date _____ | My run today felt | | Today's run was | |
| | easy | ____ | 1–20 minutes | ____ |
| Comments _____ | average | ____ | 21–30 minutes | ____ |
| _____ | difficult | ____ | 31–40 minutes | ____ |
| _____ | | | 41–60 minutes | ____ |
| | My breathing | | 61 + minutes | ____ |
| Mood _____ | came easily | ____ | | |
| _____ | was labored | ____ | Distance run | ____ |
| _____ | was labored | | | |
| _____ | throughout | ____ | | |
| | | | | |
| | Heart rate | ____ | | |
| Date _____ | My run today felt | | Today's run was | |
| | easy | ____ | 1–20 minutes | ____ |
| Comments _____ | average | ____ | 21–30 minutes | ____ |
| _____ | difficult | ____ | 31–40 minutes | ____ |
| _____ | | | 41–60 minutes | ____ |
| | My breathing | | 61 + minutes | ____ |
| Mood _____ | came easily | ____ | | |
| _____ | was labored | ____ | Distance run | ____ |
| _____ | was labored | | | |
| _____ | throughout | ____ | | |
| | | | | |
| | Heart rate | ____ | | |

[a] Comments can include such information as time of day,
weather conditions, location of the run, and companions.

Reading is also likely to increase clients' commitment to running (Joseph and Robbins 1981).

The following books for runners, some of them specifically for women runners, convey the authors' enthusiasm for running, give hints about beginning, and provide solutions to common problems. A highly recommended, entertaining, and accurate book for women clients,[3] *Running for Health and Beauty: A Complete Guide for Women,* is by Kathryn Lance (1977), who had run ten miles a week for five years before writing it. A similar book, *Marathon Mom,* by Linda Schreiber and J. A. Stang (1980), also examines topics particularly important to the novice woman runner. Joan Ullyot, M.D., a marathoner and a popular speaker at running programs, divided her book *Women's Running* (1976) into sections for the beginner, intermediate runner, and racer and includes more on the competitive aspects of running. Specific topics include training plans, aids and advice, and running medicine (physiology, injuries, treatment, etc.). In *The Sports Doctor's Fitness Book for Women,* the late Dr. John L. Marshall (1981), who was chief of surgery at New York Hospital for Special Surgery, reviewed a variety of nutrition and exercise topics. Another highly recommended, easily read, and comprehensive book on running is James Fixx's (1977) *The Complete Book of Running.* Fixx has completed more than six Boston Marathons.

FOR THERAPISTS

Clinicians who employ running as a therapeutic technique can familiarize themselves with the basic physiological considerations of exercise prescription by reading an outstanding text, *Physiology of Fitness* (Sharkey 1979). Although Sharkey's book is not readily available in bookstores, it can be ordered from Human Kinetics Publishers, P.O. Box 5076, Champaign, Illinois 61820. Portions of *Scientific Approach to Distance Running* (Costill 1979), *Implementation of Aerobic Programs* (Cundiff 1979), *Nutrition, Weight Control, and Exercise* (Katch and McArdle 1977), *Fitness: A Lifetime Commitment* (Miller and Allen 1979), and *Beyond Jogging: The Inner Spaces of Running* (Spino 1976) provide excellent information about exercise prescription, physiological considerations for the female runner, and a variety of approaches to running. Detailed information about exercise prescription is presented in *Guidelines for Graded Exercise Testing and Exercise Prescription* (American College of Sports Medicine 1980). Milvy's (1977) 1,090-page collection of papers in *The Marathon: Physiological, Medical, Epidemiological, and Psychological Studies* provides a wealth of research information.

The few books on the therapeutic aspects of running seem to benefit both client and therapist. Michael H. Sacks (M.D.) and Michael L. Sachs (Ph.D.) (1981) have presented by far the broadest and most research-oriented of the three books reviewed in this section. Their edited book, *Psychology of Running,* includes twenty-four chapters by psychologists, psychiatrists, sport psychologists, exercise physiologists, theologians, and runners. In the trade publication *The Joy of Running,* Thaddeus Kostrubala (1976), a psychiatrist who runs with his patients, discusses the physiological need for exercise, how to begin a running program, his personal views on the psychological effects of exercise, and running and therapy (see also Kostrubala, chap. 7). Frederick Harper (1979) explores the effects of jogging on physical and mental health in his monograph of sixty-one pages, *Jogotherapy: Jogging as a Therapeutic Strategy* (see also Harper, chap. 4).

### Include Some Fun in the Run

The answers to ''how fast,'' ''how far,'' and ''how often'' undoubtedly will influence the participant's affective response to running. In general, exercise must be strenuous enough to develop physiological training effects that will allow the client to adapt to the physical stress of running. This physiological adaptation will make the activity less taxing—requiring less attention—and thus more enjoyable. The fun of running can be enhanced by experimenting with location and time of day, by using a portable radio or cassette player, or by running with a companion.

### The Therapist as Runner

Therapists who have reported on their use of running as a therapeutic technique agree that the clinician needs some running experience (Barnes 1980; Buffone 1980a; Harper 1978, 1979; Kostrubala 1976). Books provide information, but experience with running is needed for personal interpretation of the facts. One of the leading psychotherapists who has used running therapy, Kostrubala (Barnes 1980), suggests that the therapist needs to run two marathons a year. Kostrubala runs *with* his clients individually and in groups to promote a closer relationship between therapist and client, to enable the therapist to shed the ''expert'' role, to promote changes in the unconscious of both patient and therapist, and to prevent ''burnout.'' Buffone (1980a,b) has noted that the therapist who runs with clients will reap the benefits of relaxation and a change of pace from the usual fifty minutes of sitting. The basic rationale for the therapist's running marathons is that it provides direct knowledge about training procedures and physiological adaptation to running and enhances self-knowledge (Kostrubala 1976).

The therapist's accompanying a client during a portion of the therapy seems to be a positive, if not ideal, situation for maximizing the therapeutic effects of running. Running tends to lessen the client's defenses and thus promotes communication. Running also may benefit the therapist and enhance therapeutic effectiveness.

The therapist's presence allows the client to ask about specific running problems as they arise and to experiment with one or more solutions when they are needed. It also provides a social model of a runner and allows the therapist to knowledgeably reinforce the client's progress (Harper 1978, 1979). However, unless the therapist approximates the amount of running Kostrubala suggests, she or he may find it physically impossible, or practically undesirable, to run with each client.

The therapist need not run with a client to make running an effective therapeutic approach. Rueter and Harris (1980) reported that running therapy combined with counseling decreased depression more than counseling alone. If the therapist does not run with clients, some minimal amount of running— perhaps of the duration, frequency, and intensity suggested for the novice runner—seems sufficient to let the therapist experience the common practical and physical problems clients encounter, experiment with their solutions, and personally observe the effects of running on mental health. Therapists who do not run with clients would use running therapy in conjunction with their customary therapeutic approaches, perhaps using part of the therapy session to monitor and guide the running program.

### Contraindications for Running

Before encouraging sedentary clients to participate in a running program, the therapist should assess their current health status. Since physiologists do not agree among themselves, a cautious approach is recommended. Running therapy may be contraindicated for *severely depressed* patients (Buffone 1979; Greist et al. 1978).

A client who is over thirty-five, without coronary heart disease (CHD) risk factors,[4] and physically inactive should have a complete medical evaluation and a graded exercise stress test before beginning to run (American College of

Sports Medicine 1980). The American College of Sports Medicine (1980, 2) does not recommend a stress test or consultation with a physician for "asymptomatic, physically active persons of any age without coronary heart disease . . . *if the current type, intensity, and duration of physical activity is maintained*" (italics added). Taken literally, this means that a fifty-year-old woman who already runs for at least twenty minutes (duration) and maintains a heart rate in her target zone (intensity) does not need a stress test before participating in running therapy. Inactive clients under thirty-five who have no CHD risk factors and no cardiovascular, pulmonary, or other diseases that might be aggravated by increased metabolic rates also can begin a jogging program with minimal risk. If there are any questions concerning the health of younger, inactive individuals, a physician should be consulted (American College of Sports Medicine 1980). If the client over thirty-five does not have a stress test, the therapist should require a statement from a personal physician supporting participation in the program. Table 2 lists clients' exercise risk by age and health status. Category A is the lowest risk; category I, the highest. Clients in categories A and B do not need medical clearance to begin running programs. Those in categories C and D should have a complete medical evaluation and a graded exercise stress test. Individuals in categories E, F, and G require a carefully supervised exercise stress test and may choose to exercise only in a closely monitored program designed for heart patients. Those in categories H and I are not suitable candidates for running therapy.

WARNING SIGNS

If any of the following occur while jogging, the client should be instructed to consult a physician:

1. *Abnormal heart action:* irregular pulse, a sudden burst of rapid heartbeats, or a very slow pulse following a rapid one.

2. *Pain or pressure in the middle of the chest, arm, or throat* that is precipitated by the running or follows exertion.

3. *Cold sweats, dizziness, lightheadedness, fainting, loss of coordination, confusion, or pallor* (Sharkey 1979, 373).

EXERCISE STRESS TESTS

Exercise stress tests are not foolproof; two types of errors may occur. "False positive" results indicating an abnormal cardiac response to exercise when none exists occur in 8 to 50 percent of the tests (Sharkey 1979). Sheehan (1979)

## Table 2. Age and Health Status Categories of Clients in a Running Program

| Category | Characteristics |
| --- | --- |

*No medical clearance needed to begin a jogging program*

    **A.** Asymptomatic, physically active clients of any age without CHD risk factors or disease

    **B.** Asymptomatic, physically inactive clients less than thirty-five years of age without CHD risk factors or disease

*Stress test and complete medical evaluation required*

    **C.** Asymptomatic, physically inactive persons thirty-five years and older without CHD risk factors or disease

    **D.** Asymptomatic, physically active or inactive clients of any age with CHD risk factors but no known disease

*A stress test and medical evaluation should be administered by a person certified in graded exercise testing with a physician in visual contact with the client during the test*

    **E.** Asymptomatic persons of any age with known disease

    **F.** Symptomatic, physically active persons clinically stable for six months or longer

    **G.** Symptomatic, physically inactive persons clinically stable for six months or longer

*In addition to the supervision listed above, these clients need a careful assessment of signs, symptoms, EKG, and medications*

    **H.** Symptomatic clients with recent onset of CHD or a change in disease status (example: recent myocardial infarction, unstable angina, coronary artery bypass surgery)

*Clients in this category should not be admitted to a jogging program until their disease has been controlled adequately to allow exercise testing to be performed safely*

    **I.** Persons for whom exercise is contraindicated

Source. American College of Sports Medicine, *Guidelines for Graded Exercise Testing and Exercise Prescription*, 1980.

reported "false positives" in 15 to 30 percent of the tests. False positives are frequent in women and in highly active people. These inaccurate results are disturbing because they may cause healthy individuals to become morbidly concerned with a nonexistent heart condition. "False negative" results occur when the text fails to reveal a circulatory problem that does exist. False negative stress test readings are less common than false positives but far more dangerous. The first symptom of a heart problem is often a myocardial infarction. Stress test results can be verified by angiocardiography (Sharkey 1979, 174), but unfortunately an undetected false negative result gives no warning of the need for this unpleasant technique.

## PERSONAL HEALTH HISTORIES

Although asymptomatic clients under thirty-five can probably begin running with no threat to their health, the therapist should take a personal medical and surgical history and a family health history and should inquire about current habits such as smoking, diet, alcohol intake, stresses, and habitual physical activity. Men and women who have had cardiovascular or respiratory problems or who have family histories of heart disease should be referred to their family physicians for stress tests. Physical problems that may preclude running therapy or require special precautions are severe anemia (hemoglobin below 10 g/dl); coronary heart disease; diabetes mellitus; severe hypertension (diastolic pressure above 110, grade III retinopathy); and neuromuscular, musculoskeletal, orthopedic, or arthritic disorders that prevent activity (American College of Sports Medicine 1980, 12–14).

## OBESITY

A walking or a walk/run exercise program in conjunction with dieting is an ideal way for obese individuals to lose weight (Sharkey 1979), but they may not reap the psychological benefits of a running program as *quickly* as those who are not overweight (Buffone 1980b; Dishman 1981). Obese clients may not adhere to exercise programs and tend to discontinue running when their supervised program ends (Buffone 1980b). The obese jogger certainly requires considerably more encouragement to continue than does her or his leaner counterpart.

## AGE

Age is not a contraindication for running. Although aerobic fitness declines with age, there is ample physiological research to support the desirability of beginning to run at any age (deVries 1974; Sharkey 1979, 18). Examples of people who began to exercise at relatively advanced ages abound. Eula Weaver had a history of congestive heart failure and poor circulation, and at age eighty-one she had a heart attack. Unable to walk one hundred feet at first, she began to run, lifted weights several times a week, and at eighty-five won a gold medal in her age group for the one-mile run at the Senior Olympics (Sharkey 1979, 18). Other outstanding runners over seventy include Mavis Lindgren (seventy-four), Walter Stack (seventy-three), who is a veteran of more than one hundred marathons, and John Kelley (seventy-three), who has run in 107 marathons, fifty-one times in the Boston Marathon (Cranston 1981; Paling 1981).

What is particularly impressive about the older women runners is that, unlike many of the men, such as Walter Stack and John Kelley, they are novice athletes. Mavis Lindgren first began running at sixty-two, ran her first marathon when she was sixty-nine and set a marathon age-group world record for women sixty-five or older when she was seventy-two (Cranston 1981). Marcie Trent (sixty) ran her first marathon at fifty-seven and also has demonstrated that performance can improve with age (Palmason 1981).

That most of the older women runners were not physically active when they were younger shows that women of all ages can begin to run if they have no signs of heart disease and few CHD risk factors. One reason there are few veteran women runners is that women have been barred from marathons and other middle- and long-distance races until very recently. As late as 1967 Jock Semple, race director of the Boston Marathon, tried to prevent Katherine Switzer from running when her gender was discovered (Thomas 1981). Olympic marathon competition for women will be held for the first time in 1984. Women who began to run late in life have helped reduce the barriers and serve as role models for sedentary women of all ages. Typical of older women runners is Ellen Pereira of Toronto, who finished second in the fifty-plus category. She remarked with pride, "When I was young, I never did anything sporting at all. Now at 53, I have become an athlete!" (Palmason 1981).

## Advantages of Running Therapy

A major advantage of running therapy is that clients accept more responsibility than in traditional approaches (Buffone 1979, 1980a,b). Running therapy provides opportunities for self-direction as clients determine how far, how long, how fast, and where they will run. Scheduling runs can be an integral element in a self-management program. In determining which days they prefer to run, the time of day that is least disruptive, and their physical functioning during the run, clients actively regulate and manage their own programs. Since running can be addicting (Glasser 1976; Sachs 1982; chap. 13 in this book), the client is likely to continue after therapy ends. Running is a time-efficient and cost-effective approach to improved mental health (Buffone 1979; Greist et al. 1978).

The self-regulatory aspects of a running program are closely associated with a client's locus of control (Dienstbier 1977). People at the *internal* end of the locus of control continuum tend to accept responsibility for their behavior; those at the external end tend to ascribe their behavior to causes beyond their control (such as luck, fate, and powerful others). Locus of control seems to be situationally specific, so clients in running therapy should be encouraged to tailor their programs to their own needs and capabilities. By focusing on their "personal best," clients can accept responsibility for their progress and thus develop a more internal locus of control. Though runners who compete in races can offer a host of "external" explanations for poor performance, since many factors determine the outcome, competing *with* one's self rather than *against* others (Dienstbier 1977) helps the client feel more responsible for success or failure. Table 3 lists responses to common problems encountered by clients in running therapy who are at the extreme ends of the locus of control continuum. Most people, of course, are near the middle and vary their responses. A client whose locus of control is internal will be more inclined to adopt a self-regulatory approach, to reap the benefits of running as therapy, and to continue running after therapy ends.

### Adherence

Adherence to exercise is a crucial concern not only for therapists who employ running as a technique but also for the directors of cardiac rehabilitation programs, physical educators, coaches, and the population in general. Morgan (1977) reports that the dropout rate of organized exercise programs ranges between 30 percent and 70 percent. Despite the significance of this issue, experimental data are just beginning to appear (Buffone, Sachs, and Dowd, chap. 11 in this book; Danielson and Wanzel 1978; Dishman 1981; Morgan 1977; Pollock et al. 1977; Wysocki et al. 1979).

#### BODY FAT, WEIGHT, AND METABOLIC CAPACITY

Dishman (1981) investigated the relation between length of exercise adherence and morphological and physiological characteristics of 181 middle-aged men over a five-year period. Some of the men participated in the exercise

Table 3. Responses to Running Problems by
Clients Who Differ in Locus of Control

| External Locus of Control | Problem | Internal Locus of Control |
|---|---|---|
| I was depressed and too tired to run. | Tiredness | Although I was depressed and had no interest in running, I jogged and walked for twenty minutes and felt a little better. |
| My boss asked me to work late, so I was unable to run. | Unexpected events | I ran early today because I worked late yesterday and had no time to run. |
| My responsibilities today prevented me from running. | Scheduling | I found time to run today by eliminating a few things that I did not absolutely need to do. |
| It was raining so I could not run | Rain | I took advantage of the few minutes today when it was not raining to run. *or* Since rain was forecast for tomorrow, my running day, I ran a day early. |
| It was too hot to run. | Heat | I ran early in the morning to avoid the heat. |
| I have decided to quit running because it is not safe to run in my neighborhood. | Muggers | I run with a friend to avoid muggers. *or* I run in a heavily populated area rather than in my favorite but deserted area because I am worried about being mugged. |

program for cardiac rehabilitation; others participated for personal reasons. Of the eleven physical characteristics tested, only *percentage of body fat, weight in relation to height,* and *metabolic capacity* together significantly differentiated between men who adhered and those who dropped out of the programs. Leaner, lighter, less fit men participated longer than others. Although these three factors were significantly related to adherence, their predictive capabilities in another sample of 181 men were low.

Dishman's (1981) explanation for the first two factors seems to disagree with that for the third. Leaner and lighter men may have persisted longer because exercise was easier for them than for their fatter and heavier counterparts. But adherence of the less fit men is the opposite of what might be anticipated if exercise ease does influence adherence. Dishman speculated that less fit men remained in the program longer because they recognized that they needed exercise to deter heart disease. If so, why did not heavier, fatter men also recognize their need for exercise? It is not surprising that in another study of sixty-six adult men in various exercise settings Dishman and his colleagues (Dishman and Gettman 1980; Dishman, Ickes, and Morgan 1980) reported percentage of body fat and weight were significantly related to exercise adherence but metabolic capacity was not.

Factors that have been related to exercise adherence in middle-aged men, some of whom had CHD, may be very different from those that influence women's adherence to exercise. But until additional information is available it seems prudent to encourage both women and men with high percentages of body fat and high weight in relation to height to continue their running. The therapist should build immediate rewards into the programs.

That excess weight tends to deter adherence has also emerged as an adherence problem in a clinical study of running therapy (Buffone 1980b) and in other physical fitness studies (Massie and Shephard 1971). But the observation that the less fit men remained in an exercise program longer (Dishman 1981) directly disagrees with Buffone's (1980b) study and the other studies by Dishman and his colleagues. Despite conflicting observations on running fitness, it is logical to encourage clients to run long enough to condition their bodies so they can run with less effort and glean the psychological benefits of running. Highly fit clients who have not run before should be helped to set challenging but attainable running goals.

SELF-MOTIVATION

Self-motivation, a general disposition to persevere, also may affect exercise adherence (Dishman, Ickes, and Morgan 1980). Self-motivation is described by Dishman and Gettman (1980) as a personality trait and thus as relatively independent of situational influences. Defined as a generalized tendency to persist without extrinsic reinforcement, self-motivation is probably socially learned and may include an ability to delay gratification. It is thought to be independent of locus of control, attributions of success and failure, achievement motivation, and approval motivation (Dishman and Gettman 1980).

Noting a need for a practical, accurate method of identifying potential exercise dropouts, Ickes (Dishman, Ickes, and Morgan 1980) constructed an initial pool of sixty objective test questions, subsequently reduced to forty. The resulting Self-Motivation Inventory (SMI) has successfully distinguished between adherers and dropouts in several circumstances. In the first study, the SMI scores of adherers on a women's varsity crew team ($N = 64$) were significantly higher than those of dropouts at each of three naturally occurring breakpoints during a thirty-two-week training season. In a second validation study the SMI was the only one of several psychological indexes that contributed significantly to separating male exercise adherers and dropouts ($N = 66$) in three twenty-week exercise programs, using discriminant and regression analysis (Dishman and Gettman 1980; Dishman, Ickes, and Morgan 1980). (The others were the Health Locus of Control (Wallston et al. 1976), the Physical Estimation and Attraction Scales (Sonstroem 1974), and the Attitude toward Physical Activity Scales (Kenyon 1968b). By noting at the outset a client's likelihood of persisting, the therapist can address the needs of the probable dropout. If the construct of a *general* disposition to persevere is accurate, scores on the SMI would indicate which clients are most likely to discontinue therapy regardless of the particular approach employed.

BEHAVIORAL CONTRACTING

In another study of exercise adherence, Wysocki et al. (1979) investigated three common problems in getting people to exercise in their natural environments: (1) equating the intensity and duration of an exercise such as running with that of another such as tennis; (2) developing a monitoring system that ensures the client has exercised, with minimal demands on the therapist or experimenter; and (3) determining the effectiveness of behavioral contracting in encouraging clients to increase their ongoing level of exercise. Cooper's (1970) aerobic point system for various activities has helped solve the first two problems. The point values guided the twelve female and male students in choosing an activity; determining and recording exercise intensity, duration, and frequency; and accurately monitoring each other (interobserver reliability across all observations was 99.2 percent).

In a behavioral contracting program that could be employed in running therapy, students and experimenters negotiated exercise goals, number of aerobic points to be earned each week, and rewards. The students deposited six valuable items with the experimenters, such as checks made out to charities, jewelry, clothing, and other personal items, then signed contracts outlining the conditions under which the deposits would be refunded. They could earn two items each week, one for attaining the aerobic point criterion and completing a form indicating the number of points, the second for recording observational data for other subjects in the study. Before the items were returned, they deposited two more items. Rules for participation were strict: those who withdrew forfeited all items on deposit, and they had to verify any illness that kept them from exercising. Forfeited items were donated to a nonprofit organization. Students and experimenters renegotiated contracts every two weeks for more aerobic points.

Although four of the twelve volunteers dropped out during the first few weeks because of time problems ($n = 3$) or because they prefered anaerobic exercise ($n = 1$) and two others were released because of medical problems, Wysocki et al. (1979) concluded that behavioral contracting was successful in encouraging the remaining participants to exercise. A follow-up questionnaire indicated that a year after the study seven participants[5] were still exercising enough to earn more aerobic points than when the study began, and three of the seven were exercising more extensively than at the end of the contract.

## ADHERENCE OF NOVICE AND TRAINED RUNNERS

Dienstbier (1977), former chairperson of the Department of Psychology at the University of Nebraska and a marathoner, has offered some practical suggestions for motivating novice joggers to become habitual runners. His major observation is that the immediate pleasures that the habitual runner experiences are not readily available to the novice. Habitual runners encounter rewards such as mood elevation, stress reduction, peak experiences, and sense of accomplishment (Carmack and Martens 1979; Glasser 1976; Kostrubala 1976; Mandell 1979), that are intrinsic to the running. But novice runners probably will not discover these joys until they have been running for the two or three months it takes the body to adapt to the physical stress of running. Novice runners tend to describe running as "painful, work, and a chore." Poor adherence rates during the first few months of training (Buffone 1980b; Danielson and Wanzel 1978) support the need for extrinsic rewards during this period of training. If running is to become a permanent component of the lifestyle rather than a transitory activity, the novice runner must experience *short-term pleasures* and rewards and anticipate *long-term benefits* such as decreases in anxiety and depression and enhanced cardiovascular fitness.

RUNNING ADHERENCE GUIDELINES

Specific suggestions that the therapist can make to help clients increase the immediate rewards of running and minimize the effort required include the following.

1. *Maintain a running log, as described in table 1*. This provides immediate, daily success. Some clients who would like to stop after ten minutes will continue ten minutes longer so they can record that they completed a minimum run. A running log also encourages clients to run *with* themselves rather than *against* other runners. Noting one's mood before and after running emphasizes the mood-enhancing results of running and can be an immediate reward.

2. *Set realistic, attainable goals*. Most clients do not feel rewarded by achieving goals set too low. Unrealistically high goals are also discouraging, provide excuses for failure, and may create a major adherence problem. Although novices need extrinsic rewards while their bodies adjust to the physical demands of running, they will observe much greater changes in their running ability than those who are highly fit when they begin. Highly fit individuals tend to set unrealistically high goals (Dishman 1981). Setting attainable but challenging goals is crucial to running adherence. In a study of dropouts, women and men who did not attain their exercise goals within six months withdrew from the program much more quickly than those who attained their objectives (Danielson and Wanzel 1978).

3. *Maintain a realistic view of running*. Do not promise too much. Some days running will be fun, challenging, or a welcome change of pace. Other days it will be painful, boring, or sheer drudgery. Novice runners should realize that committed runners often exaggerate the pleasures of running to justify their own behavior (Dienstbier 1977).

4. *Keep a decision balance sheet*. A decision balance sheet encourages the novice to systematically consider potential gains and losses resulting from a decision to jog and then to carry out that decision. This technique has been employed successfully in adult exercise programs (Hoyt and Janis 1975; Wankel and Graham 1977; Wankel and Thompson 1980) and may be especially helpful in encouraging adherence in potential dropouts identified through the Self-Motivation Inventory (Dishman, Ickes, and Morgan 1980; Wankel and Graham 1980). The general procedure includes asking clients to consider and systematically record anticipated gains and losses both to themselves and to important others that might result from their jogging. They can then read the responses to the therapist, who can respond with appropriate encouraging comments and reinforce the desirable outcomes of jogging.

5. *Dissociate from the physical effort required.* Another way for novice runners to increase short-term pleasure is to dissociate their thoughts from the physical effort by engaging in fantasy, free association, or serious productive thought while running. As Dienstbier (1977, 21) has noted, "The reduction of the perception of effort is important, perhaps essential" if the novice is to continue running. (Refer to Sachs, chapt. 16, in this book for a comprehensive examination of associative and dissociative strategies while running.) Successful world-class runners do not disassociate from their awareness of physical effort (Morgan 1978), but novice runners who are not trying to run their farthest and fastest in each run can greatly reduce the physical discomfort and boredom of running by this technique. Dissociation can be achieved most easily at a gentle, slow pace, after the body has been conditioned sufficiently so the runner is relaxed (Dienstbier 1977; Glasser 1976). Another way to dissociate from the physical effort is to talk with a companion while running (see item 8) (Dienstbier 1977).

6. *Focus on appearance.* Running will enhance most people's appearance by burning extra calories and thus reducing fatty tissue. Clients who diet while in the running program will lose more fat by running *and* dieting than by dieting alone, and a smaller proportion of the weight loss will be protein and water (Sharkey 1979, 118). Getting into shape and losing weight for the sake of appearance were the first and third most important motives for beginning to run among 315 female and male runners of various abilities (Carmack and Martens 1979; see table 4), which agrees with results reported by Campbell (1977). Appearance seems to be a particularly important goal among older women (Danielson and Wanzel 1978).

7. *Explore feelings of mastering one's body.* For novice exercisers, a majority of whom are women, feeling physically strong, powerful, and competent is often a new and exciting experience (Berger and Mackenzie 1980; Huey, 1976). Discussing these feelings will increase clients' awareness of them and emphasize the influence of running on psychological well-being.

8. *Set higher goals very gradually.* Running should be fun, not a task. Just because a goal has been met on one day does not mean it is time to raise it. Conditions differ. On one day running continuously for twenty minutes may be easy, but it may be exceedingly difficult the next time. Clients need to learn to listen to their bodies and to feel competent in interpreting physical sensations to determine the characteristics of a run on any particular day.

9. *Run with a companion.* Gregarious clients who find running boring may discover that conversing with a friend during a run makes running seem less mindless. Of course one must find a companion with comparable running

ability so both runners are content to maintain the same pace. Scheduling a definite time and place to run with another person also may increase the likelihood of running three times a week, since an obligation to meet someone may be more successful in getting the client "out the door" than a commitment to self or therapist.

10. *Experiment with behavioral contracting.* After a week or two of experimentation, therapist and client can set running goals. The client can provide three to six items of worth, as described in the preceding section on "Behavioral Contracting," and then sign a contract every two weeks or so outlining the conditions for return of one of the deposits. Refer to Wysocki et al. (1979) for additional discussion of this technique.

WHY DO RUNNERS RUN?

Integrally related to adherence is the question, Why do runners run? (Berger 1979; Berger and Mackenzie 1980; Carmack and Martens 1979; Glasser 1976). The broader question, why people spend enormous quantities of time, effort, and energy in physical activity, has interested physical educators for years (Berger 1972; Harris 1973; Kenyon 1968a,b; Slusher 1967). Answering these questions is a key to increasing exercise adherence.

Examining commitment or addiction to running, Carmack and Martens (1979) administered questionnaires to 315 runners (65 females, 250 males) aged thirteen to sixty (mean 28.8 years), in four categories from Olympic contenders to midday users of a college track. Responses were surprisingly similar in terms of comfort/discomfort, perceived addiction, and commitment to running. Reasons for *beginning* to run reflected short-term, extrinsic goals (it was not the running itself that attracted people, but its concomitants). Their reasons for *continuing* to run were more intrinsic. With running experience, enjoyment rose from 8 to 12 percent of the total responses. Competition became the third most important reason. Table 4 shows the motives of beginning and habitual runners. The runners' perceived outcomes of running, listed below, argue strongly for the therapeutic use of running:

1. physical health (cardiovascular conditioning, weight control)
2. psychological uplift (decreased anxiety, improved mood)
3. self-image (self-respect, sense of identity)
4. affiliation (fellowship with other runners)
4. achievement (success in competition) (Carmack and Martens 1979).

Studying the running motives of ten women who had been running for at least two years and who averaged between thirty and ninety-seven miles a

Table 4. Reasons for Running

| Reasons for Beginning to Run | Percentage of Total Responses | Reasons for Continuing to Run | Percentage of Total Responses |
|---|---|---|---|
| Get into shape | 14 | Maintain fitness | 19 |
| Enjoyment | 8 | Enjoyment | 12 |
| Lose weight | 8 | Competition | 6 |
| Maintain fitness | 6 | Weight control | 5 |
| Was good at it | 5 | Feel better | 5 |
| Total | 41 | Total | 47 |

Source. Adapted from Carmack and Martens 1979.

week, Hendry (1978) found that their most important motive was health. Other motives, in order of importance, included pleasure, self-esteem, appearance, influence of another person, competition, and social reasons.

LONGER RUNS MAY ENCOURAGE ADHERENCE

A running duration of twenty minutes has been suggested as an obtainable goal for a novice runner. However, there is evidence that running forty to sixty minutes may be conducive to more positive emotional states than shorter runs (Carmack and Martens 1979; Glasser 1976; Kostrubala 1976). During the first twenty minutes runners often feel pain and wonder why they are running. This dysphoria peaks between twenty and thirty minutes, and they experience an "opening up" (beginning to breathe more freely and run more easily) thirty to forty minutes after beginning. Altered states of consciousness, or "runner's highs," occur more frequently after thirty to forty minutes than in the early part of the run (Kostrubala 1976, 104–7; Mandell 1979; Sachs, chap. 15).

Carmack and Martens (1979) found that runners who ran longer than forty minutes were significantly more addicted to running than those whose runs were shorter. "Spin out" was characterized by a clearing of the mind, a floating sensation, or a detached dreaming state and was significantly related to runners' addiction only in the last quarter of the run. Their experiment supports Glasser's (1976), Kostrubala's (1976), and Mandell's (1979) contentions that the psychological "highs" occur more consistently in runs longer than forty minutes.

The psychological well-being (happiness and optimism) or uneasiness (boredom, depression, irritability) of runners who habitually ran more or less than forty minutes were compared. For the two groups different states of mind prevailed during different quarters of the run and at the beginning of the run. Those who ran longer than forty minutes reported psychological well-being during the first half and the last quarter of the run. Those who ran less than forty minutes reported psychological well-being only in the third quarter.

Adherence is a critical factor in the success of running therapy. By suggesting the preceding guidelines, by carefully monitoring the running of overweight clients, by encouraging clients to be self-motivating, and by suggesting *eventual* complete runs of forty minutes, the therapist can increase the likelihood that running therapy will be effective.

## Physiological Concerns of Women Runners

When prescribing exercise for a woman client, the therapist should discuss some of the more common myths or old wives' tales about women and exercise and address specific exercise concerns the client may have. Acknowledging, examining, and resolving personal worries about strenuous physical activity is an important aspect of the problem solving required to establish running as a daily habit. If such fears are ignored the client is likely to exercise less strenuously than desirable or to discontinue altogether.

Based on the demographic characteristics of this patient population, therapists who regularly prescribe exercise for female clients are likely to recognize certain concerns. Muscle bulk, injuries, the menstrual cycle, sagging breasts, and weight stabilization are some of the more common ones. Since most of the research on these topics has focused on women athletes rather than recreational runners, both the positive and the negative effects experienced by novice joggers will be less pronounced.

### THE MUSCLE MYTH

Women often voice concern that athletic participation will give them bulky muscles. Muscle mass is clearly related to genetically determined levels of sex hormones and the proportion of fast-twitch to slow-twitch fibers within the muscles (Harris 1973, 196; Shaffer 1972) and thus is inherited rather than developed through exercise. However, the muscle myth is perpetuated by the success of women with large muscles in strength-dependent activities such as field throwing events (discus, shot put, and javelin) and the butterfly stroke in swimming. This relationship between outstanding physical ability and muscle bulk, which unfortunately is easily observed, is one of *association* rather than *causality*. What is obvious is that muscle strength is directly related to muscle mass. Thus, women who are *born* with large muscles are far more successful in strength-based sports. Yes, women shot putters do have large muscles; but it was *not* exercise that produced their muscle. The training merely emphasized what they already had. Women with lower levels of androgen and a high percentage of slow-twitch muscle fibers, no matter how much they train, will not develop large muscles.

The prospect of a bulky, "masculine" appearance is so frightening to women who have been socialized to be thin and feminine that it may deter physical activity. A study comparing the strength and body dimensions of women and men in four different body parts before and after ten weeks of exercise indicated that women can greatly increase their strength *without* an accompanying muscular hypertrophy (Wilmore 1974). Since runners tend to have lean rather than bulky muscles, muscle development is not as strong a deterrent in some other sports. Also, stretching exercises to maintain flexibility will counterbalance any muscle hypertrophy produced by the running itself.

INJURIES

Contrary to much popular belief, the injury rates of women novice runners are comparable to those of novice males (Franklin, Lussier, and Buskirk 1979). Although differences in pelvic width and joint flexibility suggest a greater potential for running injuries in women than in men (Haycock and Gillette 1976), the actual occurrence of more injuries has not been substantiated. Since running injuries are most frequent among beginners (Glick and Katch 1970), especially within the first six weeks of training (Franklin, Lussier, and Buskirk 1979), it is particularly important to protect all novices, women and men, against injuries.

Jogging-related injuries have been positively related to the frequency, duration, and intensity of exercise. In a two-part study of male prisoners, Pollock et al. (1977) reported that for men running at between 85 percent and 90 percent of their maximum heart rate three days a week, injury rates for fifteen-, thirty-, and forty-five-minute sessions were 22 percent, 24 percent, and 54 percent respectively. Injury rates for men running at between 85 percent and 90 percent of their maximum heart rate in thirty-minute sessions increased from 0 to 12 percent to 39 percent as running frequency changed from one to three to five times a week. Although greater increases in the physiological training effects occurred in the forty-five-minute and five-day programs, this schedule is *not recommended* for beginning runners.

In a study of running injuries in women, Franklin, Lussier, and Buskirk (1979) supervised the running of thirty-six sedentary volunteers between the ages of twenty-nine and forty-seven who participated in a moderate running program similar to that suggested here. The running program consisted of four sessions a week rather than the three I have suggested for twelve weeks, and the women ran at a speed that maintained 75 percent of their maximum training heart rate. By the beginning of the fourth week each session included ten minutes of calisthenics, fifteen to thirty minutes of continuous walking/jogging, and a five-minute cool-down period. Despite the focus on stretching and muscle strengthening during the first three weeks, nine of the eleven injuries reported occurred during the first six weeks of training (82 percent). Both type and incidence of injury were very similar to those previously reported for men (Franklin, Besseghini, and Golden 1978; Pollock et al. 1977).

An interesting result reported by Franklin et al. (1979) was that the incidence of injury was similar in obese (30 percent) and in thin to normal (31 percent) women. This unexpected result apparently occurred because obese women who exercised at 75 percent of maximum heart rate often engaged only in brisk walking rather than running. If exercise intensity is monitored by heart rate, therefore, women with a high percentage of body fat seem no more prone to injury than leaner women.

To reduce the likelihood of injury, novice runners should:

1. begin slowly
2. remain within the suggested duration, frequency, and intensity
3. wear well-cushioned, properly fitted running shoes
4. perform at least five minutes of stretching exercises after running (muscles are more limber at this time) or at some other time whenever they run
5. avoid running in only one direction on hard surfaces (paved roads generally are banked, placing excess stress on one hip and knee)
6. avoid running on uneven or irregular surfaces (to avoid ankle injuries)
7. follow recommended foot placement (strides should be relatively short and one should strike the ground gently, landing on the heel before rotating to the toes).

INJURY TO THE REPRODUCTIVE SYSTEM

Another concern often voiced is that the jarring as the feet hit the ground may injure a woman's reproductive organs. Little mention is made in the media of danger to men's reproductive organs, which are less well protected than women's. An example of the common message to women is the large headline that appeared in the *Houston Post:* "PHYSICIAN TELLS WOMEN JOGGING NOT BENEFICIAL."

Chicago (UPI)—The female body is not constructed for jogging so women joggers should switch to other sports, a gynecologist says. "Women are not built for jogging," says Dr. Allan G. Charles of Michael Reese Hospital and Medical Center. "I will be accused of being a male chauvinist, but the facts are that the female bony pelvis is much wider than the male's." (*American Medical Joggers Association Newsletter,* 1979, p. 28)

He notes that muscular and connective tissues are often weakened by childbirth, resulting in a prolapsed uterus and stress incontinence, in which the pressure of the uterus on the bladder causes dribbling of urine at each impact. Articles like this are difficult for many women and men to interpret and undoubtedly do prevent some women from running. In a few rare ailments, running may be detrimental to health; but I wonder why Dr. Charles did not simply advise that women with such stretched pelvic muscles do regular Kegel exercises to correct the condition rather than merely accept it. For the "normal" female, the doctor's caution is not supported by experimental evidence.

### The Menstrual Cycle

In general, research evidence indicates that menstruation has a slight negative effect on coordination (Shangold 1980) but no effect on perceived exertion, work capacity, or anaerobic threshold (Stephenson, Kolka, and Wilderson 1980). As might be expected, women with histories of dysmenorrhea may not perform at their best during menstruation (Bonen 1981; Shangold 1980), but many athletes have reported less dysmenorrhea than usual while training (Dale, Gerlach, and Wilhite 1979; Shangold 1980) and a lighter menstrual flow (Dale, Gerlach, and Wilhite 1979). In fact, it has been substantiated by a series of studies that dysmenorrhea is more prevalent in women who are physically inactive (Gendel 1978). There is no evidence that women should not run while menstruating (Parlee 1976; Thomas 1971; Ullyot 1976, 119–20; Wells 1971).

Menstrual irregularity or disappearance of a woman's monthly cycle (amenorrhea) is experienced by *some athletes* who engage in strenuous training (Dale, Gerlach, and Wilhite 1979). The type of amenorrhea most frequently experienced by athletes is termed "secondary amenorrhea" and may be related to the loss of body fat that often accompanies strenuous training rather than to a hormone deficiency. "Secondary amenorrhea" refers to missing three regular cycles or ceasing to menstruate for six months ("Menstrual Changes in Athletes" 1981). "Primary amenorrhea" indicates that a woman has not begun her menstrual cycle by the age of sixteen (Frisch and McArthur 1974; "Menstrual Changes in Athletes" 1981). "Oligomenorrhea" is used to describe infrequent menstruation ("Menstrual Changes in Athletes" 1981). In a study of 557 Hungarian female athletes, Erdelyi (1962) reported that strenuous training had an adverse effect on menstruation in 12 percent, no effect in 83 percent, and a beneficial effect in five percent. Since athletes competing in strenuous sports such as skiing and tennis experienced secondary amenorrhea and oligomenorrhea more frequently than those competing in less strenuous activities (Erdelyi 1976), it is unlikely that women who run for therapeutic purposes will notice any change in their menstrual patterns.

Since a small amount of body fat is necessary to maintain normal menstrual functioning, amenorrhea is a common symptom of anorexia nervosa (Dale, Gerlach, and Wilhite 1979; Sours 1980, 1981). A regular menstrual cycle usually follows when these women gain enough so that fat constitutes about 22 percent of total body weight (Frisch and McArthur 1974). This percentage seems high, since obesity for women has been reported to be 30 percent body fat (McArdle, Katch, and Katch 1981, 406). In fact, others have reported that lower percentages of body fat (12 to 18 percent) maintain regular menses (McArdle, Katch, and Katch 1981, 370–71). Sharkey (1979, 114) reported the minimum amount of body fat needed for good health and nutrition to be about 7 to 10 percent for women and 5 percent for men.

Strenuous exercise does reduce the percentage of body fat. An average woman's body weight is approximately 25 percent fat (Katch and McArdle 1977, 102–4; Wilmore, Brown, and Davis 1977). As Wilmore (1979) noted in comparing the physical capabilities of female and male athletes in a variety of sports, the mature woman's average percentage of fat is considerably above the ideal. Wilmore blames the sedentary lifestyle of the average woman for her undesirable level of fat. Very thin women have about 15 percent body fat, and one woman runner has been reported to have 5.9 percent body fat (McArdle, Katch, and Katch 1981, 371).

Amenorrhea tends to occur when body fat falls below 10 to 12 percent of body weight. Among women runners who have secondary amenorrhea, reducing training to under fifty miles a week usually reestablishes regular monthly cycles (Bonen 1981). Dale, Gerlach, and Wilhite (1979) also reported that amenorrhea frequently is reversed when training is reduced, as in injury or at the conclusion of a competitive season. It is not certain, however, whether the return of menses is caused by an increase in adipose tissue or by the decrease in training itself (Dale, Gerlach, and Wilhite 1979). Speculating on the cause(s) of changes in menstrual patterns, Dale and his colleagues reported,

> The response to physical and psychological stresses may be reflected through changes in body weight, percentage of body fat, hormone secretion, subtle changes in body-core temperature, and emotional makeup, all of which may influence hypothalamic function and be expressed as alterations in menstrual patterns. (Dale, Gerlach, and Wilhite 1979, 51)

Dale, Gerlach, and Wilhite (1979) studied the menstrual cycles of women runners who ran more than thirty miles a week, those who ran between five and thirty miles a week, and a control group who did not run. Speroff and Redwine (1980), by contrast, noted no correlation between miles run per week and amenorrhea in their study of 859 women runners. Only 18.6 percent of these women ran more than twenty miles a week, well below the fifty miles suggested by Bonen (1981) as the critical distance that causes a pronounced loss of body fat and an increase in amenorrhea. Speroff and Redwine concluded in their study of low-mileage women that low initial weight and weight losses of more than ten pounds while running were more closely related to the development of menstrual irregularity than were age, height, or duration of running.

Amenorrhea in exercisers tends to be reversible (Dale et al. 1979; Dale, Gerlach, and Wilhite 1979) and also is unrelated to future childbearing (Dale et al. 1979). However, as Shangold (1980) cautioned, athletes with menstrual dysfunction should be evaluated as thoroughly as nonathletes so major medical problems can be diagnosed and treated. *"No problem should be presumed to be either exercise related or insignificant"* (p. 68; italics added).

Most women clients will not be running enough to reduce their body fat below 10 to 12 percent (McArdle, Katch, and Katch 1981; Sharkey 1979). Despite the *association* between low body fat and amenorrhea, it should not be presumed that exercise *causes* amenorrhea. In the absence of infertility, a menstrual interval of twenty to sixty days requires no attention (Shangold 1980). If a woman's menstrual interval is less than twenty days or more than sixty, or if she has intermenstrual bleeding, she should consult a specialist. Special attention to the diet and the running mileage of extremely thin clients can prevent many cases of secondary amenorrhea. Should any of the problems above occur the client should be examined by a specialist, since studies indicate they normally are not exercise-related.

*Pregnancy and Childbirth*

There is no evidence that vigorous exercise is detrimental to a woman or her fetus during a normal, uncomplicated pregnancy (Dressendorfer and Goodlin 1980; Hutchinson, Cureton, and Sparling 1981; Ullyot 1976, 120–21), and some studies indicate that strenuous exercise benefits the pregnant woman by improving her physical work capacity (Collings, Curet, and Mullin 1981; Dressendorfer 1978) or maintaining her prepregnancy fitness level (Ruhling et al. 1981).

Patricia Hutchinson and her colleagues (1981) reported a case study of a thirty-two-year-old pregnant runner; her metabolic, respiratory, and circulatory responses to running during pregnancy were similar to those of nonpregnant women. She had run between three and five miles three to five days a week for eight years preceding her pregnancy and continued to run the same distance until the ninth month of her pregnancy, when she chose to walk three miles a day. In monthly testing sessions during the third to the ninth month of pregnancy the experimenters observed that as body weight increased running became increasingly stressful, as indicated by substantial increases in oxygen uptake, heart rate, and ventilation. They recommend that pregnant women progressively decrease their running speed to maintain a constant level of physiological strain.

In their study of 859 women runners, Speroff and Redwine (1980) noted that 7.3 percent of the respondents were pregnant and running, 3.3 percent were breastfeeding and running, and 14.2 percent had run during pregnancy. It seems that women and their physicians are increasingly recognizing that running enhances rather than harms physical health during pregnancy.

SAGGING BREASTS AND BREAST DISCOMFORT

Great attention has been focused on this minor problem. For women who wear a B cup or larger, running a mile or two several times a week *without* a supportive bra probably will increase the likelihood that the breasts will lose support from the connective tissue. Although the effect may be more readily apparent in large-breasted women who are already beginning to sag, the woman runner whose breasts are large enough to bounce should wear a highly supportive bra if she cares whether her breasts sag. There are ''sport'' and even ''running'' bras designed to be particularly supportive.

Noting that 72 percent of women athletes experienced sore or tender breasts after exercise (Haycock and Gillette 1976), Gehlsen and Albohm (1980) examined the support offered by eight sports bras, the range of breast movement acceptable for comfort while jogging, and the effects of binding the breasts while running. The large and significant differences in vertical displacement of the breasts allowed by the eight bras show that the buyer should jog in place to test several bras before purchasing one. Breast mass, in conjunction with velocity of vertical displacement, significantly differentiated between women who had experienced breast discomfort from running and those who had not. Thus, women who experience discomfort should wear effective support bras.

My own experience is that the popular see-through nylon bras do not provide enough support for running comfort, but many of the more substantial styles provide as much support as the specially designed sport bras. Women who normally experience no breast discomfort may use any bra or go braless while running; if they experience some breast tenderness before their menses they might wear support bras at these times. Each woman should experiment to determine what is best for her.

## WEIGHT LOSS OR WEIGHT GAIN

That a person must run for thirty minutes (burn approximately three hundred calories) on eleven occasions to lose one pound of fat (3,500 calories) has deterred many prospective exercisers. But if one diets in conjunction with exercise, the loss of body fat and the conservation of lean tissue are far superior to what is accomplished by dieting alone (Sharkey 1979, 116–28; Stalonas, Johnson, and Christ 1978; Thompson et al., 1982). Chapters 7 to 11 in the *Physiology of Fitness* (Sharkey 1979) provide additional information. As noted by Wilmore, Brown, and Davis (1977, 764), "Recently, it has been established unequivocally that exercise is a primary factor in both the control and alteration of body composition. This has been demonstrated in the normal population as well as in various athletic populations for males and females alike."

Another misleading idea is that thin persons will become even thinner if they exercise. However, exercise tones muscles and thus contours the body and produces a more pleasing shape whether a person is thin or fat. Sedentary clients with little muscle who begin running may gain weight as they replace fat with heavier muscle tissue. Such overweight clients may conclude that exercise is useless and stop running. But in spite of their weight gain, heavy persons will appear lighter or thinner after running because of their firmer, more muscular body contours.

## Conclusion

Regardless of a client's age, physical condition, or weight, a properly prescribed running program is safe and will be psychologically beneficial. Adherence to the prescribed exercise program will be enhanced by the skill with which the therapist guides the client through the maze of myth and into the reality of well-being through running.

## Notes

I wish to thank Dr. Jerome Winter for his thoughtful suggestions on this chapter. Most of the material applies equally to women and men. Where special considerations for women exist, they will be noted separately.

1. Duration can also be measured in the number of calories burned or the distance run. For example, a person may run or walk two miles regardless of the time required.

2. Running one and a half to two miles is equivalent to running for twenty minutes for the "average" beginning runner.

3. I think women novices will find books by women more helpful than those by men as they begin and continue their running. Men certainly are not excluded from reading books by women.

4. Coronary heart disease risk factors include elevated blood cholesterol, smoking, electrocardiographic abnormalities, and family history of CHD (Hartung 1980).

5. If six dropped out of the study, it is not clear how seven of the original twelve subjects were continuing to exercise a year after its conclusion. Perhaps one of those who had had medical problems began to exercise again after the experimental portion of the study.

## References

American College of Sports Medicine. 1980. *Guidelines for graded exercise testing and exercise prescription.* 2d ed. Philadelphia: Lea and Febiger.

*American Medical Joggers Association newsletter.* 1979. Physician tells women jogging not beneficial. September, 28.

Bahrke, M. S., and Morgan, W. P. 1978. Anxiety reduction following exercise and meditation. *Cognitive Therapy and Research* 2:323–34.

Barnes, L. 1980. Running therapy: Organized and moving. *Physician and Sportsmedicine* 8(6):97–100.

Berger, B. G. 1972. Relationships between the environmental factors of temporal-spatial uncertainty, probability of physical harm, and nature of competition and selected personality characteristics of athletes. Ph.D. diss., Columbia University. *Dissertation Abstracts International* 33:1014A; University Microfilms no. 72-23689, 373.

————. 1979. The meaning of regular jogging: A phenomenological approach. In *American Alliance for Health, Physical Education, and Recreation research consortium symposium papers,* ed. R. Cox, vol. 2, book 2. Washington, D.C.: American Alliance for Health, Physical Education, and Recreation.

Berger, B. G., and Mackenzie, M. M. 1980. A case study of a woman jogger: A psychodynamic analysis. *Journal of Sport Behavior* 3:3–16.

Blue, F. R. 1979. Aerobic running as treatment for moderate depression. *Perceptual and Motor Skills* 48:228.

Bonen, A. 1981. The menstrual cycle and the female athlete. *Track and Field Journal* 8:15–16.

Brown, R. S.; Ramirez, D. E.; and Taub, J. M. 1978. The prescription of exercise for depression. *Physician and Sportsmedicine* 6 (12):34–37, 40–41.

Buffone, G. W. 1979. The use of running as therapy. *Racing South* 1(10):14–15.

————. 1980a. Exercise as therapy: A closer look. *Journal of Counseling and Psychotherapy* 3:101–15.

————. 1980b. Psychological changes associated with cognitive-behavioral therapy and an aerobic running program in the treatment of depression. Ph.D. diss., Florida State University.

Burke, E. J. 1979. Individualized fitness program. *Journal of Physical Education and Recreation* 50(9):35–37.

Campbell, G. 1977. Women of marathoning. *Runner's World,* September, 40–43.

Carmack, M. A., and Martens, R. 1979. Measuring commitment to running: A survey of runners' attitudes and mental states. *Journal of Sport Psychology* 1:25–42.

Collings, C. A.; Curet, L. B., and Mullin, J. P. 1981. Acute and long term effects of aerobic exercise during pregnancy on maternal and fetal well-being. *Medicine and Science in Sports and Exercise* 13:105 (abstract).

Cooper, K. H. 1970. *The new aerobics.* New York: Bantam Books.

————. 1977. *The aerobics way.* New York: Bantam Books.

Costill, D. 1979. *Scientific approach to distance running.* Los Altos, Calif.: Track and Field News.

Cranston, A. 1981. Science slows aging. *Runner's World,* May, 36–40.

Cundiff, D. E., ed. 1979. *Implementation of aerobic programs.* Washington, D.C.: American Alliance for Health, Physical Education, and Recreation.

Dale, E.; Gerlach, D. H.; Martin, D. E.; and Alexander, C. R. 1979. Physical fitness profiles and reproductive physiology of the female distance runner. *Physician and Sportsmedicine* 7(1): 83–86, 88–91, 94–95.

Dale, E.; Gerlach, D. H.; and Wilhite, A. L. 1979. Menstrual dysfunction in distance runners. *American College of Obstetricians and Gynecologists* 54:47–53.

Danielson, R. R., and Wanzel, R. S. 1978. Exercise objectives of fitness program dropouts. In *Psychology of motor behavior and sport, 1977,* ed. D. M. Landers and R. W. Christina. Champaign, Ill.: Human Kinetics Publishers.

deVries, H. A. 1974. *Physiology of exercise.* Dubuque, Iowa: Brown.

Dienstbier, R. A. 1977. Running motivation: A psychological perspective. *Today's Jogger* 1(1):18–21, 56–57.

Dienstbier, R. A.; Crabbe, J.; Johnson, G. D.; Thorland, W.; Jorgensen, J. A.; Sadar, M. M.; and LaVelle, D. C. 1981. Exercise and stress tolerance. In *Psychology of running,* ed. M. H. Sacks and M. L. Sachs. Champaign, Ill.: Human Kinetics Publishers.

Dishman, R. K. 1981. Biologic influences on exercise adherence. *Research Quarterly for Exercise and Sport* 52:143–59.

Dishman, R. K., and Gettman, L. R. 1980. Psychobiologic influences on exercise adherence. *Journal of Sport Psychology* 2:295–310.

Dishman, R. K.; Ickes, W.; and Morgan, W. P. 1980. Self-motivation and adherence to habitual physical activity. *Journal of Applied Social Psychology* 10:115–32.

Dressendorfer, R. H. 1978. Physical training during pregnancy and lactation. *Physician and Sportsmedicine* 6:74–80.

Dressendorfer, R. H., and Goodlin, R. C. 1980. Fetal heart rate response to maternal exercise testing. *Physician and Sportsmedicine* 8:91–96.

Editors of Consumer Guide. 1978. *The runner's almanac.* New York: Beekman House.

Erdelyi, G. J. 1962. Gynecologic survey of female athletes. *Journal of Sports Medicine and Physical Fitness* 2:174.

———. 1976. Effects of exercise on the menstrual cycle. *Physician and Sportsmedicine* 4:79.

Fixx, J. F. 1977. *The complete book of running.* New York: Random House.

Folkins, C. H., and Sime, W. E. 1981. Physical fitness training and mental health. *American Psychologist* 36:373–89.

Foster, C. 1980. Exercise and coronary artery disease. In *Exercise physiology: Exercise and heart disease and analysis of body composition,* ed. R. H. Cox and J. K. Nelson. AAHPERD research consortium symposium papers. Washington, D.C.: American Alliance for Health, Physical Education, Recreation, and Dance.

Franklin, B. A.; Besseghini, I.; and Golden, L. H. 1978. Low intensity physical conditioning: Effects on patients with coronary heart disease. *Archives of Physical Medicine and Rehabilation* 59:276–80.

Franklin, B. A.; Lussier, L.; and Buskirk, E. R. 1979. Injury rates in women joggers. *Physician and Sportsmedicine* 7(3):105–7, 110–12.

Frisch, R., and McArthur, J. W. 1974. Menstrual cycles: Fatness as a determinant of minimum weight for height necessary for their maintenance or onset. *Science* 185:949–51.

Gehlsen, G., and Albohm, M. 1980. Evaluation of sports bras. *Physician and Sportsmedicine* 8(10):89–90, 92–96.

Gendel, E. S. 1978. Lack of fitness a source of chronic ills in women. *Physician and Sportsmedicine* 6(2):85–87, 90–91, 94–95.

Glasser, W. 1976. *Positive addiction.* New York: Harper and Row.

Glick, J. M., and Katch, V. L. 1970. Musculoskeletal injuries in jogging. *Archives of Physical Medicine and Rehabilitation* 51:123–36.

Glover, B., and Shepherd, J. 1978. *Runner's training diary*. New York: Penguin Books.

Greist, J. H.; Klein, M. H.; Eischens, R. R.; Faris, J.; Gurman, A. S.; and Morgan, W. P. 1978. Running through your mind. *Journal of Psychosomatic Research* 22:259–94.

Harper, F. D. 1978. Outcomes of jogging: Implications for counseling. *Personnel and Guidance Journal* 57:74–77.

———. 1979. *Jogotherapy: Jogging as a therapeutic strategy*. Alexandria, Va.: Douglass.

Harris, D. V. 1973. *Involvement in sport: A somatopsychic rationale for physical activity*. Philadelphia: Lea and Febiger.

Hartung, G. H. 1980. Major risk factors associated with development of coronary heart disease. In *Exercise physiology. Exercise and heart disease and analysis of body composition*, ed. R. H. Cox and J. K. Nelson. AAHPERD research consortium symposium papers. Washington, D.C.: American Alliance for Health, Physical Education, Recreation, and Dance.

Hartung, G. H., and Squires, W. G. 1980. Exercise and HDL cholesterol in middle-aged men. *Physician and Sportsmedicine* 8:74–79.

Haycock, C. E., and Gillette, J. V. 1976. Susceptibility of women athletes to injury: Myths versus reality. *Journal of the American Medical Association* 236:163–65.

Heaps, R. A. 1978. Relating physical and psychological fitness: A psychological point of view. *Journal of Sports Medicine and Physical Fitness* 18:399–408.

Hendry, C. H. 1978. Motivation and female distance runners. *Running* 3(3):16–17.

Hoyt, M. F., and Janis, J. L. 1975. Increasing adherence to a stressful decision via a motivational balance sheet procedure: A field experiment. *Journal of Personality and Social Psychology* 31:833–39.

Huey, L. 1976. *A running start: An athlete, a woman*. New York: Quadrangle Books.

Hutchinson, P. L.; Cureton, K. J.; and Sparling, P. B. 1981. Metabolic and circulatory responses to running during pregnancy. *Physician and Sportsmedicine* (8):55–61.

Joseph, P., and Robbins, J. M. 1981. Worker or runner? The impact of commitment to running and working on self-identification. In *Psychology of running*, ed. M. H. Sacks and M. L. Sachs. Champaign, Ill.: Human Kinetics Publishers.

Katch, F. I., and McArdle, W. D. 1977. *Nutrition, weight control, and exercise*. Boston: Houghton Mifflin.

Kenyon, G. S. 1968a. A conceptual model for characterizing physical activity. *Research Quarterly* 39:96–105.

———. 1968b. Six scales for assessing attitudes toward physical activity. *Research Quarterly* 39:556–74.

Kirby, M. S. 1980. Secondary risk factors related to coronary heart disease. In *Exercise physiology: Exercise and heart disease and analysis of body composition*, ed. R. H. Cox and J. K. Nelson. AAHPERD research consortium symposium papers. Washington, D.C.: American Alliance for Health, Physical Education, Recreation, and Dance.

Kostrubala, T. 1976. *The joy of running*. Philadelphia: J. B. Lippincott.

————. 1981. Running: The grand delusion. In *Psychology of running,* ed. M. H. Sacks and M. L. Sachs. Champaign, Ill.: Human Kinetics Publishers.

Lamb, L. E., ed. 1974a. Jogging, exertion, sudden death. *Health Letter,* vol. 4.

————. 1974b. Osteoarthritis: Degenerative or wear and tear arthritis? *Health Letter,* vol. 4.

————. 1974c. Rheumatoid arthritis. *Health Letter,* vol. 4.

————. 1975. Varicose veins. *Health Letter,* vol. 5.

————. 1976a. Playboy's jogging prank plus other topics. *Health Letter,* vol. 7.

————. 1976b. Heat stress: Cramps, exhaustion, stroke. *Health Letter,* vol. 7.

————. 1976c. Asthma. *Health Letter,* vol. 8.

————. 1977. Fatigue: Feeling tired and weary. *Health Letter,* vol. 9.

————. 1978. Your feet and how to care for them. *Health Letter,* vol. 11.

————. 1979. A perspective on jogging deaths. *Health Letter,* vol. 13.

Lance, K. 1977. *Running for health and beauty: A complete guide for women.* New York: Bantam Books.

McArdle, W. D.; Katch, R. I.; and Katch, V. L. 1981. *Exercise physiology.* Philadelphia: Lea and Febiger.

Mandell, A. J. 1979. The second second wind. *Psychiatric Annals* 9:57, 61–63, 66–69.

Marshall, J. L. 1981. *The sports doctor's fitness book for women.* New York: Delacorte Press.

Massie, J. F., and Shephard, R. J. 1971. Physiological and psychological effects of training. *Medicine and Science in Sports* 3:110–17.

Menstrual change in athletes. 1981. *Physician and Sportsmedicine* 9(11):98–104, 107–9, 112.

Miller, D. K., and Allen, T. E. 1979. *Fitness: A lifetime commitment.* Minneapolis: Burgess.

Milvy, P., ed. 1977. The marathon: Physiological, medical, epidemiological, and psychological studies. *Annals of the New York Academy of Sciences,* vol. 301.

Morgan, W. P. 1977. Involvement in vigorous physical activity with special reference to adherence. In *Proceedings of the National Association for Physical Education of College Women/National College Physical Education Association for Men national conference,* ed. L. Gedvilas and M. Kneer. Chicago: University of Illinois at Chicago Circle.

————. 1978. The mind of the marathoner. *Psychology Today* 11:38–40, 43, 45–46, 49.

————. 1979. Anxiety reduction following acute physical activity. *Psychiatric Annals* 9:36–45.

Noakes, T. D., and Opie, L. H. 1979. Heart disease in marathon runners. *Physician and Sportsmedicine* 7:141–42.

Paffenbarger, R. S.; Wing, A. L.; and Hyde, R. T. 1979. Physical activity as an index of heart attack risk in college alumni. *American Journal of Epidemiology* 108:161–75.

Paling, D. 1981. John Kelley's golden race: Fifty years at Beantown. *Runner's World,* April, 68–69.

Palmason, D. 1981. In praise of older women athletes. *Track and Field Journal* 1(8):4–5.

Parlee, M. B. 1976. The premenstrual syndrome. In *Beyond sex-role stereotypes: Readings toward a psychology of androgyny,* ed. A. Kaplan and J. Bean. Boston: Little, Brown.

Pollock, M. L.; Gettman, L. R.; Milesis, C. A.; Bah, M. D.; Durstine, L.; and Johnson, R. B. 1977. Effects of frequency and duration of training on attrition and incidence of injury. *Medicine and Science in Sports* 9:31–36.

Rueter, M. A., and Harris, D. V. 1980. The effects of running on individuals who are clinically depressed. Paper presented at the annual convention of the American Psychological Association, Montreal.

Ruhling, R. O.; Cameron, J.; Sibley, L.; Christensen, C. L.; and Bolen, T. 1981. Maintaining aerobic fitness while jogging through a pregnancy: A case study. *Medicine and Science in Sports and Exercise* 13:93 (abstract).

Sachs, M. L. 1982. Compliance and addiction to exercise. In *The exercising adult,* ed. R. C. Cantu. Lexington, Mass.: Collamore Press.

Sacks, M. H., and Sachs, M. L., eds. 1981. *Psychology of running.* Champaign, Ill.: Human Kinetics Publishers.

Schreiber, L., and Stang, J. 1980. *Marathon mom: The wife and mother running book.* Boston: Houghton Mifflin.

Shaffer, T. E. 1972. Physiological considerations of the female participant. In *Women and sport: A national research conference,* ed. D. V. Harris. University Park, Pa.: Pennsylvania State University.

Shangold, M. M. 1980. Sports and menstrual function. *Physician and Sportsmedicine* 8(8):66–70.

Sharkey, B. J. 1979. *Physiology of fitness.* Champaign, Ill.: Human Kinetics Publishers.

Sheehan, G. A. 1978. *Running and being.* New York: Simon and Schuster.

———. 1979. Medical advice. *Runner's World,* June, 20–22.

Slusher, H. S. 1967. *Man, sport and existence: A critical analysis.* Philadelphia: Lea and Febiger.

Sonstroem, R. J. 1974. Attitude testing examining certain psychological correlates of physical activity. *Research Quarterly* 45:93–103.

Sours, J. A. 1980. *Starving to death in a sea of objects: The anorexia nervosa syndrome.* New York: Jason Aronson.

———. 1981. Running, anorexia nervosa, and perfection. In *Psychology of running,* ed. M. H. Sacks and M. L. Sachs. Champaign, Ill.: Human Kinetics Publishers.

Speroff, L., and Redwine, D. B. 1980. Exercise and menstrual function. *Physician and Sportsmedicine* 8(5):42, 44–47, 50, 52.

Spino, M. 1976. *Beyond jogging: The inner spaces of running.* New York: Berkeley.

Squires, W. G. 1980. Exercise, diet and blood lipids in coronary heart disease. In *Exercise physiology: Exercise and heart disease and analysis of body composition,* ed. R. H. Cox and J. K. Nelson. AAHPERD research consortium symposium papers.

Washington, D.C.: American Alliance for Health, Physical Education, Recreation, and Dance.

Stalonas, P. M.; Johnson, W. G.; and Christ, M. 1978. Behavior modification for obesity: The evaluation of exercise, contingency management and program adherence. *Journal of Consulting and Clinical Psychology* 46:463–69.

Stephenson, L. A.; Kolka, M. A.; and Wilderson, J. E. 1980. Anaerobic threshold, work capacity, and perceived exertion during the menstrual cycle. *Medicine and Science in Sports and Exercise* 12:87 (abstract).

Thomas, C. L. 1971. The female sports participant: Some physiological questions. In *DGWS research reports: Women in sports,* ed. D. V. Harris. Washington, D.C.: American Association for Health, Physical Education, and Recreation.

Thomas, E. 1981. The marathon: Past, present and future. *Track and Field Journal* 8:27–30.

Thompson, K. J.; Jarvie, G. J.; Lahey, B. B.; and Cureton, K. J. 1982. Exercise and obesity: Etiology, physiology, and intervention. *Psychological Bulletin* 91:55–79.

Ullyot, J. 1976. *Women's running.* Mountain View, Calif.: World Publications.

Wallston, B. S.; Wallston, K. A.; Kaplan, G. D.; and Maides, S. A. 1976. Development and validation of the health locus of control (HLC) scale. *Journal of Consulting and Clinical Psychology* 44:580–85.

Wankel, L. M., and Graham, J. H. 1980. The effects of a decision balance-sheet intervention upon exercise adherence of high and low self-motivated females. Paper presented at the annual conference of the Canadian Society for Psychomotor Learning and Sport Psychology, Vancouver, British Columbia, 22–25 October.

Wankel, L. M., and Thompson, C. 1977. Motivating people to be physically active: Self-persuasion vs. balanced decision making. *Journal of Applied Social Psychology* 7:332–40.

Wells, C. 1971. The menstrual cycle and physical activity. In *DGWS research reports: Women in sports,* ed. D. V. Harris. Washington, D.C.: American Association for Health, Physical Education, and Recreation.

Wilmore, J. H. 1974. Alterations in strength, body composition and anthropometric measurement consequent to a ten week weight training program. *Medicine and Science in Sports* 6:113–38.

———. 1979. The application of science to sport: Physiological profiles of male and female athletes. *Canadian Journal of Applied Sport Sciences* 4:103–15.

Wilmore, J. H.; Brown, C. H.; and Davis, J. A. 1977. Body physique and composition of the female distance runner. *Annals of the New York Academy of Sciences* 301:764–76.

Wilson, V. E.; Berger, B. G.; and Bird, E. I. 1981. Effects of running and of an exercise class on anxiety. *Perceptual and Motor Skills* 53:472–74.

Wysocki, T.; Hall, G.; Iwata, B.; and Riordan, M. 1979. Behavioral management of exercise contracting for aerobics points. *Journal of Applied Behavior Analysis,* 12:55–64.

# 3

# Beginning and Continuing Running: Steps to Psychological Well-being

## Introduction

Over the past fifteen years we have worked with several hundred people who, for a wide variety of reasons, have wanted to become runners. Our main virtue as running therapists lies in what we have learned from working with others. In the past two years, the dropout rate among people coming to us to begin running has been 11 percent. This includes many with diagnoses of depression and some with diagnoses of schizophrenia. Most patients are overweight, and many are smokers. What follows is a description of the techniques we have evolved and are currently using in our running program.

Although many of the physical effects of exercise are apparent to others, the emotional benefits that are more directly perceived by each individual often have an even more telling effect on our lives. Depression diminishes, anxiety abates, anger attenuates, solutions to difficult intellectual problems mysteriously materialize, and exercisers generally "feel good." The discovery of the positive psychological effects of physical activity represents a rediscovery in our culture of the psychological benefits of the ancient disciplines of hatha yoga, tai chi, akaido, zazen, meditation, and sufi dancing. These activities share a number of factors that, when applied to a running program, increase the likelihood of a positive effect on psychological and physical well-being. These common factors are (1) intent, (2) regularity, (3) approach to limits of capacity, and (4) concentration.

Our culture places great emphasis on goal-directedness and measurable accomplishments. If healthful physical activity is to have a secure place and meaning in our lives, the *intent* should be simply to do the activity itself. If your goal is to run a marathon rather than simply to run, you may give up in disappointment or with a sense of failure if the marathon distance is too great; or you may stop running after finishing the marathon and achieving that narrow goal. The running we describe is not incompatible with racing—each of us races. But if all the races were canceled, we would continue running because of the way we feel each day before, during, and after our runs. Try to recognize and accept running as what it is for you: training for racing, calorie expenditure for weight loss, reduction in risk of coronary artery disease, psychological benefit, or a combination of these and other values.

REGULARITY

Adherence (in terms of both dose and duration) is a critical factor in the success or failure of any treatment. You must schedule running time as an important treatment activity. When you first include running in your life, all tactics promoting regularity should be brought to bear. After running becomes a stronger influence, you can become somewhat more casual about scheduling. (See chap. 11, by Buffone, Sachs, and Dowd, for more on adherence to exercise.)

## Approach to Limits of Capacity

Our emphasis is on a constant discovery of individual physiological and psychological limits: the application of a stimulating but manageable stress and the conscious avoidance of distress. Concentration on running form, attention to feedback from breath, muscles, and bowel, and relation to terrain, temperature, and humidity are new experiences for many of us. Learning how and when to rest is an important part of creating the run.

At times we all exceed our adaptive capacity, take on too much stress, and find running difficult. As we err in this way, smoothness fades, fatigue builds, our minds drift to negative thoughts and feelings. This feedback is an important part of the running experience, and learning to attend and respond to it is a critical step in the growth of every runner. Each run is different, and the task is to create each run in sensitive response to other aspects of our experience.

There are many approaches to running. We may deceive ourselves for a time into thinking we are automatons, but the reality of our constantly changing equilibrium inevitably intrudes. Contrary to common lore and misnomers such as "Heartbreak Hill," Boston is really an easy marathon course, as demonstrated by the fast times consistently run there. But there is an old saw about Boston that rings true: "Run with the course and you will have a good time [meant both literally and figuratively]—try to break the course and it will break you." In a similar vein, Sir Edmund Hillary spoke of "conquering" Mount Everest. Tensing, the Sherpa guide who carried more weight without auxiliary oxygen and was acknowledged by all as the expedition's most capable climber, concluded that "together, the mountain and I achieved great heights."

CONCENTRATION

Attention to your environment, running form, and both bodily and metal feedback form the essence of running—an openness to the experience of the run. Developing the capacity to concentrate and learning how and when to concentrate and not concentrate are important steps on the path to psychological well-being. Concentration can be intense yet relaxed and joyful.

HOW TO BEGIN

To begin is simple. Set aside some time, buy some running shoes that feel good on your feet, and go out the door. The five lessons described below should help you learn from your most important master, the intimate relationship between yourself and the run.

Each lesson is written for the beginner, a person with little physical fitness. The lessons are also suitable for fit individuals, who can work through them and then repeat them at a higher level of capacity. To progress through these five lessons will require at least five weeks; properly used, with variations developed by each person, they can provide the foundation for a lifetime of running and physical activity.

**Lesson One**

GOALS

To fill thirty minutes with comfortable activity: walking, running, and stretching. To begin to concentrate on breathing and smoothness of rhythm, and to learn not to overdo. To establish a pattern of regular physical activity.

In the first days, weeks, and months you must prepare yourself to run regularly. This means increasing the flexibility and strength of your feet, ankles, knees, and hips and developing a running form that is smooth and rhythmic. Smoothness and rhythm are your objectives, not distance or speed.

## SELECTING A PLACE

Select an area that is relatively flat. At first, hills place too much strain on tendons, ligaments, and muscles unaccustomed to the motions of running.

## STRETCHING

Although the core of your program is walking and running, it is desirable to include activities that increase flexibility and strength in muscles opposing those that are naturally shortened and strengthened by running. The stretching we suggest should be done comfortably — go to the point of first discomfort and then ease up slightly to a more comfortable position. Perform each activity from one-half minute to one minute — no more is necessary, and excessive stretching (like excessive running) can produce injuries. We suggest the following four stretches:

1. *Ankle and shin*. Kneel with your knees together, toes pointing backward and heels together. Slowly lower yourself until your buttocks are resting on your heels. This exercise increases flexibility of the front of the ankle and stretches the muscles of the shin. A word of caution — your ankles may be very tight, so be careful about resting your full weight on your heels — place your hands on the ground for support and proceed gently.

2. *Dolphin*. Take a position on your hands and knees, this time with your toes curled forward. Your hands should be slightly ahead of your shoulders and shoulder-wide. Slowly straighten your legs to lift your buttocks high in the air and without bouncing bring your heels toward the ground. Emphasize keeping your buttocks high so you feel the stretch along the length of your legs. This position stretches muscles all along the back of the leg (calf, thigh, buttocks) that are strengthened but shortened by running.

3. *Pelvic stretch (inner thigh)*. Sit on the floor with legs straight ahead. Bend your knees and bring both heels back toward your buttocks as far as you comfortably can. Grasp your feet with your hands and then let your knees fall outward toward the ground while keeping your back erect.

4. *Lotus (leg extension)*. Sit on the floor with your legs straight in front. Keep

your back erect throughout this exercise. Place your right hand, palm down, on the inside of your right knee. Slide your hand down your calf toward your arch and grasp your calf, ankle, or foot (depending on how far you can comfortably reach). Pick up your leg and very gently raise it as high as you comfortably can. Try to relax the hamstring muscle (the large muscle group in the back of your thigh). Return your leg to its original position and then bend the knee and bring it to your chest. Wrap both arms around your bent leg and gently draw the knee closer to your chest. Return your leg to its original position. Repeat with other leg.

Although many other stretching positions are possible (some proponents advocate forty-nine stretching exercises *before running*), these four stretch the most important muscle groups that tend to be shortened by running.

The purpose of these exercises (yoga practitioners call then asana) is not only to warm you up to run — walking and slow jogging are an effective warm-up. The goal of stretching is to increase flexibility, strength, and awareness of the limits of stress.

WALK/RUN

Today you want to fill thirty minutes with comfortable walking and running (reduce the time if thirty minutes seems too much). It's important to do enough to energize or tire yourself slightly (or both), but not so much that you feel fatigued. It is better to do too little than too much.

Start at a brisk walk. Concentrate on your breathing. You should be aware of a slight increase in rate. Without resisting this quickening, make each breath slightly deeper. Don't concern yourself with mechanics; simply breathe more deeply. Be aware of your movement — put energy into every step. When you feel loose, smooth, and relaxed (often after five to ten minutes of brisk walking and for some people not at all during the first few days of movement), do your first running segment.

Running is a natural movement and differs from walking only in the brief instant when both feet are off the ground. Concentrate first on your breathing. It will increase in rate even more as you begin running, and as this happens you should deepen it as well. Next shift your attention to rhythm and smoothness and let them dictate pace. Think of moving lightly over the ground.

Today you will tie the distance you run to your breathing. To do this, count each complete breath cycle as one, counting on either inhalation or exhalation. Run for five to fifteen complete breath cycles. Don't worry about whether it is far enough — simply experience the run.

How fast should you go? Don't try to run fast or hard. Try to be smooth and rhythmic and let the pace determine itself. If you sense your breath getting out of control, slow down. If it seems easy, do the full fifteen breath cycles.

After five to fifteen breath cycles, return to brisk walking and evaluate the run. Did you tire at all? If so, do not increase and consider decreasing the number of breath cycles in the next running segment. During the next running segment, again begin by deepening your breathing as it quickens and run as smoothly and rhythmically as you can, putting energy into each stride. Energetic striding is more an attitude than a movement. Try to feel that each step is vigorous. Do not alter your pace or tempo or run jerkily or bouncing up and down. Flow smoothly along the ground. Repeat walking and running segments until thirty minutes have passed or until you begin to tire. Midway through the walk/run you may wish to stop and repeat some of the stretches you performed before starting.

After the run, finish up with the same stretching that began your activity.

### COMMENT

Concentrating on breathing, smoothness, and rhythm helps maintain and enhance awareness of your movements. Concentration will help you focus on what is happening in you, through you, and around you. Concentrate on different elements of running to keep from being carried away by nonrunning thoughts, worries, or even a beautiful view. Give each of these experiences their due, but keep in touch with feedback from yourself. You've taken your first run and begun to learn about your present capacity. Ideally, you will feel pleasantly energized—even if a bit tired.

The positive aspects of the run are produced by the rhythm and smoothness of movement and the effort to be energetic, not to lag or drag through any part of the run. To be energetic while running, you must be rested, and the walking segments are essential energizers. When Bill Rodgers set an American Marathon record at Boston in 1975, he walked four times and stopped to tie his shoe once. He has run all the way in marathons many times since then, but never completed the course as fast.

The most important thing is to begin—to act on your intention to make running a healthful part of your life. Next in importance in regularity. If you run regularly, your capacity will grow naturally. It is important not to rush through any session. Fatigue is a suble intruder, so you should take no chances.

The next question is How often should I run? From the beginning to the end of a running career, it is important not to let fatigue build up. Here are three options for tomorrow that will guard against excessive fatigue:

1. Do only stretching for flexibility and strength.
2. Do flexibility and strength exercises and walk (don't run) for twenty minutes.
3. Do flexibility and strength exercises and walk/run for fifteen minutes.

Exercise physiologists have now shown that alternating "hard" with "easy" days leads to the most rapid increase in strength—thus confirming what many experienced exercisers had already worked out for themselves (see Sharkey 1979 for more on the physiology of fitness).

Why wasn't a day of complete rest recommended? It is usually easier to make changes in lifestyle stick if we perform the new activities frequently.

You should feel very little stiffness or soreness when you awaken tomorrow. If you are sore or stiff, decrease the amount of exercise.

Repeat lesson one for a minimum of one week.

**Lesson Two** (do not begin before the second week)

INTRODUCTION

The activity we select for recreation must be done regularly. Well-being, like wisdom, is not a lasting state but must be continually renewed through practice. We must recognize both our strength and our fragility and consider our daily physical activity an important factor in our well-being.

In lesson two the emphasis is on further development of concentration, smoothness and rhythm, and extension (straightening) of your spine. You will also begin increasing the distance covered in some running segments.

Distance and pace are simply related. The farther you want to go, the slower you go. At this point in your running program, the prime concern is to develop an easy, rhythmic style. Endurance will grow naturally as you continue to do thirty minutes of comfortable walking and running.

Running slightly faster may help you run more smoothly. "Slightly faster" does not mean very fast—you should still be breathing easily. Running smoothly is a skill that develops with practice. Don't be disappointed if you feel slow, awkward, ungainly, and unbalanced. The important thing is to make the effort to walk and run. The periods of coherent and concentrated running that occur before tiredness and lack of concentration interfere will grow in length as you grow in capacity.

WALK/RUN

As usual, begin with flexibility and strength exercises, then walk, concentrating on breathing and putting energy into each step. When you feel relaxed and smooth, proceed as follows:

*Run:* Fifteen to forty breath cycles (or, if counting is not for you, a specific number of seconds or to a point *before* you tire). Concentrate on your breathing and deepen it. Try to make your running smooth, then turn your concentration to your spine. Feel the base of your spine and extend your spine upward from it, feeling yourself lighten as you run more erectly. Relax your shoulders. Extending your spine can be difficult—again, therefore, making the effort is the most important thing.

*Walk:* It is important to walk before tiredness forces you to do so. Walk briskly and continue to concentrate on your spine and breathing, walking smoothly but with energy. Once you have recovered, run again as you have done before. Repeat the walk/run sequence for the rest of the session.

COMMENT

You may notice that the first run is more difficult than later ones. It often takes several minutes for our bodies to warm up.

Slow recovery, stiffness, and soreness are signs of fatigue and overstress. If these signs persist, accept them as clear messages that you should do less for now and allow more time for adapting to the stresses you are experiencing.

Continue this lesson for several weeks. Continue, as well, to alternate "long hard" days with "short easy" ones.

## Lesson Three (may begin fourth week)

INTRODUCTION

Just as varying the amount of stress from day to day is helpful, changing the activities within each session often heightens awareness of the variety of experiences available through running. However, some people find that repeating a specific course, pace, and distance is reassuring. This pattern can work well for some, particularly if the distance is short enough so that the run can be done at a good pace and rhythm and is not fatiguing.

WALK/RUN

Begin with flexibility and strength exercises and move next to a walking segment. The emphasis in this lesson is on adjusting pace and distance. If you are counting breaths, the first running segment might be ninety breaths at a slow pace, the second sixty breaths at a quicker pace, and the third running segment thirty breaths at a fairly fast but smooth and comfortable pace. If you are timing segments, appropriate durations might be three, two, and one minutes. If you are simply responding to tiredness, all you need to attend to is tiredness at different paces, making certain you return to a walking segment *before* fatigue begins.

Repeat this sequence for thirty minutes and conclude with stretching. If you notice tightness as a result of your faster running, you may wish to do some stretching at some point during the thirty minutes of movement.

COMMENT

This lesson is fun for most people, and its purpose is to provide a variety of feedback from your body as you run at different paces. You should always be able to maintain rhythm and smoothness in your breathing and running motion.

As always, alternate intense with less intense days. If you begin a session feeling tired and don't feel stronger after the first walk/run cycle, reduce the intensity and/or duration of the session.

**Lesson Four** (may begin fifth or sixth week)

INTRODUCTION

This lesson deals with the relation between pulse rate and stress. The heart, like all muscles, is strengthened by tolerable stress followed by rest. This lesson helps you define the relation between the stress of running and heart rate.

If you have been able to maintain a comfortable, steady breathing rate during your run segments, your heart will naturally be in the range of healthful stress — between 110 and 160 beats per minute (See Berger, chap. 2, for more on heart rate and exercise.) Take your pulse rate at rest by feeling for your pulse either in the front of your neck (beside your windpipe) or on the inside of your wrist behind the base of your thumb. You will need a watch with a second hand or a digital display. Count the number of beats in ten seconds and multiply by six to obtain the number of beats per minute.

Do your usual flexibility and strength exercises and take your pulse rate again. You will probably notice an increase in rate, although if you have had an intense, activity-filled day the rate may decrease.

WALK/RUN

Walk briskly and check your pulse rate again. It will probably rise. Run, doing a comfortable running segment, and check your pulse rate again. It will rise still further. When you return to walking, note your pulse rate just before your next running segment. It will have fallen.

Add thirty breath cycles or one minute to the next running segment and check your pulse rate. It will probably be higher than at the end of the previous running segment unless you have slowed your pace. Continue varying distance and pace as in lesson three and note the effect of different paces on pulse rates and length of time required for your rate to return nearer a resting level during the walking segment.

COMMENT

During your runs, pulse rate should have reached 110 to 160 beats per minute. If it is below this level, don't worry. It will eventually reach a higher rate as you gradually lengthen your runs. The most important thing in each lesson is that you keep moving and concentrate on running for thirty minutes or more unless you feel tired. You are also learning to be aware of feedback from your movement and to use it to control intensity of stress created by walking and running.

Much of the positive psychological effect of running is tied to the style, rhythm, and pace of your movement. These elements can be incorporated into your program from the beginning. A few people develop a running program in which they simply go out and run a distance easily and naturally. More often this approach does not work, and beginning runners drift or struggle through the same slow, uncomfortable, unfocused run each day. By creating each day's run out of a variety of distances and paces and points of concentration, you can avoid boredom and creatively use the run to regenerate a positive emotional state.

The important thing is to be aware of yourself in the activity—this requires effort and concentration. Your rhythm, breathing, spine, and style are all accessible to your attention, and as you become more aware of them you can take control of your movement.

**Lesson Five** (may begin sixth through eighth week)

INTRODUCTION

How you move affects your emotional state as much as the distance you move. In lesson five your emphasis should be on a controlled, vigorous stride, paying attention to spine extension, head position, leg and foot movement, and arm position and action. You can approach running in a relaxed yet energetic manner and develop greater awareness of your physiological responses to stress. Try to avoid a tense, analytic approach to form—an attempt to rigidly copy the style of another runner. Let your run develop as a freely flowing pattern—a relaxed yet energetic and intense expression of your being. The joy of movement lies within the activity itself, not in analysis by experts. If you pay close attention to different aspects of your technique and experience in each of your sessions, they will slowly but certainly become a natural part of your running.

The goal of lesson five is to focus on specific aspects of running in each segment. Begin with flexibility and strength exercises.

WALK/RUN

Walk, concentrating on feeling the base of your spine and then extending your spine. Feel yourself lighten, and find the ease with which your legs move through beneath you in the running movement.

Check again to see that your spine is extended and your shoulders relaxed. Then begin running and maintain awareness of your spine as sensations change with the changing pace of running.

When you return to walking, focus on the movement of your legs and feet—the movement of your ankles, the position of your foot as it meets the ground (usually heel first, although you may feel you're landing flat-footed and a few people land naturally on the ball of the foot), rolls over, and leaves the ground. Next, emphasize the pushoff for several steps, straightening the foot fully (you may find it helpful to think of pushing off the ground with your toes).

Begin running and retain your focus on your feet, ankles, and legs. Vary your pace within this running segment to see what effect pace has on how your legs feel and function.

During the next walking segment, check the position of your arms. They should not be high but should be carried comfortably low, with natural movement at the elbow. Carrying your arms too high can cause tension and tiredness in your neck and shoulders, and exaggerated arm swinging interferes with balance. Again, focus on your arm movement as you do the next running segment. Rotate your focus through the different physical elements of running as you move through lesson five.

It is important to realize the extent of your awareness. Even while focusing on your foot or spine, you can sense your breathing and remain open to the environment. The essence of the run is to concentrate on the activity.

## Consolidation of Your Running Program

General principles of your program include:
1. All sessions begin and end with flexibility and strength exercises.
2. More- and less-intense days should be alternated.
3. Concentrating on form and style should be a part of all your runs. Set aside one day a week to emphasize each element of the running activity in turn.
4. At least one day a week should include several faster pace/shorter distance running segments, unless you are feeling tired or ill.
5. Whenever you run long segments, maintain a vigorous style. Avoid dragging through the last part of a run segment; if you feel tired, start to walk sooner than you had planned.

After reaching thirty minutes of comfortable movement of which most is running, you may wish to increase the total amount of time you are moving. This will usually not occur in the first six months of a beginning program. Try adding ten minutes to *one* day of the week. After two to three weeks, add ten minutes to a second day (again, be sure you are adding time to alternate days rather than consecutive days). Avoid fatigue and overstress. If you feel ill or sense an approaching illness, a day off or a walk will usually speed recovery and lead to the highest overall level of fitness.

Beginning and continuing running is a pleasure and satisfaction almost everyone can enjoy. To be successful, one must decide that physical activity is important and establish a regular pattern that is immediately reinforcing as well as providing long-term benefits. Failures (and they are unhappily common) result from ignoring feedback from our bodies (it takes time for adaptation to occur and physiological capacity to grow). Moving comfortably today ensures enthusiasm for movement tomorrow. Even more failures result from our mind's unrealistic expectations. We have become a culture of shortcuts and expect instant change and success, often in blatant defiance of the laws of nature. Comfortable daily physical activity will produce fitness and the physiological and psychological benefits we seek. Too much, to paraphrase Schumacher, produces less.

The lessons presented for beginning and continuing running help one attain psychological well-being. They are designed for use by therapists and by individuals interested in progressively and safely developing their running capacity. The antidepressant effects this running may provide have been amply documented in past research as discussed in other chapters (see chaps. 1 and 9) and in earlier work we have conducted (Greist et al. 1978, 1981). We have identified several factors that may be important in determining why running works, when it works: mastery, patience, capacity for change, generalization, distraction, positive habit or "addiction," symptom relief, consciousness alteration, and biochemical changes.

The second section of this chapter provides some general principles associated with any medical treatment for depression. These are designed to identify certain basic criteria to be followed in specifically applying the running treatment for depression. The treatment plans offered should be considered in conjunction with the lessons presented earlier, in providing the most effective treatment possible for the depressed patient.

## General Principles

Some general principles associated with any medical treatment also apply to the running treatment of depression.

### PREPARATIONS

Just as one undergoes tests to identify unforeseen problems before an operation, clients should be evaluated for certain potential problems before they begin running. First, it is important to determine that their depression is the kind that is likely to respond to running treatment. About 75 percent of all depressions fall into this category—these are the minor to moderate neurotic-reactive depressions. But for the major depressions (endogenous-psychotic) there is at present no evidence that running is helpful, and our limited attempts at using running for patients with major depression have produced no beneficial effects.

For depressed people who have lost contact with reality (often expressing delusions of bodily illness and feeling totally helpless, hopeless, or worthless), who are severely physically retarded or agitated, who have substantial weight loss or sleep disturbance, who have lost their sense of humor and interest in all activities, who are not cheered even momentarily by good news, or who are actively suicidal, running is not indicated. In fact, at present we feel running is contraindicated for patients with severe depression unless it is used as an adjunct to other demonstrably effective drug or electroconvulsive therapies.

Our second concern is the integrity of the cardiovascular system. Sudden strenuous exercise in deconditioned people has on rare occasions been associated with heart attack or death owing to loss of normal heart rhythm. While the running treatment we use is not suddenly strenuous, some people grow so enthusiastic about their improvement that they exceed the treatment prescription and place a substantial stress on their cardiovascular systems.

We recommend (and carry out with patients who are over forty years of age, smoke, or have a family history of heart disease or any complaints that suggest heart or lung problems) a careful cardiovascular history, resting electrocardiogram, and maximum exercise stress test on a treadmill. All three procedures can easily be completed in an hour and a half. Some people ask, "What happens if the tests show that I have heart trouble?" Of course the answer depends on the kind of heart trouble found. For most of the problems encountered exercise would be prescribed as part of the treatment. Additional supervision to ensure that stress is carefully monitored and that help is available if symptoms appear are prudent precautions for those with recognized heart problems. Although lack of exercise is one of the factors producing heart problems, the same heart problems seldom require abstinence from exercise.

Assuming that the cardiovascular system is not diseased and no extra precautions are needed during the running treatment of depression, we are next concerned with the "mechanical apparatus" of toes, feet, ankles, legs, knees, thighs, hips, and back.

Most of us have some inequality in the length, girth, and joint structure of our lower extremities, and some minor differences that are unnoticed in ordinary movement can become problems as one begins to run. Many of these problems are so minor that a good pair of running shoes protects against discomfort and injury. Others can easily be remedied by shoe inserts of various kinds. At times, specific exercises will be prescribed to overcome weakness or imbalance.

Unless you have an obvious problem, it is usually reasonable to begin running without a specific examination of your legs and to seek help if problems appear. For those with known foot, leg, or back problems, a consultation with a podiatrist or orthopedic surgeon known to be interested in running (preferably a runner) is certainly advisable. Take a pair of old, worn shoes with you, since the pattern of wear often reveals specific problems.

### Primum Nil Nocere—First, Do No Harm

It is a fundamental principle in medicine that treatments should not leave the patient worse off. Treatments come and go, waxing and waning in popularity, and more often than not prove the dictum, "When many treatments are available for a condition, none is effective." Certainly, physicians should not give and patients should not take a treatment whose result may be worse than the disease itself. Even effective treatments are double-edged swords, capable of curing and killing. Antibiotics, for example, have dramatically altered our health experience, but a few individuals have serious allergic reactions to them. While running can relieve depression, it can also cause physical injury, usually to the legs, and can even contribute to depression in those who run too hard or too much.

### The Right Treatment

Correct diagnosis is of first importance in medical practice; but correct selection of treatment is also important to a favorable outcome. There are some disorders for which diagnostic precision is low, and depression, unhappily, remains one of them. When many treatments have been reported to be effective for a disease, physicians may conduct clinical trials to determine which will provide the best results, be safest and easiest to take, and be least costly for the patient.

When conducting these clinical trials, it is important to continue each treatment long enough to determine whether it will work. No single treatment is ever effective for all cases of a particular disease, and it is fortunate that there is usually more than one treatment available.

### The Prescription Should Be Simple

In some studies up to 50 percent of psychiatric outpatients fail to take any of their prescribed medication. The problem of treatment "compliance" or "adherence" is fascinating. (See chap. 11, by Buffone, Sachs, and Dowd, for more on this area.) No matter how effective the treatment, it must be taken before it can work. The prescription should be tailored, whenever possible, to the patient's lifestyle. For example, it is much easier to take medication once a day than to remember to take it every four hours around the clock, and it is far simpler to take one medication than several.

## Give the Right Dose

Too little antidepressant medicine will not relieve symptoms, and too much may cause so many side effects that the treatment becomes intolerable. With running, there is for each individual an *adaptive range* within which that person can, by regular running, increase physical capacity. Beneath a critical minimum level (typified by the largely sedentary individual), physical fitness will not increase and depression will not be relieved. Above a critical maximum the individual exceeds adaptive capacity and the side effects (injuries, fatigue, "stale athlete syndrome") may actually cause greater depression and will certainly make the treatment less tolerable.

## Monitoring

It is always helpful and usually necessary to carefully monitor both the treatment itself and the patient's response. For major depression, we want to know how much medication the patient has taken, when it was taken, and whether the symptoms of depression are changing. In the running treatment of depression, we also need to know when the treatment was taken, how much was taken, and whether depressive symptoms are increasing, decreasing, or staying the same. A running log or diary can be helpful with this. See Berger's table 1 and the accompanying discussion (chap. 2), for more on running logs.

### SPECIFIC INSTRUCTIONS

If you've decided you are moderately depressed and that you would like to try running as a treatment, you might follow the specific instructions and other suggestions we have used to treat patients with moderate depression. But if you feel you may have a major depression, or if you feel suicidal, discuss your problem with your physician. We have not adequately evaluated running by itself as a treatment for major depression, and our limited experience suggests that it would only delay the onset of effective treatment with medication or electroconvulsive therapy.

We present two alternative treatment plans, each of which has been effective with different depressed patients. They represent the maximum and minimum extremes of treatment we use. See the first part of this chapter for further details of our current techniques.

*Treatment Plan 1*

1. Set aside a minimum of thirty minutes and a maximum of sixty minutes each day for seventy days for your running therapy.
2. Go out each day and walk/jog/run for thirty to sixty minutes in such a way that you are never gasping for breath (if you can sing to yourself or talk out loud or under your breath while running, you are not going too fast).
3. Run in a way that feels natural to you. Most people land either on their heels or on their heels and toes at about the same time. Running on the toes is fine for sprinting, but you can't sprint for thirty minutes. (A few people run naturally on their toes—if you are a natural toe runner, don't force yourself into the more common heel-toe routine).
4. If your legs become sore, increase the amount of walking and decrease the amount of running to half the amount run the previous day. Continue decreasing your running to half the amount done the previous day until you are no longer sore.
5. Reasons to skip a day:
   a. fever
   b. broken bones
   c. chest pain that increases with activity (consult your physician)
   d. leg pain made worse by walking for thirty minutes (The emphasis is on taking your treatment every day for seventy days; there should be very few if any missed days.)
6. What if I miss a day? Try not to! If you start running at 11:30 P.M. you can still get your run in for that day. If you do miss a day, record it and note the reasons and use them as guides not to miss another day.
7. Once you've found the number of minutes of running that does not make you sore when you are running at a comfortable pace (can sing or talk to yourself or others), try to increase your minutes of jogging/running by 12 to 15 percent from one week to the next. Thus, if you're able to jog thirty-five minutes the first week (about five minutes a day out of thirty minutes spent walking/jogging/running), try to *comfortably* jog/run about forty minutes (roughly six minutes per day) the second week. If you become sore, increase more gradually. Beware the temptation to "run forever." Running sometimes causes euphoria, even in those who are depressed, and exceeding your

body's adaptive capacity will surely lead to pain, fatigue, interruption of running and a possible worsening of depression.

8. Keep track of the number of minutes you are jogging/running and record that and any other special observations in a diary (see Berger's table 1, in chap. 2, for some suggestions on putting together a running log).

9. If you aren't feeling less depressed after ten weeks of running, consult your physician for consideration of alternative treatments.

*Treatment Plan 2*

1. Set aside a minimum of thirty minutes and a maximum of sixty minutes three days a week for ten weeks for your running therapy.

2. Go out on each of your scheduled treatment days and walk/jog/run for thirty to sixty minutes in such a way that you are never gasping for breath (if you can sing to yourself or talk out loud or under your breath while running, you are not going too fast).

3. Run in a way that feels natural to you. Most people land either on their heels or on their heels and toes at about the same time. Running on the toes is fine for sprinting, but you can't sprint for thirty minutes. (A few people run naturally on their toes — if you are a natural toe runner, don't force yourself into the more common heel-toe routine.)

4. If your legs become sore, increase the amount of walking and decrease the amount of running to half the amount you ran on the previous treatment day. Continue decreasing your running to half the amount done on the previous treatment day until you are no longer sore.

5. Reasons to skip a scheduled treatment day:
   a. fever
   b. broken bones
   c. chest pain that increases with activity (consult your physician)
   d. leg pain made worse by walking for thirty minutes. If you miss a scheduled treatment day for any of these reasons, try to make it up the next day. Three times a week is the minimum number of treatments we have found to be effective for alleviating depression (and three thirty-minute sessions is less than 1 percent of your week).

6. Once you've found the number of minutes of running per treatment day that does not make you sore when running at a comfortable pace (can sing or talk to yourself or others), try to increase your minutes of jogging/running by 20 percent from one week to the next. Thus, if you are able to jog approximately twenty minutes the first week (seven minutes of jogging/running out of

thirty minutes spent walking/jogging/running on each of three days a week), try to comfortably increase to about twenty-five minutes the second week. If you become sore, increase more gradually. Beware the temptation to "run forever." Running sometimes causes euphoria, even in those who are depressed, and exceeding your body's adaptive capacity will surely lead to pain, fatigue, interruption of running, and possible worsening of depression.

7. During the third week, add a fourth day of running to your treatment prescription. If you are enjoying running a great deal and missing it on the days when you are not running, you may add an additional day per week beginning the fifth week. Do not add more than one day in any given week and do not hesitate to drop back one or more days per week if you grow fatigued. Remember, though, that fatigue is also a symptom of depression and can frequently be relieved by running. Try very hard to run at least three times a week.

8. Keep track of the number of minutes you are jogging/running and record that and any other special observations in a diary (see Berger's table 1, in chap. 2, for some suggestions on putting together a running log).

9. If you aren't feeling less depressed after ten weeks of running, consult your physician for consideration of alternative treatments for your depression.

Plan 1 has been used by a few single-minded patients whose hard-driving style may actually be a part of the problem leading to their depression. Nevertheless, this approach has had antidepressant value for them, and we have later been able to suggest that the rigid routine they establish for themselves rapidly becomes a rut it is difficult to climb out of.

Far more generally therapeutic is plan 2, which emphasizes prescription flexibility tailored to varying needs and schedules. The nine points described above are a stark outline that depressed patients can use to treat their own depressions with running. Far from being an exclusively physical therapy, running provides a solitude that permits emotional as well as physiological introspection and feedback. For an expanded presentation of these aspects of running, you may wish to read *Run to Reality* (Eischens, Greist, and McInvaille 1978).

### Conclusion

Running as a treatment for depression shares many features with other medical treatments. It has been shown to be effective for some but not all cases of moderate depression. Its usefulness in the treatment of major depression has not been studied, but happily, other effective treatments for this disorder are available.

For running to be effective, one must do it often enough (at least three and ideally five or more times a week) and in a comfortable manner that will lead to an increase in physical fitness. It is possible to run too much, and what is "too much" varies from person to person. It is especially important to recognize that it also varies for each person from time to time.

Most people with moderate depression who run in this way begin to feel better within a week and feel virtually well within three weeks. Obviously, this is an average, and not all patients have responded so quickly. Indeed, some have not responded to running at all. On the other hand, in our experience, no moderately depressed patients have grown *more* depressed while running, and the few who have remained depressed appreciate the improvements in their physical functioning. As with other medical treatments, it is wise to obtain competent screening before treatment begins.

If there is any secret to the success people have had in treating their depression with running, it is to run each day in such a way that they will want to run again the next day.

### References

Eischens, R.; Greist, J. H.; and McInvaille, T. 1978. *Run to reality*. Madison, Wisc.: Madison Running Press.

Greist, J. H.; Eischens, R. R.; Klein, M. H.; and Linn, D. 1981. Addendum to running through your mind. In *Psychology of running*, ed. M. H. Sacks and M. L. Sachs. Champaign, Ill.: Human Kinetics Publishers.

Greist, J. H.; Klein, M. H.; Eischens, R. R.; Faris, J.; Gurman, A. S.; and Morgan, W. P. 1978. Running through your mind. *Journal of Psychosomatic Research* 22:259–94.

Morgan, W. P. 1977. Involvement in vigorous physical activity with special reference to adherence. *Proceedings, NCPEAM/NAPECW National Conference*. Chicago: University of Illinois at Chicago Circle, Office of Publications Services.

Sharkey, B. J. 1979. *Physiology of fitness*. Champaign, Ill.: Human Kinetics Publishers.

# 4

# Jogotherapy: Jogging as Psychotherapy

The theoretical approach of "jogging as psychotherapy" is predicated on the supposition, supported by empirical evidence, that jogging can alter both psychological states and psychological traits. At this time there is more research support and promise for altering states of behavior than lasting traits (Fixx 1977; Harper and Adams 1977; Wood 1977). For example, the internal mechanisms of psychophysiology suggest that sustained jogging can alter biochemical levels in the brain and thus change psychological mood or state. More specifically, there is research, however limited, indicating that jogging can increase levels of certain biochemical neurotransmitters, such as the catecholamines, whose increased output at synaptic junctions within the brain is associated with a lift in mood or a decrease in depression (Greist et al. 1978; Ismail and Young 1977; Mandell 1979. See also Dienstbier, chap. 14 and Sachs, chap. 15). In other words, sustained jogging can modify the chemical actions at brain-cell connections, thus influencing our psychological state or simply "upping our mood." A more recent study suggests that jogging, or sustained, intensive exercise, may have psychotherapeutic value in treating manic-depressive patients because it can alter blood levels related to mood or "affective illness" (Lykouras et al. 1979).

Iversen's (1979) article "The Chemistry of the Brain," in *Scientific American*'s special issue "The Brain," explains the numerous ways chemical states of the brain are related to psychological disorders and moods. Moreover, Ismail and Young (1977) have documented the association of personality state with levels of biochemicals in the brain and blood and shown that exercise can affect personality by altering biochemical levels within the body. The implied challenge for psychotherapy rests in using jogging programs to alter brain states and therefore influence the quality of psychological consciousness and the quality of life itself.

Another argument for using jogging as psychotherapy is related to its value in regulating sensory states. Examples include reports that jogging decreases the sensation of hunger after a long run on an empty stomach, and runners' self-reports of heightened taste immediately after a vigorous run. However, improved taste quality does not imply increased hunger drive. It is possible that jogging might be useful in sexual therapy to enhance both the drive for and the sensory appreciation of the sexual experience.

In a recent experiment with college students (Harper 1978), we observed a number of psychotherapeutic outcomes based on four to five miles of jogging, five days a week, over a fourteen-week semester (students started out at a half mile and worked up to four to five miles over several weeks). Post-test measures indicated a significant decrease in state anxiety, a moderate decrease in trait anxiety, and a moderate improvement in self-concept. Moreover, self-reports from the students themselves indicated improved ability to sleep and relax, increased physical and mental energy, improved sexual appreciation, ability to cope with stress, mental alertness, and self-confidence, increased capacity for work, and greater appreciation for health. Consistent with these findings, studies by Hartung and Farge (1977), Renfrow and Bolton (1979), and McCutcheon (1978) have also documented positive psychological effects from jogging or positive personality traits associated with joggers. (See also Dienstbier, chap. 14, on the effect of exercise on personality.)

Although there is not a sizable body of robust empirical studies on jogging and psychotherapeutic outcomes, there is sufficient evidence to conceptualize a theoretical framework for applying jogging to psychotherapy. This deliberate and systematic therapeutic process is referred to here as "jogotherapy."

## Assumptions of Jogotherapy

Jogotherapy is a therapeutic as well as a preventive process that can be employed within a treatment or helping setting. The psychotherapist may systematically apply a program of jogging to correct or prevent various human problems. The psychotherapist, with input from the client, delineates specific goals that are measurable and that can be attained through a program of jogging, alone or in combination with another therapeutic technique. The success of psychotherapy depends upon a jogging regimen that specifies distance, speed, time, frequency, and place. This general principle is conceptualized within the following list of theoretical assumptions about jogotherapy (Harper 1979).

1. A systematically designed jogging program can provide specific therapeutic benefits for specific human problems.
2. Particular goals are enhanced by a prescribed jogging program that systematically manipulates distance to be run, time of day for jogging, place or setting, frequency per week or day, and the state or activity before and after jogging.
3. Jogotherapy is a "treatment-training" approach (Gazda 1971) in that treatment benefits occur during the training program. Training the physical organism is psychologically therapeutic.
4. Sustained jogging improves the efficiency of glands and organs, therefore improving the level of psychophysiological functioning and the general quality of life.
5. Physical health and mental health are interdependent and inseparable; to improve one's physical health through jogging is to improve one's mental health and vice versa.
6. Jogotherapy is an adjunct to counseling and psychotherapy, both for preventing and for treating human problems.
7. Unlike the traditional "talk therapies" such as psychoanalysis and client-centered therapy, jogotherapy can guarantee observable and measurable changes in behavior and performance.
8. Jogotherapy ensures clients' active physical participation; "talk therapy" alone often limits the client to the role of passive listener or passive responder to the psychotherapist's communication cues.

## Role of the Psychotherapist

What is the psychotherapist's role in jogotherapy? This question can have a variety of responses, since the role of the psychotherapist is not fixed. The general purpose of the psychotherapist in the helping process is to define problems or concerns that may be appropriate for jogotherapy; translate such problems into achievable, observable, and measurable goals; and design a systematic jogging program to achieve these goals. The psychotherapist, of course, seeks input from the client in this diagnostic/planning stage. The administration of the jogging program dictates the psychotherapist's role. Jogotherapy can be carried out within individual or group psychotherapy. The psychotherapist may serve the following functions:

## FACILITATOR/MONITOR

In this role the psychotherapist functions in a one-to-one relationship or within individual psychotherapy. After designing and prescribing the jogotherapy program, the psychotherapist monitors the client's progress from week to week (Harper 1979) and also motivates and promotes the client's consistent participation and follow-through. The client keeps a progress chart, and the psychotherapist assesses ongoing problems and evaluates changes and progress toward defined behavioral goals.

## LEADER OF JOGOTHERAPY GROUP

The psychotherapist can serve as a leader or co-leader of a jogotherapy group. The content and the process of the group may vary according to the needs of the clients. It might be a *common problem group,* with all clients having the same problem or needs—for example, college students who are anxious and tense, people suffering from chronic depression, or alcoholics. Gary and Guthrie (1972) employed jogging with alcoholics for physical rehabilitation and self-concept improvement. A *general jogotherapy group* may enlist clients with different goals and problems, and the psychotherapist can also use individual counseling and additional therapeutic techniques (such as biofeedback, relaxation therapy, diet therapy, and meditation) to focus on each client's individual problem or needs (e.g., see table 1).

The group leader or co-leaders may choose to hold a formal group counseling session before or after jogging at least once a week to give clients a structured and scheduled opportunity to discuss their needs and their jogging. Gazda (1978) refers to this type of group arrangement as "activity group counseling." In our study (Harper 1978) of college students we held a formal group counseling session at the end of the week (Fridays), preceding the day's jogging. The students benefited from exchanging ideas and sharing needs, jogging experiences, and successes. (The sessions were held before jogging since group members found it difficult to shower and reassemble afterward—especially since some took much more time to complete their distance.)

Table 1. Jogotherapy Programs for Specific Problems

| Problem | Goals of Jogotherapy | Distance [a] in miles | Speed [b] | Frequency in days per week | Time of Day | Place or Setting | Before/After Conditions |
|---|---|---|---|---|---|---|---|
| Anxiety/ tension | Reduce anxiety, tension, and stress | 3+ | Moderate | 5 to 7 | Midday, late afternoon, or when tense | Scenic trail; quiet park or track | After: relaxation techniques (relaxation exercises, meditation, etc.) |
| Loneliness | Alleviate loneliness; meet others | 2+ | Moderate-slow | 4 or more | When lonely or when convenient | Popular place for jogging; jogging events | After: chat with other joggers; get involved in meaningful activity |
| Alcoholism | Provide an alternative to drinking; improve self-concept and attitudes toward health | 2+ | Slow | 4 or more | Morning or when convenient | NA | Before or after: AA meeting or group counseling session |
| Depression | Alleviate depression; increase productivity | 6+ | Brisk-moderate | 5 to 7 | When depressed or when convenient | Scenic trail; popular jogging site | After: group counseling, reading, or relaxation exercises |
| Overweight | Reduce body weight; improve self-concept (especially physical self) | 3+ | Moderate | 5 to 7 | Midday or when convenient | NA | Before or after: fast or follow low-calorie diet |

[a] Beginning joggers should gradually work up to the recommended minimum distance and speed.

[b] Speed defined: brisk, less than eight minutes per mile; moderate, eight to nine minutes per mile; slow, more than nine minutes per mile.

NA = Not applicable.

In this role the psychotherapist runs along with a single client or several clients while counseling on the run about any problem or concern. The jogging itself does not necessarily play a major part in the therapy, although it can. The primary idea is to counsel in a relaxed and natural setting as an alternative to the formal and possibly inhibiting atmosphere of an office. The relaxed state generated by jogging also promotes psychotherapist-client rapport and client self-disclosure. (See suggestions for therapist as fellow jogger in Kostrubala, chap. 6. and Kostrubala 1976.)

REFERRAL

The psychotherapist may refer the client to appropriate jogging activities, information, and specialists. Such sources may include doctors who specialize in jogging injuries, places that administer treadmill tests and other fitness tests, books and articles on jogging, and jogging groups and clubs for ongoing company and support. The psychotherapist should know about various resources related to jogging.

## Problem Areas for Jogotherapy

Table 1 lists five psychotherapeutic problems along with suggested jogotherapy programs for each in terms of jogging conditions. These common problem areas—anxiety and tension, loneliness, alcoholism, depression, and overweight—are presented to demonstrate how jogging conditions can be manipulated to optimize therapeutic outcomes. A systematic program based on jogging can help alter psychophysiological states and even traits. The psychotherapist should encourage the client to progress gradually in distance and rate, run regularly, remain relaxed (as much as possible), and take precautions to prevent accidents and injuries. A physical examination should be recommended before the client starts a jogotherapy program, especially if it has been some time since the last one or if age or medical history suggest the need. If the psychotherapist is not an active jogger, he or she should at least be well read on the physiology of jogging and related topics.

ANXIETY AND TENSION

State anxiety (situational anxiety) and trait anxiety (anxiety proneness) are common psychotherapeutic problems (Levitt 1967). There is research evidence that jogging or sustained exercise can reduce anxiety levels, especially in state anxiety (Harper and Adams 1977). (See Berger, chap. 9, for a review of the running and anxiety literature.) A jogotherapy program for anxious clients seeks to reduce the level of anxiety, tension, and stress that they experience or perceive. It is recommended that clients jog at least three miles each time, at the moderate rate of eight to nine minutes per mile, as frequently as five to seven days a week. Jogging should be done in a scenic, relaxing, or soothing setting, at the time of day when the client is most tense. Midday and late afternoon are good times, since anxiety and tension often arise from fatigue, pressure, and hurry on the job and since people are often free to jog during lunchtime and after work and find that jogging relaxes and energizes them. The psychotherapist may recommend relaxation techniques to be used after jogging. Relaxation programs with exercises for tense muscles can be purchased, packaged with audiotapes or records and explanatory booklets. Various meditation regimens and biofeedback programs can also reinforce a jogotherapy program for reducing anxiety and tension.

## LONELINESS

A jogotherapy program for loneliness seeks to move clients from an isolated residential environment to an outdoor setting where they can relate to others who are interested in jogging. Clients should jog at least two miles at each outing, at a moderate to slow rate, at least four times a week. The client should jog upon feeling lonely, if possible, and should seek to run with others or in a setting other joggers favor (such as a park, school or university track, or indoor track). After or during jogging, the client may want to chat with other joggers. The client may be referred to a regular jogging group that runs together on a fixed schedule. When the client returns home, he or she may prevent or alleviate further feelings of loneliness by such activities as reading, letter writing, professional work, or some hobby. Healthy and enjoyable activities involving others are another alternative to relapsing into loneliness.

## ALCOHOLISM

Alcoholism is the most prevalent drug-related illness in the United States (*Alcohol and Health* 1974). Gary and Guthrie (1972) found jogging a minimum of one mile a day for twenty consecutive days influential in improving the fitness, self-esteem, and sleep of alcoholics. The goals of a jogotherapy program for alcoholics are consistent with Gary and Guthrie's (1972) findings, traditional treatment goals for alcoholics, and psychophysiological outcomes of jogging. Specifically, this program aims to improve self-concept and attitudes toward health. It also aids in the physical rehabilitation of alcoholics while speeding detoxification (since jogging improves metabolism). Moreover, jogging can provide a positive alternative to heavy drinking. A jogotherapy program for alcoholics recommends a distance of two miles or more at each outing, at a slow speed (can be gradually increased with increased fitness or rehabilitation), four or more times a week. Jogging should be done in the morning, followed by an Alcoholics Anonymous group meeting or a group counseling session. Another time of day can be substituted, but morning jogging lets the alcoholic start the day with a positive activity that provides a sense of achievement and supports abstinence through the day. For encouragement and consistency, jogging in a group is best for alcoholic clients. The place or setting for jogging is not a significant condition for treatment. (See Summers and Wolstat, chap. 5, for further insights into this area.)

DEPRESSION

Depression is a widespread psychological problem, mood, or mental disorder, characterized by sadness, anxiety, lethargy, and inability to find self-fulfillment in meaningful activity (Bourne and Ekstrand 1976). The use of jogging to alleviate depression has been supported by recent research (Ismail and Young 1977; Greist et al. 1978). The underlying physiological factor that elevates mood seems to be the ability of sustained exercise to alter biochemical levels in the brain. Since a "jogging high" takes longer distances at a steady pace, it is recommended that the depressed client run six miles or more at each outing, at a brisk to moderate pace, at least five days a week. The goal of such a program is to alleviate depression while increasing activity and productivity. A scenic or popular jogging site may aid in lifting mood, and group counseling, relaxation exercises, or reading are appropriate supportive activities. (See Buffone, chap. 1, and Berger, chap. 9, for more about depression and running.)

OVERWEIGHT

Obesity is a common problem among clients who seek help. It can be a direct concern, or it can be an indirect factor in expressed problems such as interpersonal conflict, poor self-image or self-concept, and health difficulties. The equation for weight reduction is based on burning calories while reducing intake. A jogotherapy program for weight reduction suggests three miles or more at each outing, at a moderate speed, five to seven days a week. The client should fast once a week for about eighteen hours, follow a regulated diet with low-calorie foods and smaller portions, or do both. The setting for jogging is not nearly as important as the regularity and amount.

## Applications of Jogotherapy for Career Improvement

Clients frequently come to counseling and psychotherapy with serious concerns about "lack of job satisfaction" or "lack of high-level job performance" in work of which they are capable. Job satisfaction and performance are often related to mood, energy level, and physical and mental stamina. Since jogging can influence all these behavioral characteristics, it may help with career problems. Jogotherapy may be employed in vocational counseling, career counseling, and placement counseling, and even in personal-social counseling where the client's job is indirectly related to the expressed problem. Police and firefighters may undertake regular vigorous jogging coupled with weight training to build the physical stamina required in their work. Fashion models can jog to attain or maintain optimum weight and muscle tone. Salespersons may jog before work to acquire the "up" or psychic energy necessary for high-powered selling. Health professionals can surely employ jogging to improve their own health and fitness and thus project themselves as positive models for their patients. Even college students, preparing for a career, can jog to relax after a fatiguing day of sitting in classes and studying, or to improve stamina for study.

Jogotherapy can also reduce stress in high-level executives and managers, provide year-round basic fitness for professional and amateur athletes, and serve as an outlet and therapy for depressed, lonely, or overweight homemakers. It can relax persons carrying on stressful psychological work in the helping professions, maintain basic fitness for military personnel and professional dancers, and reduce stress for air traffic controllers. Jogotherapy can increase performance and satisfaction in numerous other careers, if the program is fitted to the nature and goals of the client's work.

## References

*Alcohol and health.* 1974. Rockville, Md.: National Institute on Alcohol Abuse and Alcoholism.

Bourne, L., and Ekstrand, B. 1976. *Psychology: Its principles and meanings* 2d ed. New York: Holt, Rinehart and Winston.

Fixx, J. F. 1977. *The complete book of running.* New York: Random House.

Gary V., and Guthrie, D. 1972. The effect of jogging on physical fitness and self-concept in hospitalized alcoholics. *Quarterly Journal of Studies on Alcohol* 33: 1073–78.

Gazda, G. M. 1971. *Group counseling: A developmental approach* 1st ed. Boston: Allyn and Bacon.

———. 1978. *Group counseling: A developmental approach* 2d ed. Boston: Allyn and Bacon.

Greist, J. H.; Klein, M. H.; Eischens, R. R.; and Faris, J. W. 1978. Antidepressant running: Running as a treatment for non-psychotic depression. *Behavioral Medicine,* June, 19–24.

Harper, F. 1978. Outcomes of jogging: Implications for counseling. *Personnel and Guidance Journal* 57:74–78.

———. 1979. *Jogotherapy: Jogging as a therapeutic strategy.* Alexandria, Va.: Douglass Publishers.

Harper, F., and Adams, R. 1977. An experimental course in jogging. *Journal of Physical Education* 74:64–65.

Hartung, G., and Farge, E. 1977. Personality and physiological traits in middle-aged runners and joggers. *Journal of Gerontology* 32:541–48.

Ismail, A. H., and Young, R. J. 1977. Effect of chronic exercise on the multivariate relationships between selected biochemical and personality variables. *Multivariate Behavioral Research* 12:49–67.

Iversen, L. L. 1979. The chemistry of the brain. *Scientific American* 241:134–49.

Kostrubala, T. 1976. *The joy of running.* Philadelphia: J. B. Lippincott.

Levitt, E. E. 1967. *The psychology of anxiety.* Indianapolis: Bobbs-Merrill.

Lykouras, E.; Garelis, E.; Varsou, E.; and Stefanis, C. N. 1979. Physical activity and plasma cyclic adenosine monophosphate levels in manic-depressive patients and healthy adults. *American Journal of Psychiatry* 136:540–42.

McCutcheon, L. 1978. Personality traits of distance runners. *Running Times,* July, 9–11.

Mandell, A. 1979. The second second wind. *Psychiatric Annals* 9:154–60.

Renfrow, N. E., and Bolton, B. 1979. Personality characteristics associated with aerobic exercise in adult males. *Journal of Personality Assessment* 43:261–66.

Wood, D. T. 1977. The relationship between state anxiety and acute physical activity. *American Corrective Therapy Journal* 31:67–69.

# 5

# Creative Running

Dr. Wolstat is a psychiatrist in private practice who has been running for more than ten years and has completed more than a dozen marathons. Dr. Summers, a clinical psychologist, specializes in hypnotherapy and has run for three years and competed in several races. Working as a team, we have synthesized an approach using various psychological techniques applicable in both training and treatment (Wolstat and Summers 1980a,b). Both of us have been trained in hypnosis and Gestalt imagery as well as in more traditional psychological techniques. Since running is a repetitive exercise, it lends itself readily to hypnotic techniques that use repeated suggestions to achieve an altered state of consciousness.

The theoretical background of our approach involves a holistic health model as opposed to the traditional dualistic model. Therefore we will first discuss some assumptions of the holistic health model. We will then examine a number of psychological techniques that have been useful for training runners and finally consider running as a treatment modality in psychotherapy.

## The Holistic Health Model

The holistic health model approaches the organism as a total process of being (as opposed to the traditional dualistic view of the separation of mind and body). If the person is to function as a whole, healthy organism, it is important to evaluate both physical and psychological processes. Because the person is a whole system, a change in any part of the system also affects the other parts. An intervention on the psychological level also affects the physical level and vice versa. A change in one aspect of the system, no matter how positive, is also a disruption. And a disruption in the system, even if productive, creates stress. Therefore, a new approach (running, for example) will be accompanied by stress.

For one of our clients running was very beneficial, but it was also disruptive and she initially gained weight because of this change in lifestyle. She had never thought of herself as athletic, and she needed to integrate the new information when, in fact, after several months she was running five or six miles at a time.

Another client found running a panacea for a faltering marriage. He used running as an escape hatch—as many do—to avoid destructive confrontations with his spouse. Only after his self-esteem had been reestablished was he able to deal effectively with the marital stresses and work toward resolving the conflicts.

A third client (a situation more frequently seen) became obsessed with the newfound sport of running. He literally "ran away" from responsibility. His job, friends, and family saw less and less of him as he increased his mileage dramatically over a short period. As could be expected, a muscle injury slowed him down enough so he could begin dealing again with the conflict in his life. (See chap. 13, by Sachs and Pargman, for further insights into this area.)

Thus, if the organism is to be an effective whole, running must be integrated into a therapeutic program. Using running and psychotherapy together makes it possible to release new creative energy. Together they create a synergistic union, demonstrating a basic tenet of Gestalt psychology—the whole is greater than the sum of its parts.

## Psychological Techniques Used in Running

What are some of the psychological techniques used in running? There has been much discussion of the "runner's high" that some runners report about forty-five minutes into a run. (See chap. 15 by Sachs.) This altered state of consciousness can be used to induce deep concentration, attention, and relaxation.

There are many ways to induce this altered state. Meditation, yoga, and sensory deprivation are some examples. The methods we use are hypnosis and deep muscle relaxation. The latter process involves learning how to relax at a very deep level, which can be done over several weeks of practice and repetition. It can be done first apart from running (for example, in an office) by systematically and consistently contracting and relaxing one's muscles. As one learns to do this more efficiently and effectively it can be done while standing, walking, and eventually running. The runner not only is more relaxed but breathes more efficiently, which leads to a better style of running. Eventually the runner may integrate these methods into speed work and endurance.

Hypnosis is also an effective way to enhance running performance (Wolstat and Summers 1980b). The hypnotist, ideally also a runner, is a trained mental health professional and will screen out those for whom hypnosis is contraindicated. For example, in a latent schizophrenic hypnosis could precipitate a psychotic break. In most cases, however, hypnosis is safe and effective.

The subject is acquainted with hypnosis and taught self-hypnosis before running. Then, during a run, the hypnotist accompanies the runner and institutes a light hypnotic state with guided imagery. Many images can be suggested, depending on the personality of the runner and using environmental images. For example, evergreen trees and running water are particularly "energetic" as well as relaxing images. By running with the client, the hypnotist can suggest images using stimuli present in the environment. An example is suggesting that the road is a giant conveyor belt carrying the runner along. Other images are sailboats gliding before the breeze, a well-oiled machine moving rhythmically, or (in a group run) being attached by a rope to the runner in front.

It is also helpful to use passive as well as active imagery. In active imagery the presenter continues to talk and expand upon the visual suggestions. After training in this area, runners may be taught passive imagery—they can be given the beginnings of an image and then expand upon it themselves. For example, the hypnotist can suggest seeing oneself running effortlessly across the plains, then let the runner continue to "roll that film before the eyes" while running. With any of these psychological approaches the trainer should be a runner who can present images that are particularly effective in running. It is a subtle art to know when to actively push and encourage and when to hold back so as not to strain the runner.

### Running as a Psychological Technique

Running itself can be used as a treatment modality or as an adjunct treatment in psychotherapy. Running not only affects the psyche in such areas as depression and anxiety, but also changes people's approach to caring for their bodies. Nutrition and lifestyle are often radically modified as runners realize that nutritious, low-calorie foods (often approaching vegetarianism) are essential to maintaining health. The early-morning runner decides on earlier bedtimes, and drugs and alcohol may be essentially eliminated. Since it is essential to breathe easily, runners rarely continue to smoke. But most important, the runner experiences a subjective sense of well-being and increased energy for all life tasks.

In depression, the individual often withdraws inward. The therapist intervenes with psychological techniques that will enable the client to reactivate in terms of work, relationships, and physical momentum. Therefore running is a logical approach to mobilization. The therapist can begin by suggesting walks and perhaps running (individually or in an organized program), and the client can build skills by reading books and keeping a journal. Next the client can contract with the therapist to keep records of running experiences, to get weekly feedback, and to receive support and encouragement in accomplishing goals.

Another approach is to form a group of individuals at various stages of running to give mutual support and share knowledge. Often people who are very depressed are also isolated. Using a running group psychotherapeutically serves two functions. It allows the person who needs to be alone to fulfill that need in a constructive manner. Even when running in a group we basically are self-aware. But the group setting also makes it possible to share one's experiences and to develop friendships and relationships around social aspects of running. Many of our clients have described what we consider a unique social aspect of group running. They have developed close friendships with other runners, yet for the most part these friendships have been restricted to running activities. For the individual who values aloneness, such relationships are nonthreatening and nonintrusive. These new friends have whetted the appetites of ''isolates'' for other friendships, which has led to fuller, more gratifying social lives.

The anxious person has an extremely high activation level (see Berger, chap. 9, for more on anxiety), and it is often necessary to channel that high level of excitement to a positive use. Running can do this, and it also is extremely calming, often enabling people to discharge frenetic, destructive energy.

One of the earliest clients with whom we used running as an adjunct therapy was a young woman who was severely alcoholic and also troubled by a chronic situational depression. For some time she had participated in Alcoholics Anonymous with varying degrees of success, and though she had consulted several psychotherapists she continued in self-destructive patterns. She had run on her own, so we suggested she attempt to keep a journal of her runs and tie this in with her psychotherapy as well as continuing with Alcoholics

Anonymous. After several weeks she found that her depression was lifting and that she had gained much more control of her drinking. Her journal showed a great variety of feelings (such as exuberance, grief, and contentment). At the same time there was a general improvement in her physical health; she lost weight and ate a more balanced, nutritious diet. She soon became an "addicted" runner (see Sachs and Pargman, chap. 13) and realized in therapy that she had substituted running for alcohol. She terminated therapy much improved, still running, and firmly committed to the Alcoholics Anonymous program. This is similar to cases reported by Glasser (1976).

A second case illustrates a more common usage of prescribed running, for reactive depression. The client was an outdoor-oriented man in his early thirties who was physically fit but severely depressed and anxious. (Incidentally, it is important to make sure that those entering a running program are in good physical health. If there is any question, they should consult their family physicians.) This man was going through a divorce and found himself eating and drinking to excess and having difficulty with important decisions. Although the marriage had not lasted long, it had met his dependency needs and given him some stability. We suggested a graduated program of running, beginning with one mile a day three days a week. Within a month he was up to three miles a day five days a week. As part of his once-weekly psychotherapy he was taught deep muscle relaxation and self-hypnosis, which he applied to his runs with various guided images. As he became more involved in running he became more decisive and began to reorient his life goals.

Since running is a process of self-mastery, it enhances self-esteem and can increase the ability to make important life decisions. After allowing clients to see that for once they can control something, the next logical step is to transfer this ability to work, relationships, and other important areas of life. Not only does running increase decisiveness, it seems to promote creativity in people's approach to life, demonstrated in the ability to generate new solutions to problems. Often, while running, people can sharply focus their cognitive processes so as to solve problems, organize their schedules, write letters, or generally clear up confusion or fogginess (see Sachs, chap. 16, on the mind of the runner).

A third client was a former college athlete, thirty-six years old, who had achieved the limelight in college as a champion ski racer, almost making the United States Olympic team. After two disastrous marriages, several business failures, severe bouts of alcoholism that necessitated hospitalization, and untold other psychological miseries, he ended up living at home under the care of his aging parents. He found many ways to defeat his therapists until a highly structured program was instituted involving Alcoholics Anonymous, behavioristic therapy, and Antabuse. Stability of some sort was achieved for more than six months, but he — literally — was going nowhere. He stayed home, not working, with few relationships and little stress in his life. We prescribed running, and he immediately threw himself into this physical outlet. His lost self-confidence began returning. He began to question his exile from life. Now he has started to move. We expect no miracles, but there is a new quality to his optimism.

Alcoholism played a prominent role in all these cases. Because we have gained a reputation for working with difficult cases like these, one of our main sources of referral is the local Alcoholics Anonymous program. If one accepts that one of the causes of alcoholism is faulty habit formation, it follows that running's "positive addiction" qualities (as formulated in the excellent book by William Glasser, *Positive Addiction;* see also Sachs and Pargman, chap. 13) can substitute for the "negative" addictions of drugs and alcohol. Several competitive runners have claimed that running helped them cope with drinking and drug problems (personal communication).

A final client helped in this way was a twenty-nine-year-old graduate student. After a youthful marriage ended in divorce in his early twenties, he attempted suicide by asphyxiation. The short period of anoxia left some residual brain damage that did not affect him intellectually but acted as a physical and emotional stop valve when he was under too much stress. His energy level was chronically low, he became flooded with anxiety during stressful times (especially in his relations with women), and he depended increasingly on stimulants that had been prescribed early in his treatment. Several years of intensive psychotherapy allowed him to pursue his career (with great academic success) and remarry. But many of his original symptoms, though diminished, continued. We prescribed running mainly to give his sedentary body a good physical outlet. After six months he reported a radical change in his energy level, a marked diminution of anxiety, and a tapering off of medication (on his own initiative).

### Conclusion

It is apparent that running, whether as a primary or an adjunct technique, is an effective and valid therapeutic tool. The creative energy that is released helps transform insight into integrated action. Our techniques, such as hypnosis, represent a structured, controlled presentation, in contrast to the spontaneous trancelike experience ("runner's high") that some runners report. We believe this is a synergistic experience that combines an altered state of consciousness with the physical state of running, forming a joyful new experience for the runner.

It is said that running enhances creativity. There have been numerous anecdotal reports about runners solving problems, writing reports, or composing poetry, prose, or music during a run (see Sachs, chap. 16). George Sheehan (1978) wrote extensively about this. We find that the creative process of runners also enables them to create their own imagery and, subsequently, their own altered states of consciousness during a run. Many runners report having developed the use of imagery on their own, without formal training. This release of creative energy lets us use the synergy of running as a therapeutic tool. The runner begins to feel a sense of self-mastery that enhances self-esteem, and the release of creativity that follows permits insight gained in conventional psychotherapy to be emotionally integrated into the psyche. Emotional blocks are removed, options are discovered, and the runner begins to solve problems of daily living. These creative solutions seem to work in both intrapsychic and interpersonal life, alleviating neurotic symptoms. Thus movement mobilizes the individual to work toward "self-actualization."

Our program is a prescription for health. A number of investigators have previously discussed running as a prescription for specific mental disorders (Brown, Ramirez, and Taub 1978; Driscoll 1976; Greist et al. 1978; Lion 1978; Orwin 1974; see also Berger, chaps. 9 and 10). We are concerned with the broader definition of health as a sense of well-being, both psychological and physical. These combined aspects themselves lead to a "synergistic experience," a totality of "wellness." Our program thus creates energy for living through creative psychotherapeutic techniques aimed at integrating movement and imagery, enabling clients to extend themselves beyond their limits and find again, or for the first time, a zest for living.

### References

Brown, R. S.; Ramirez, D. E.; and Taub, J. M. 1978. The prescription of exercise for depression. *Physician and Sportsmedicine* 6(12):34–37, 40–41, 44–45.

Driscoll, R. 1976. Anxiety reduction using physical exertion and positive images. *Psychological Record* 26:87–94.

Glasser, W. 1976. *Positive addiction*. New York: Harper and Row.

Greist, J. H.; Klein, M. H.; Eischens, R. R.; Faris, J.; Gurman, A. S.; and Morgan, W. P. 1978. Running through your mind. *Journal of Psychosomatic Research* 22:259–94.

Lion, L. S. 1978. Psychological effects of jogging: A preliminary study. *Perceptual and Motor Skills* 47:1215–18.

Orwin, A. 1974. Treatment of a situational phobia: A case for running. *British Journal of Psychiatry* 125:95–98.

Sheehan, G. 1978. *Running and being: The total experience.* New York: Simon and Schuster.

Wolstat, H., and Summers, J. 1980a. Creative running. Paper presented at the meeting of the American Medical Joggers Association, Boston, Massachusetts.

————. 1980b. Running and hypnosis. Paper presented at the meeting of the American Society of Clinical Hypnosis, Minneapolis, Minnesota.

# 6

# A Psychoanalytic
# Perspective on Running

Any effect of running in part depends on the meaning the runner attaches to it. What distinguishes George Sheehan's religious-mystical approach to running from J. B. McEvoy's widely quoted remark—"The secret of my abundant health is that whenever the impulse to exercise comes over me I lie down until it passes away" (1938, 166)—is most likely to be found in the personal meanings of physical movement, breathlessness, muscular exertion, perspiration, and so forth, which derive from one's own experience. These historically derived meanings combine with processes of the endocrine, muscular, cardiovascular, respiratory, and neurological systems to produce a total effect, but none by themselves can explain running. In the following essay I will use psychoanalysis to explore one aspect of running: the meanings runners attach to it.

The primary assumption of psychoanalytic theory is that behavior is motivated by a dynamic unconscious—those aspects of memory, knowledge, cognition, and perception that are "out of awareness" and cannot be retrieved by attention or concentration (Rado 1969). In specifying that these unconscious processes are dynamic I emphasize their motivating influence in all our activities, thoughts, and feelings. Every aspect of behavior is in large part determined by factors outside our awareness. The material we are aware of is often compared to the visible tip of an iceberg, the submerged part representing the unconscious. A second assumption of psychodynamic theory is that childhood fantasies and events occupy a significant place in the dynamic unconscious (Brenner 1974). A third assumption, multiple determination, states that an activity or behavior can have many meanings, including the expression both of conscious and unconscious wishes and of the unconscious prohibitions against them.

A psychoanalyst sees as simplistic and naive studies that seek to understand why people run by exploring runners' conscious motivations. For example, when runners are asked why they run, fitness is given as principal motivation. But what is meant by fitness? Does it relate to health, fear of illness or aging, concern about physical attractiveness or sexuality, a wish to be superior to others, fear of inner deadness or decay—physical or spiritual—uncertainty regarding masculinity or femininity that is fueled by work or personal disappointments, or to some combination of these and many other possibilities?

Even if we asked runners these specific questions we might not be satisfied with their answers, because people often do not tell the truth about themselves to investigators or even to themselves. We like to behave properly not only for authorities such as parents, teachers, employers, and psychological investigators of running behavior, but for that internal authority, our own standards or conscience. Some runners might run for sexual reasons such as wanting to look at other people's bodies or to show off their own. But it is unlikely that most people would feel comfortable admitting to such voyeuristic or exhibitionistic reasons.

A colleague reported that a patient of his, a competitive runner, often ran against the flow of runners during workouts because when running behind men he felt an uncomfortable impulse to stare at their buttocks. Running against the flow, he experienced pleasure at feeling that people would admire his strong and graceful stride and might even notice the bulge of his genitals in his skimpy briefs. After some reflection on this and on related feelings it became evident that he was struggling with unacknowledged homosexual impulses that frightened him because he feared that if they emerged into full awareness he might become a practicing homosexual. These conflicts contributed to his vague discomfort at the sight of men's buttocks and his pleasure in proving how masculine he was. Although this man is a psychiatric patient, it is generally true that the anxieties and symptoms of the neurotic represent failures to successfully master universal conflicts; this patient's discomfort concerning male runners expressed a universal concern about bisexuality (Kubie 1974). Although this in no way implies that running is always a way of warding off or expressing sexual impulses, it does suggest that for *some* runners it might represent *an aspect* of a complexly determined behavior. It is precisely this capacity of running to represent so much that makes it so rich an experience for so many people.

Let me illustrate a psychoanalytic approach to the antidepressant effects of running, utilizing Freud's (1957b) theory of depression as presented in his essay "Mourning and Melancholia," which views depression as a response to the loss of an ambivalently loved object. Such an "object" can be a personal relationship, an important ideal, or an aspect of one's self-image such as being brilliant or physically strong. Though the lost object was both loved and hated, the hated aspect was disavowed or repressed from conscious awareness. As a result the relationship, ideal, or aspect of one's self is viewed only in idealized or favorable terms, while its undesirable aspects are "ignored" or pushed into the unconscious because of their unacceptability. When the loss occurs this process is intensified, and one identifies with or internalizes in the unconscious an image of the lost object; the shadow of the lost object falls on the ego (Freud 1957b). In this way one can symbolically deny the loss by maintaining the relation to it on an unconscious level. Bereaved individuals frequently manifest this unconscious identification by taking on characteristics or traits of the lost person (Lindemann 1944). The previously repressed negative feelings toward the lost person are now directed to the altered self. The result is the painful self-recriminations of the depressive. This discharge of negative feelings toward one's self also provides a masochistic appeasement of the punishing superego, which believes that the object was lost because of some failure by the depressed person.

Running might act as an antidepressant on a simple level by discharging the repressed aggression in physical activity. Similarly, the physical pain suffered during long runs or races might replace the superego punishment for causing the loss. The feeling of being inadequate or unable to survive without the lost object might be countered as the runner demonstrates self-sufficiency and gains a realistic increase in self-esteem. Another way we might explain why running relieves depression is to invoke a total denial of the loss. The independence and self-sufficiency fostered by the running might on an unconscious level be equated with the statement, "I am so self-sufficient that I don't need anyone and therefore have not suffered a loss." In this dynamic the running does not relieve the depression by aiding the process of grieving but defends against it by denying the loss through an illusory self-sufficiency.

For example, Mr. A lost his father after a prolonged illness. During the final stages of the illness, Mr. A began to run, and he soon became an addicted runner. During runs he frequently felt a pleasurable sense of mastery, strength, and personal efficacy. At his father's death he did not experience any grief, but he felt driven that day to run for an unusually long period. In later psychoanalytic treatment it became clear that the running was an attempt to recapture an aspect of his early relationship with his father, during which they would playfully try to catch each other. The running and the weight loss that attended it were secondarily reinforced by an identification with the father's illness and consequent weight loss. The running also represented Mr. A's wish to strengthen his father's failing health by making himself strong so his father could borrow his strength; he would "breathe life" into his father. After his father's death Mr. A was able to deny the loss by continuing the unconscious fantasy that his father was running with him. This became clear when after a particularly joyous run he began to cry uncontrollably. In therapy he was able to recall that just before crying he had had a memory of his father and the strange sensation that somebody was running alongside him. When he looked and saw no one, he felt a profound sense of loss and began to cry.

The role of running in this patient is complex. It represented a denial of the grief associated with the impending loss, then death, of his father. By identifying with his father in his failing health and increasing his own strength by running, Mr. A symbolically attempted to restore his father's strength. This was reinforced by the pleasurable unconscious repetition of their chasing each other when Mr. A was a child. During this game the child experienced intense delight at being powerful enough to catch his father or playfully flee from him. This example not only illustrates how running can be an antidepressant but also demonstrates the three assumptions of psychoanalysis listed earlier and shows the richly complex meanings running can begin to assume.

Over time Mr. A gradually appreciated the fantasies his running enacted and learned to accept and fully grieve over his father's death. He continued to run, though less compulsively, and the conscious memory of his childhood games with his father added to his pleasure. These fantasies now began to include thoughts of someday playing running games with his own children.

We can use this case as a springboard to a more general psychoanalytic consideration of running. Several questions I would like to consider are: (1) Does running therapeutically influence mental conflict, or is it simply a readily available activity that can express psychological conflicts but has no lasting psychological benefit? (2) Is running distinguishable from other sports on psychoanalytic principles? (3) Are the psychological effects of running compatible with psychotherapy, with its emphasis on expressing feelings and conflicts verbally in the context of a therapeutic relationship?

Let us examine the first question. The determinants that motivate sport can derive from all phases of development; they can be narcissistic, dependent, hostile, or sexual. Sport seems to have no specific or exclusive intrapsychic meanings, and the psychoanalytic literature on the subject reports numerous dynamics. Freud (1957c) noted masturbatory elements in running, and Klein

(1923) drew attention to its aggressive aspects as well as its possible oedipal significance. Fenichel (1939) and Deutsch (1926) have emphasized counter-phobic elements in sportsmen; Deutsch cites an athlete who used baseball in an attempt to master his intense fear of retaliation for his own aggressive and assertive wishes. In a study of cricket and other bat-and-ball games, Adrian Stokes (1956) illustrated how all aspects of the activity, including the equipment, the playing field, and the other players, can become elements in an unconscious drama. For runners this can include the terrain, the weather, their bodies, their running shoes, or their times in a race.

*Example:* A patient preparing for a marathon daydreamed that he would reach the twenty-four-mile mark in two hours and forty minutes, which meant he could attain a much-sought-after goal of running a marathon in three hours. However, in the fantasy he either never completed the marathon or else he fell dead at the finish line. Certainly a curious fantasy. Why should the runner create this particular daydream when he might have fantasized running the marathon in three hours or, if he wished, in the world-record time of two hours and seven minutes to the acclaim of thousands of spectators? The explanation for the often curious choices we make in daydreams is to be found in the unconscious wishes and fears that the fantasy expresses in a symbolically disguised way. For this runner psychoanalysis revealed that the twenty-four-mile mark was where he entered the oval terrain at the Central Park area where he frequently trained. In his dreams it became clear that the oval represented the female genitalia and that the part of the park where he would enter this area was associated with danger—it was an area of frequent muggings. The early part of the marathon represented innocent, childlike sexual play before entering the dangerous and forbidden area of adult sexuality where he would have to run the risk of castration and death. The ''wall'' for this runner had the unconscious meaning of childhood prohibitions against being sexual.

An interesting aside is the similarity between this runner and the runner who carried to Athens the news of the Athenian victory over the Persians. On reaching the gates of the city he cried ''Rejoice, we conquer'' and fell dead. Both runners, the patient in fantasy and the legendary Greek runner, success-fully complete their races, the one in less than three hours and the other with the news of the young Greek nation's victory over the oppressive older Persian empire. The oedipal dynamics of the patient are implicit in the legendary run from Marathon to Athens—the price of victory is death.

Not only oedipal elements are found in running, but also narcissistic ele-ments. Fears of an inner deadness and hypochondriasis can often be countered by intense physical activities. Also, an image of self-perfection in which the body is viewed as possessing incredible endurance or as totally devoid of fat can become a quest in itself. Some runners, like people with anorexia nervosa, starve themselves and even induce vomiting after heavy meals to maintain their leanness (DeFries 1981; Sours 1981). Fantasies of total self-sufficiency, invincibility, and immortality attach to these perfect bodies in which the ravages time wreaks on the musculoskeletal and cardiovascular systems are reversed.

It is important to distinguish a pathological body stimulation from more socially integrated forms of athletic body stimulation. An example of pathological body stimulation is one patient who would stay in bed all day except to rouse himself from a stuporous, almost catatonic state to run fifteen to twenty miles. Another patient responded to humiliating hurts by taking long and physically exhausting runs. The physical pain he experienced during these runs was a welcome respite from his mental anguish and inner deadness. As he recognized his oversensitivity to being hurt by people, his toleration for emotional pain increased without the need to "run" from it by substituting painful body stimulation. He now runs less compulsively and no longer needs to experience exhaustion.

That running lends itself to representing a broad range of psychological feelings and conflicts says nothing about whether it can help the runner creatively master such distressing feelings and conflicts. In many of the examples given thus far the runners were running addicts: the running addict is characterized by a *compulsive* need to run at least once and sometimes twice a day. If for some reason he is prevented from running, he becomes irritable, restless, sleepless, and preoccupied with guilty thoughts that his body will decondition or deteriorate. He is logically able to recognize the irrationality of these feelings and thoughts, but they are inescapable and can be relieved only by running. Scheduled daily runs often preempt important vocational and social commitments so that work, family, and friendships suffer. A frequent response to stress is to run or to daydream about running. In such cases running has become a symptom of underlying psychopathology that represents a miscarried attempt at relieving psychological distress. Compulsive or addictive running can be contrasted to playful running (Sacks 1981; see also Sachs and Pargman, chap. 13).

Playful running has none of the compulsive or preemptory qualities of addictive running. Though important, it is one of many activities in a life that finds the average expectable gratifications and disappointments from family, friends, and work, but its importance is not of the same order. Missing a day's run is not the same as missing an important business meeting or neglecting one's wife, children, or friends. In a critical way these activities are real—the substance of adult life—while running is a diversion, a welcome respite— time off from the real world. It is precisely because it is not important in the real world that it is special. Once we run to accomplish a specific end or goal such as fitness it becomes like work and loses this quality. When we make it utilitarian, it is no longer playful running and becomes subject to the demands and limitations of reality.

The importance of playful running lies in its freedom from the real world. Erikson (1963) called play a "vacation from the superego," that agency within the mind that represents the real world. Mark Twain made the same point when he said that play is an activity full of meaning but no purpose. Running as play evokes a special form of mental activity, because within play everything is possible. We can win the five thousand-meter, ten thousand-meter, and marathon races in Los Angeles in 1984 in world-record times; we can murder our opponents; we can do anything we wish, because reality is not relevant.

From a psychoanalytic perspective play can inform and energize the rest of our lives by providing opportunities in fantasy, conscious or unconscious, for expressing otherwise inhibited or even forbidden feelings or wishes so we can return to real life refreshed and perhaps a little wiser about ourselves. In this way running may influence our behavior by providing a regular opportunity for adult play.

In response to the first question then, running is an activity that nonspeci-fically lends itself to representing any feeling or psychological conflict. This ability can be used adaptively in playful running or nonadaptively in compul-sive or addictive running. In playful running, its playfulness gives it special properties that allow the expression and creative mastery of inner conflicts.

The second question asks if running can be distinguished from other sports on psychoanalytic principles. A simple and practical advantage of running is the ease of doing it. The runner does not need expensive equipment, court time, or a partner, but only a pair of running shoes and a place to run. Running requires no new motor skills; one simply remembers what it was like to run as a child (Perry and Sacks 1981). Running may provide a wide range of pleasur-able emotions such as power, strength, invincibility, and efficacy. In this regard it seems very similar to the "practicing period" described by Mahler (1966). A child taking its first steps experiences intense elation. With the ability to move away from its parents and explore the world comes a new feeling of independence and of invincibility. Falls do not hurt.

This is not the only form of elation achieved by running. Some runners experience fusion or flow described as oneness with the environment or with the motion of running itself (Altshul 1978). Such experiences are often accompanied by a sense of timelessness and mystical awe. For others, the pleasures of control or of competition contribute to these peak experiences or to the runner's high. One runner said at the completion of a marathon: "I wasn't first, but I beat thousands; and if you include all the others who can't run a marathon I beat billions." These different kinds of peak experiences are not mutually exclusive. (See also Sachs, chap. 15.)

We can therefore answer the second question with a qualified yes. The ease of learning to run and its closeness to the practicing period and the mastery of the upright position may lend it a special significance, though I suspect every sport in some way captures the infant's joy in beginning to master its body and the world. For example, the eye-hand coordination of an infant three to six months old is an early achievement of physical mastery that may be significant in racket sports.

The third question regards the role of running in psychotherapy and brings us to the question of "acting out." The patient described earlier used running as resistance to recalling his dependent and intimate relation to his father. He "acted out" the memory and fantasy rather than recalling them. This also represented a transference wish, since it represented his knowledge that I was a runner and also the unacknowledged wish to run with me as he had once run with his father. The running thus served several psychic functions; it was overdetermined. In the analysis, these feelings were intensified by the father's illness.

Freud's original notion was that "acting out" was a resistance to the forward progress of the psychotherapy. For example, Dora's abrupt termination of treatment was an unconscious repetition of her wish to take revenge on Herr K. "She acts out an essential part of her recollections and fantasies instead of producing it in the treatment" (Freud 1957a). Further development of the theory of acting out has increased its use in treatment as an additional valuable source of information about the patient. The therapist is now inclined not to prohibit acting out, but to study it.

The concept of acting out has been expanded beyond the analytic situation and is used to describe physical activity in a general sense as a means of dealing with impulses and conflicts. This includes behaviors seen in a wide group of diagnostic entities, including impulse disorders, psychosomatic disorders, drug addiction, and so forth. Patients in these diagnostic groups may be said to "act out," or more accurately "to enact" unconscious impulses and memories in physical activity rather than in mental activities such as fantasy (Sandler,

Dare, and Holder 1978). Greenacre (1950) emphasized that the activity is motivated by a memory, and that exhibitionism and a belief in the "magic of activity" are essential elements. She suggested that predisposition to this psychic pattern may be found in trauma associated with the first two years of life, the ability to verbalize.

These ideas readily integrate with the idea that running is related to the practicing period in infancy. People who regularly turn to a physical activity to express psychological conflict and feelings may have developed this characteristic coping style because they had not yet developed the requisite verbal skills. When they seek to master stress as adults, they may turn (return) to physical expression rather than verbal expression. Implicit in this view is the assumption that using physical activity to represent or express feelings or conflict is less mature than using thinking or fantasy, which are detached from actual physical activity. I disagree. The playful use of the body in a sport such as running may be a regression to a more primitive mode of problem resolution, but like other forms of regression it must be judged by its outcome. If it provides a symbolic mode of experience that permits one to energize and creatively inform one's life, then it can be a "mature" behavior. Some confirmation for the existence and importance of physical activity in the mature adult is to be found in George Vaillant's (1977) work. Although he focused on the defense mechanisms that characterize the mature adult, he noted that participation in physical activity distinguished the mature from the immature subjects in his study.

In answer to the third question, in some individuals who have a tendency to use physical activity as a means of coping, running seems to provide a readily available way to master psychological distress. When running occurs as acting-out in therapy it can provide information about the patient's behavior and insight into problems and conflicts; for many people it is a creative way to deal with conflict by learning about the self.

In summary, psychoanalysis provides a valuable perspective for understanding the rich complexity of meanings and feelings found in running. Contrary to the popular notion that running is a lonely and dull sport, this physical activity is part of an intense internal drama, both conscious and unconscious, in which people express significant past experiences as well as current wishes and fears. This can be done pathologically in compulsive running or creatively in playful running. In either case, examining the mental behavior can provide access to the significance of running in the internal life of the runner.

## References

Altshul, V. A. 1978. The ego-integrative (and disintegrative) aspects of long distance running. *Current Concepts in Psychiatry* 4(4):6–11.

Brenner, C. 1974. *An elementary textbook of psychoanalysis*. New York: Anchor Books.

DeFries, Z. 1981. Running madness: A prelude to real madness. In *Psychology of running*, ed. M. H. Sacks and M. L. Sachs. Champaign, Ill.: Human Kinetics Publishers.

Deutsch, H. 1926. A contribution to the psychology of sport. *International Journal of Psychoanalysis* 7:223–27.

Erikson, E. 1963. *Childhood and society*. New York: W. W. Norton.

Fenichel, O. 1939. The counter-phobic attitude. *International Journal of Psychoanalysis* 20:263–74.

Freud, S. 1957a. Fragment of an analysis of a case of hysteria. In *The collected works of Sigmund Freud*, ed. J. Strachey, vol. 7. London: Hogarth Press.

———. 1957b. Mourning and melancholia. In *The collected works of Sigmund Freud*, ed. J. Strachey, vol. 14. London: Hogarth Press.

———. 1957c. Three essays on sexuality. In *The collected works of Sigmund Freud*, ed. J. Strachey, vol. 7. London: Hogarth Press.

Greenacre, P. 1950. General problems of acting out. *Psychoanalytic Quarterly* 19:455–67.

Klein, M. 1923. Infant analysis. In *Contributions to psychoanalysis*. London: Hogarth Press.

Kubie, L. S. 1974. The drive to become both sexes. *Psychoanalytic Quarterly* 43:349–426.

Lindemann, E. 1944. Symptomatology and management of acute grief. *American Journal of Psychiatry* 101:141–48.

Mahler, M. 1966. Notes on the development of basic moods: The depressive affect. In *Psychoanalysis—A general psychology: Essays in honor of Heinz Hartmann*, ed. R. M. Lowenstein, L. M. Newman, M. Schur, and A. J. Solnit. New York: International Universities Press.

McEvoy, J. B. 1966. *American Mercury*, December 1938. Quoted in *Familiar medical quotations*, ed. M. B. Strauss. Boston: Little, Brown.

Perry, S. W., and Sacks, M. H. 1981. Psychodynamics of running. In *Psychology of running*, ed. M. H. Sacks and M. L. Sachs. Champaign, Ill.: Human Kinetics Publishers.

Rado, S. 1969. *Adaptational psychodynamics*. New York: Science House.

Sacks, M. H. 1981. Running addiction: A clinical report. In *Psychology of running*, ed. M. H. Sacks and M. L. Sachs. Champaign, Ill.: Human Kinetics Publishers.

Sandler, J.; Dare, C.; and Holder, A. 1978. *The patient and the analyst*. New York: International Universities Press.

Sours, J. A. 1981. Running, anorexia nervosa, and perfection. In *Psychology of running,* ed. M. H. Sacks and M. L. Sachs. Champaign, Ill.: Human Kinetics Publishers.

Stokes, A. 1956. Psychoanalytic reflections on the development of ballgames, particularly cricket. *International Journal of Psychoanalysis* 37:185–92.

Vaillant, G. 1977. *Adaptation to life.* Boston: Little, Brown.

# 7

---

# Running and Therapy

In March 1973 I first began running with a group of my psychiatric patients. We walked, jogged, and ran for one hour, then had an hour of group therapy. The ambulation rate was determined by a cardiovascular formula based on the target pulse rate of each patient. Each had a cardiovascular stress test carried to maximum performance, and each patient's goal was to eventually ambulate at 75 to 80 percent of a target rate expressed as pulse rate over ten seconds. The patients carried diagnoses of schizophrenia, multiple drug abuse, depression, and anorexia nervosa. Of the six, four had been hospitalized. Except for the multiple drug abuse patient, all were on medication.

Five of the six patients responded favorably to therapy. One experienced a severe exacerbation of paranoid schizophrenia and had to be rehospitalized for electroconvulsive treatment. As of March 1982, all but that one had maintained their recovery. One, a paranoid schizophrenic, sporadically requires a therapy session (once every three to six months). All the others are living without medication.

### The Tools of Psychotherapy

In March 1973, in my fifteenth year as a physician, I employed a new tool in psychiatry. Instead of the consulting room or the couch, I began to employ one of the most fundamental biomechanical behaviors of our species—walking/jogging/running—with a specific definition based upon cardiovascular criteria. I chose the time of one hour, based upon data that after approximately forty-five to fifty minutes of exercise growth hormone was measurable in the peripheral blood, a clue that the pituitary was involved and so the stimulus might arise from the hypothalamus. If so, I was getting at the brain from the bottom up. I also noticed that somewhere around the fifty-minute level my own feelings differed from the response at twenty, thirty, and fifty to sixty minutes. Thus the formula was to run one hour, at 75 to 80 percent of maximum cardiac output, three times a week. If nothing else happened, at least the patients would be improving their cardiovascular apparatus.

My experiences using this tool were described in my book *The Joy of Running*, written in 1975 and published by Lippincott in 1976.

We can often clarify a concept through contrast. Here I will contrast the couch, the chair, and running as therapeutic tools. "Running" will be used to mean walk/jog/run. The couch and the chair are symbols of the psychotherapeutic acts associated with their use.

### THE COUCH AS A TOOL OF THERAPY

The patient face up on the couch, with the therapist out of sight behind it, is a physical acting out of the psychological positions of patient and analyst. In the supine position humans are at their most vulnerable, since the abdomen has no bony cage to protect it. This is reflected in the American slang term "belly up."

Psychoanalysis is consistently done in an office, indoors and enclosed. Some analytic offices have two doors, one for entering and one for leaving, to ensure "confidentiality," and some have soundproofed or double doors for the same reason. The entire concept is one of enclosure—of a box. The analyst, who must remain in the box from patient to patient, may attempt to alleviate this by windows or photographs or special sound and lighting techniques.

These features are not necessarily in the conscious conceptual framework of either the patient or the therapist during psychotherapy. But the setting does communicate to both of them aspects of the relationship that are both overt, such as the need for secrecy—described as the protection of confidentiality— and covert, such as the effect of the patient's supine position.

Another feature of the couch is its use in intensive "one to one" psychotherapy. Thus the Freudian therapeutic goal is to analyze the transference. The dynamics and material of such a therapeutic focus are consistent with an enclosure where human beings are placed in intimate proximity.

Freudian contributions to our understanding of such interpersonal dynamics have become an established part of our conceptualizations in both the culture at large and the broader reaches of psychotherapy. Insights into human behavior gained by the techniques of the couch and free association are assumed to be valid, and transference and countertransference, unconscious factors apparent in interpersonal dynamics, are considered observable dimensions of human behavior.

## THE CHAIR IN PSYCHOTHERAPY

As a tool, the chair is similar to the couch in many respects. It is indoors, passive, and implicitly constrictive of movement. Therapists generally do not object if their patients wiggle about or occasionally get up and move about the room, but the expectation is that therapy will be carried on in a virtually sedentary fashion.

Much has been written about the differences in dynamics when the chair is substituted for the couch. The patient's ability to see the therapist's face provides a whole new dimension. The therapist's ability to maintain a neutral posture is lessened, since the patient is able to discern minute expressions, usually nonverbal. Many therapists solve the issue by having both chair and couch in their offices.

## RUNNING IN PSYCHOTHERAPY

The setting is outdoors, mobile, and expressly nonrestrictive of physical movement. Both patient and therapist are on their feet. The internal—physiological—state of the patient is mobilized with the movement of large muscle groups, and the cardiovascular, endocrinological, and neurophysiological states are also activated by the aerobic running. The literature is replete with studies of the effects of running upon the total organism. There are documented changes in perception—in hearing, for example—and in other parameters such as lipid distribution in circulating blood, endorphins, and rapidity of neuronal transmissions (Riggs 1981).

These data form the physiological baseline for the tool of running as used in psychotherapy (Baekeland 1970). Most techniques of psychotherapy are designed to alleviate pain—whatever the cause. If the ''cause'' is thought to be in the sociocultural or interpersonal realm, the search for that cause usually ''uncovers'' conditions that were, or are, painful. The physiological response to a noxious event, in all forms of mobile life, is flight or fight. Only if a mobile creature is trapped does it attempt to adapt to the noxious stimulus.

When therapy discovers a noxious stimulus, the appropriate physiological responses to flee or fight will occur as the endocrine, neurological, and musculo-skeletal systems are activated. When running is employed, large muscle groups appropriately discharge the fight/flight stimulus in a physiologically beneficial manner.

## Running Therapy

Certain features are peculiar to running as a therapeutic technique, but the fundamental principles of therapy are maintained.

Masserman (1955) felt that the therapeutic process could be understood by the "Ur delusions"—the notion that each individual carries three belief systems that allay fear and anxiety. These are the belief that the individual organic unit—the biological machine of each person—is inviolate and will function to serve our needs forever; the belief that our interpersonal rela-tionships will last and secure comfort and support for us; and a transcendent belief that our individual existence has a purpose beyond the sphere of our own influence. We depend on the body, others, and God.

Analyzing the effects of running upon my patients, I have found that running can both support and challenge those inner beliefs (Kostrubala 1981). For example, improvement in the physical workings and appearance of the body is very important to my patients. Running therapy is body-oriented. The cardio-vascular aspect directs the patient's and the therapist's attention to the workings of the body in a manner that helps them understand the patient's inner function-ing. The further emphasis on locomotion focuses attention on feet, legs, breathing, and other physical features. This attention to the body, with the virtual guarantee of physical improvement, is the foundation of this form of therapy. The focus upon the body is continuous; the improvement is visible and measurable; and the technique has tangible effects.

Thus the physiological aspect does focus upon that first delusion—that one's body will go on and function well and improve. Of course this is not always true, and patients who use this technique do suffer injuries, breakdowns, and terminal illnesses. When the patient's body is functioning well and improving, the anxiety level is low, but an injury can exacerbate the underlying pathologi-cal state.

Because this form of therapy focuses upon the body, the running therapist needs continual updating of information on diet, vitamins, liniments, shoes, foot and leg problems, electrolyte replacement fluids, injuries of all sorts, training schedules, and a wide array of other "body" situations that become daily business (Kostrubala 1978).

In the interpersonal realm running therapy also includes transference and countertransference. Since in this modality it is impossible and unnecessary to maintain the notion of the therapist as a blank screen, the dynamics of transference and countertransference are altered. In most instances the process appears to be accelerated when the therapist is physically visible.

Striated muscle is the major medium of communication available to the brain, and movement is the most overt aspect of interpersonal communication. In this form of therapy, however, the less voluntary systems such as breathing and heart rate play an equal role in interpersonal dynamics. The action of the autonomic system is highly visible in some patients as flushing, sweating, piloerection, salivation, and so forth. Metabolic states can often be detected by odor. Bits of personal history may emerge in the smell of foods such as garlic, cigarette smoke, or the breakdown products of alcohol and other drugs. Patients in ketosis, as when depleted for a marathon, also can be identified by smell.

It has been my experience that it is critical to maintain an open attitude in the therapy session. This has been a major problem in training running therapists. The nature of the process encourages expression of whatever lies within, and the therapist is as subject to that process as is the patient. After nine years of employing this technique in group and individual therapy, I find that therapy sessions are regularly ninety minutes long and are conducted totally outdoors. There is no need to sit down and talk indoors unless the weather dictates it. Indoors, I recommend using an indoor track, or any area where therapy can proceed while patient and therapist walk/jog/run.

As in Freudian dynamics, analysis of the transference begins immediately. However, since transference and countertransference never end, they are considered givens in the therapy situation, and the patient's stated goals are continually addressed as the direction therapy will take.

In my years of using running as a tool of psychotherapy, I have also noted the apparently spontaneous appearance of transcendent belief systems. The urge to express a belief that is manifestly "transcendent" can emerge in formal religious practice or the inner belief in God, or in a heightened sense of social responsibility that leads to altruistic behavior. This last of the Ur delusions often means therapy is nearly completed.

## Physiological Stages in a Therapy Session

A "typical" therapy session is accompanied by physiological "stages" that the running therapist can make use of. We can distinguish four stages (Andrews 1978).

## Stage 1

The first twenty minutes constitute stage 1. Dysphoria is most common in this stage, and the patient may express this by overt resistance to movement, by depression, by anger, by crying—or by all of these. The therapist should keep the patient moving. I have found it best to walk at the very beginning, then slowly begin to jog. I do not usually do stretching exercises as part of the therapy session; I expect the patients to do these on their own. During this "warmup" period we may simply talk about the weather or such. After fifteen to twenty minutes of slow jogging or fast walking the dysphoria begins to lessen. Often the most difficult work for the therapist occurs in stage 1, but gentle encouragement and the knowledge that in most cases this dysphoria will lessen at thirty minutes makes it easier. The techniques used to get through this period will reflect the therapist's personality. I prefer the slow warmup and the willingness to walk at any time, with the eventual goal of target-rate walk/jog/run.

## Stage 2

Stage 2 occurs at thirty to fifty minutes. Patients often talk a great deal and think more rapidly, and many experience euphoria. They may sprint, and laughter is common. The most apparent change is usually the marked increase in verbalization. During this period the therapist can obtain much historical material. Often the patient's talk appears driven or pushed, as in amphetamine states. This stage is the one referred to in the lay literature as the "runner's high." (See Sachs, chap. 15, for more on this.) During this stage insight is virtually nil.

## Stage 3

This stage lasts from fifty minutes to ninety minutes. Often the patient experiences feelings akin to those associated with opiates or hallucinogens (Kostrubala 1976). Here the effect of the run, producing changes in the brain itself, can be used to great advantage. It is the stage of gold. Patient and therapist are together in a state that at times resembles a shared dream. Deep affect states are often mobilized, anhedonia is relieved, and depression is virtually impossible for patient or therapist. Insight and other forms of comprehension become available to the therapeutic process.

There are varying degrees of this stage. When it is fully "on" it is as if the limbic brain is mobilized, and the therapist may notice that the subject matter of therapy is devoted to the patient's perception of fight, flight, food, and sex. The therapist should be alert for the spontaneous discussion of one of these, which often leads to the exploration of psychodynamics.

### Stage 4

The therapy session ends at ninety minutes or more and the run ceases. The therapist now can select from the material presented certain concepts, features, insights, and suggestions to emphasize and support. Often the therapist's comments may appear droll—such as suggesting that the patient can expect to feel this way again—without depression, or anhedonia, cheerful and alert— by simply going out for a run and recalling the material discussed and explored.

Early in therapy it is difficult to expect patients to do this on their own, since the resistance of stage 1 often is too strong; it is of major importance that the therapist assist the patient in maintaining the three-times-a-week training pattern. This initial period is usually six weeks, with some major variations dependent upon factors such as age, genetic background, and cultural and social influences. The usual pattern is a formal therapy session once a week. I make it a practice to suggest that patients participate in social runs such as the San Diego Marathon Clinic and in informal group or family runs.

The mutual sharing of inner life is reflected in the openness of the therapist's family life, if the patient wishes it. The model most closely allied to this aspect is the stereotype of the general practitioner in an American small town early in this century. Doctor and patients mingled socially as friends. In the way I conduct running therapy, a patient is considered in this light. This pattern has changed for a variety of reasons: for example, late-twentieth-century urban lifestyle, persistence of the notion that psychotherapy is a covert process, and the stigma attached to various mental states such as schizophrenia.

### Summary of Therapy

Running therapy is basically physical and thus, represents a major departure from the established concepts of traditional couch/chair psychotherapies. I have met mental health professionals who feel that running therapy is not, and never can be, a form of psychotherapy. Coaches may feel it is not an adequate form of physical therapy. Perhaps it is at some stage in between.

Using running as a tool of psychotherapy makes the therapist a kind of psychopharmacologist, able to induce changes in the patient's neurochemical apparatus. The difference is in how those changes are wrought: by physical activity or by an introduced substance. Indeed, the therapist may also prescribe medications.

The running therapist is someplace on a scale where the coach is at one end and the sedentary psychotherapist at the other. Coaches certainly have long recognized the psychotherapeutic effects of exercise as they have intuitively applied their skills as lay psychotherapists. They deal with human behavior, whether it means finding an effective way to stop fumbling or altering a depressive pattern.

The sedentary psychotherapist, who may be philosophically polarized by the jock/intellectual dichotomy, has something to offer as well. Either applying the many successful techniques of psychotherapy within the framework of running therapy as described above will enhance their effectiveness, or the therapist will be forced to abandon some cherished professional beliefs. Conventional therapists need not be threatened by the use of running as a tool in psychotherapy, for if the premise I offer is correct, virtually any belief system will do as long as it reflects common sense.

Just as psychotherapists of differing cultures, with differing concepts of the basic condition of man's psyche, use the couch and the chair, so too the use of running should transcend cultural, philosophic, and language differences. Human culture reached its hunter-gatherer peak ten thousand years ago. Agriculture, then urbanization, changed the conditions imposed upon the species, in most instances catastrophically. When I use running as a tool in psychotherapy, I am struck by the rapid appearance of "new behaviors" in some patients. This basic biological form of locomotion may resonate with dormant cerebral responses established over four million years and now "reawakened" by this technique. The aerobic effect of running should also be evident in children and research animals.

Shipman (see chap. 8) has noted significant changes in the children in his running program, including reduction in their need for medication and in their aggressive behavior. Pysh and Weiss (1979), in their experiments with laboratory rats in three groups—sedentary, control, and exercised—have shown that the exercised rats have changes in myelinization of peripheral nerves. More startling is their finding of increased dendritic proliferation of the Purkinje cells in the cerebellum, which shows organic change in nerve tissue in the brain itself.

T. Bassler (personal communication) has been in the forefront of the pathologists who feel that the lifestyle of the marathoner, coupled with a proper nutritional base (e.g., adequate vitamin C and plenty of fluids, including beer) will physiologically alter the microscopic features of cardiovascular tissue. The high-density lipoprotein/low-density lipoprotein findings support the theory that runners are profoundly altering their inner environment. We should expect those same changes in the rest of the runner's body—especially the brain.

Jokl (1977) has persistently proposed that sports—by which he means gymnastics and other Olympic sports—are a clue or model for a profound understanding of human behavior. In Jokl's perspective, sport and art intermingle and become indistinguishable.

Greist and his colleagues (Greist et al. 1978; see also chap. 3) have published studies on running therapy with depressed patients. The problem with all such studies is the effect of the therapist. Though a running therapist may be called for in a treatment protocol, there is as yet no agreement on exact qualifications. Most running therapists that I have certified are physicians—and marathoners. Several are psychologists. All are requested to consider themselves certified only if they complete two marathons a year as the minimum physical requirement (Kostrubala 1978). Yet even that baseline is not a sufficient indicator of the effectiveness of a running therapist. Many techniques of diagnosis and therapy are taken directly from traditional medical disciplines.

For example, one of the most active "tools" of the running therapist is the patient's nonverbal communication. As one works with a patient, that person's particular postures, small muscle movements, and running style will all translate into a gestalt. The subtle signs of anhedonia, depression, anxiety, anger, withdrawal, mania, catatonia, and other states not yet collected within a syndrome complex become glaringly evident to the trained running therapist. I have found that such subtle nonverbal cues are exceedingly important to those dealing with the severely mentally ill in large institutions. The same nonverbal signs and postures occur in running therapy. The same processes operate here as in other situations, but they begin to be expressed during the run.

## Case Reports

Let me describe some cases in which I have used running therapy.

### Case 1

G. A. is a twenty-four-year-old white female who had been in running therapy for four months. Her initial complaint was discomfort in social situations, a generalized perception of being withdrawn and isolated, episodes of immobile, fixed gaze at irrelevant objects, and anhedonia. She lost spontaneity and seldom spoke. She often stood in one position for long periods. Her expression was generally flat, and little small muscle movement was visible in her face. Her upper torso also appeared rigid.

As therapy progressed, often in stage 3, I would coach her on her style, focusing especially on the shoulders. She would respond, and her style would become much easier. It is clear after many such episodes that she can obtain relief from her symptoms, even during an exacerbation of her problems, by running and at the same time consciously loosening her shoulders. She is now aware that holding her shoulder girdle rigid is directly connected to her fear of being beaten by her father. Both parents are emotionally disturbed, with periods of depression, anger, multiple illnesses, alcohol abuse, and repeated double-bind interactions with each other and their children.

This patient can also bring her immobile faces into consciousness, and with the help of the therapist and other patients during stages 3 and 4 she can mobilize those small muscle structures. When this happens the interlocking behaviors that make up the symptom complex are loosened, and she experiences a generalized sense of well-being. She begins to talk readily and openly, and her body movements are less stilted. This patient is currently in therapy and has shown moderate improvement.

### Case 2

I was called in the summer of 1981 by B. B. J., a thirty-year-old white female from New York seeking help for depression. She said she had been overtly depressed for more than a year. The depression was triggered by her husband's imprisonment and her subsequent loss of her home, her income, and her community standing. She sought psychiatric aid and found a psychotherapist she liked and trusted. He prescribed antidepressive medication and had her evaluated, but she did not improve and so he recommended electroconvulsive treatment. Her husband suggested she call me.

After many telephone calls, in which the patient fully communicated her distress, she made arrangements to come to Encinitas, California, for two weeks. Before she flew to the West Coast I had telephone conversations with the major parties on the East Coast: friends, physicians, husband.

When she arrived she was frightened, demonstrated massive dependence, was highly anxious, tremulous, and cried often. She was housed by the minister of a local church and his wife.

She was five feet two inches tall and was thin. She had not "run" before, and it soon became clear that her depression was based in a family environment that had culminated in her father's suicide. She had two children, ages three and one, each staying with a different relative. The patient had been unable to care for them, since she herself was being cared for by an apparently resentful mother-in-law.

I saw the patient twice a day in morning and afternoon sessions on the beach in Encinitas. The first morning out I walked, jogged, and ran with her for nine miles. During that session crying, depression, dependency, and other features of her history appeared. Most significantly, for one brief period—after ninety minutes of therapy in that first session—she experienced relief from her depression. This did not last long, and she immediately regressed, with a continual outpouring of depressive symptoms: anger, crying, pleas for assurance and comfort, and avowed inability to function. The vivid story of the unfortunate events leading to her husband's imprisonment was tragic—it was riches to rags, honor to dishonor, social approval to opprobrium.

The afternoon session was again devoted to therapy, but we used the ocean and boogie-boarding as a way to continue the activity without further strain on the running muscles. Her behavior was much the same. It required the efforts of myself and another therapist to get her to run and to enter and stay in the ocean.

On the third day, after the long morning run, she was depression free. Her affect had changed, and she began to make plans to reassemble her life. She left on the sixth day, depression free.

She returned to New York and immediately resumed caring for her two children. She continued to run, and six months later she was still running and free of depression. She is not in psychotherapy and not on medication.

Depression often self-remits. Thus this may have just been a spontaneous remission that was on the way. The next criticism would be the value of the running as a therapeutic tool as opposed to the effect of such an intensive psychotherapeutic encounter. It is possible that the same result would have occurred had we sat in the office for comparable periods of time. In a single case study there is no way to calculate the influence of these factors.

## Conclusion

The biological function of depression appears to be related to healing processes. Severely injured animals may appear profoundly depressed while recovering. They move as little as possible and consume minimal food and water. Thus severe injury may be the causative agent leading to depression. In a profoundly social animal such as man that severe injury can be an interpersonal loss. Loss of love object, infantile miasma, and the vulnerability of primates to loss of mothering in infancy would be considered the correlates of severe physical injury. (See also Little 1969; and Sachs and Pargman, chap. 13, on running addiction.)

I began using running as a therapeutic tool with little expectation of anything unusual. I decided to investigate this technique because of my perception that the initial group of patients were victims of nature or nurture or both. Their future was grim. Some had been institutionalized several times, and all had gentic histories of aberrant behavior in parents and grandparents. Many had childhood experiences that were explicitly traumatic, such as sexual assault. My own diagnoses were often confirmed by other mental health professionals, psychiatrists, psychologists, psychiatric nurses, psychiatric social workers, referring internists, family, and friends. All the patients were on medication when group therapy began, and all were responding to medication in an expected manner. The drugs I used were Elavil, Stelazine, Thorazine, and Valium. I did not then use large doses of medication but tried to manage potential exacerbations with temporary increases of medication, extra psychotherapy, and hospitalization as a last resort.

I had had experience with group psychotherapy (McGee and Kostrubala 1964), and the first breakthrough was an alteration of the expected pattern. I did not have high therapeutic hopes for the effect of a group process upon this particular group of patients. All were in individual therapy before joining the group. Had they been selected as patients who might benefit from a group I would have expected more.

The changes I observed in that group have been confirmed by subsequent patients of mine and by patients who have treated themselves using running as the therapeutic tool. The range of diagonostic categories include schizophrenia, depression, organic brain syndrome, alcoholism, anxiety states, and acute depression following severe interpersonal loss. Running has even helped alleviate the effects of imprisonment.

Since March 1973 I have gradually modified my use of running. I have found that the office is no longer necessary; I conduct the entire therapeutic process outdoors. This, I am sure, self-selects certain patients. I conduct evaluations the same way; all are expected to dress for walking on the beach. Sessions last ninety minutes, and at times I cover about fifteen miles a day. In most sessions we jog at a slow pace; some patients only walk; a few run hard, and many of these become faster runners than I am. Completing a marathon is a significant therapeutic event, and I often run marathons with my patients. Most often we finish separately.

The effect of the tool of running is still being determined. There are patients who find any form of activity, even walking, a threat. Some patients will never exert themselves beyond walking; they do not seem to do much better than in sedentary therapy. There are patients who show full remittance of a disease process but stop running when symptoms reappear. Other patients stop running after therapy, yet their symptoms do not reappear.

I have attempted to examine running as a tool of therapy. It is, after all, only a tool—the basic processes of therapy remain intact. If we think of psychotherapy as being like gardening, then the psychotherapist is the gardener. And gardeners use many tools: mechanical, chemical, heuristic, and at times spiritual. Running is a new psychotherapeutic tool that may change both the garden and the gardener.

## References

Andrews, V. 1978. *The psychic power of running.* New York: Rawson Associates.

Baekeland, F. 1970. Exercise deprivation: Sleep and psychological reactions. *Archives of General Psychiatry* 22:365–69.

Greist, J. H.; Klein, M. H.; Eischens, R. R.; Faris, J.; Gurman, A. S.; and Morgan, W. P. 1978. Running through your mind. *Journal of Psychosomatic Research* 22:259–94.

Johanson, D., and Edey, M. 1981. *Lucy, the beginnings of mankind.* New York: Simon and Schuster.

Jokl, E. 1977. Running, psychology, and culture. *Annals of the New York Academy of Sciences* 301:970–1001.

Kostrubala, T. 1976. *The joy of running.* Philadelphia: J. B. Lippincott.

———. 1978. The training of a running therapist. *Medicine and Sport* 12:111–15.

———. 1981. Running: The grand delusion. In *Psychology of running,* ed. M. H. Sacks and M. L. Sachs. Champaign, Ill.: Human Kinetics Publishers.

Little, J. C. 1969. The athlete's neurosis: A deprivation crisis. *Acta Psychiatrica Scandinavica* 45:187–97.

Lorenz, K. 1977. *Behind the mirror.* New York: Harcourt, Brace, Jovanovich.

Masserman, J. 1955. *The practice of dynamic psychiatry.* Philadelphia: Saunders.

McGee, T., and Kostrubala, T. 1964. Neurotic equilibrium in married couples applying for group psychotherapy. *Journal of Marriage and Family Living,* 78–82.

Pysh, J., and Weiss, G. M. 1979. Exercise during development induces an increase in Purkinje cell dendritic tree size. *Science* 206 (4415):230–32.

Riggs, C. E., Jr. 1981. Endorphins, neurotransmitters and/or neuromodulators and exercise. In *Psychology of running,* ed. M. H. Sacks and M. L. Sachs. Champaign, Ill.: Human Kinetics Publishers.

# 8

# Emotional and Behavioral Effects of Long-Distance Running on Children

The thoughts were not new to me; they were simply playing with each other and inventing a new game. Their game opened a door to allow an idea to emerge—I would find out what effects slow long-distance running might have on the behavior and emotions of emotionally disturbed children. During my four years of running I had become aware of many of its effects upon myself and upon my running friends and colleagues, and I had become familiar with the literature on the subject. But my unique opportunity to study children and running had never occurred to me before, at least not so clearly as it did on that summer dawn in 1980 on the beach in Encinitas, California. I was into the second hour of running with a friend, Craig Silberman. The caption of a poster that had impressed me years before flashed into focus: "Children see what we can only look at, and feel what we can only touch." The picture above the words showed an infant sitting at the water's edge, mesmerized by a fistful of wet sand. "How do we lose it?" I thought. "What happens to adults that renders them less sensitive to everything?

I focused for a while on how I, as a psychiatrist, had at first doubted claims about the emotional and behavioral effects of running. Now, after five years and ten thousand miles of recreational running, I was deeply impressed with the emotional, sensory, behavioral, and mental changes I had seen in myself and in my running friends. There is an increased sensory awareness from running that appears to be connected with tranquillity and lack of fear. This is different from the tranquillity that comes from a *decrease* in sensory awareness—a disturbing aspect of much human functioning. This increased sensory awareness, along with other changes, may differ in quality and in time of onset between age groups.

A seventy-one-year-old woman who has been running thirty miles or more a week for four years recently talked to me after one of her ten-kilometer competitons. She said she now has difficulty identifying herself as the same person she was before she started running. When I asked what was the single most significant emotional or mental change she had observed in herself, she said, "problem solving. After I am twenty to thirty minutes into my daily run, answers to problems I have been pondering seem to appear from nowhere. What had been difficult now becomes obvious and clear."

I present this particular case because of the time factor of twenty to thirty minutes—a shorter time span than would be associated with this type of mentation change in young or middle-aged adults, who undergo similar experiences at forty-five minutes to an hour. Other older runners seem to concur with the experiences of this woman. I am of course curious about what, if any, time-related change differences will be observed as we learn more about the effects of running on the emotions and mentation of children. There could well be significant time-related changes coincidental with stages of central nervous system development.

It is also possible that regular sustained running (with children, even within weeks) has an effect upon glandular functions and the efferent as well as sensory and integrative components of the human nervous system. Perhaps sustained firing of the muscle-contracting component affects our glandular and sensory integrative and perceptual functioning.

With these thoughts and questions in mind, my friend and I were "fired up" to design and conduct a running study with children. Craig Silberman, as a special education teacher in the local school system and a recreational runner with several years' experience, volunteered to act as project coordinator. We had self-observations and reports from others attesting to heightened sensory awareness (Could it be that a great deal of slow long-distance running would affect the sensory, motor, perceptual, and integrative functions of the learning-disabled child?), ease of creative problem solving while running, reduced depression, increased rate of associative thoughts, and reduced frequency of aggressive acting out. We certainly could not investigate more than a few of these areas, so we went to the literature to see what our predecessors and contemporaries had found.

## Research Literature

Solomon and Bumpus (1978) reported that for some hyperactive children with minimal brain damage running seemed to provide ego enhancement and support. Their conjecture was that "running reduces the general stress syndrome, allows them [the children] to work off excess energy, and sublimates dependent, sexual and aggressive energy" (p. 590). Johnson, Fretz, and Johnson (1968) reported improved self-concept in seventy-four disturbed children in a six-week physical development program. More specifically, they described improvements in social adjustment, schoolwork, finger skills, speech, and functional intelligence, as well as greater response to psychotherapy. John Greist's survey article (Greist, et al. 1978), concludes regarding children's running, "In a number of uncontrolled studies, children seem to respond to improved neuromuscular control and fitness with generalized improvement in many intellectual and psychological spheres" (p. 263). The literature, though sparse, was definitely encouraging.

## Children

If I were to select one quality in children that has special value, it would be optimism. In observing understimulated, neglected, and emotionally abused children, I have been amazed by their persistent optimism in the face of contrary reality. To me this reflects an underlying growth potential that augments their chances for a better future. In addition, their drive toward maturation raises the self-esteem of those who work with them, since doing even a little bit right pays off heavily. Giving children opportunities for expression is casting seed on extremely fertile soil.

Joseph Pearce (1977), speaking of the experientially inhibited child who has been prevented by lack of stimulation from making use of this enormous optimistic potential for growth and creativity, says: "A shallow dimensional world view based only on the long-range senses of sight and sound is often the kind of knowledge constructed by the child. Direct physical contact with the world—taste, touch, even smell—[is] often even discouraged or actually forbidden in the parents' anxiety over the hazards of germs and imagined threats. Without a full dimensional world view structured in the formative years, no earth matrix can form. No knowledge of physical survival can develop and no basis for abstraction and creativity can arise."

In the terms of economics, I often see adults mired and having great difficulty in living above the "break-even point." Their emotional overhead is so high that they constantly experience diminished returns from their investments and are left with a negative emotional "cash flow." Given even minimal opportunity, children avoid this type of morass. They possess enormous creative energy to invest in whatever activity or interest we adults come up with next.

Running is a "natural" as such an activity. I suspect it promotes the creative mode of operation and fuels the already smoldering fire of optimism and satisfying creative energy available to the child. Imagine running as having the potential to lift anyone (perhaps most easily a child) out of the closed and muddy view from the trenches into the comprehensive and stimulating perspective of the air.

## More "Evidence"

Anecdotal information on children's running was abundant, essentially reports that children who participated in organized sustained running for more than half an hour at a time showed reduced hyperactivity, improved internal control, increased acceptance and support within their families, and enhanced self-esteem.

Pete Saccone, an avid local runner in San Diego and a fifth-grade teacher, has encouraged running among his pupils. He recently reported that twenty-seven of them were running in organized races. He strongly believes that they are all happier and healthier because of their involvement in running. He has seen low achievers become much less of a problem in the classroom. Absenteeism is markedly reduced among these running students, and he is enthusiastic about the "fringe benefits," such as their sense of accomplishment, their improved peer relation, and the positive identification with the group's running activities by children and parents alike.

It was schoolteachers who first let us know we had hit on something meaningful in our own running study. In my years as medical director at the San Diego Center for Children, I have seen many projects and activities undertaken. Enrichment programs and specialty therapeutic approaches were open for voluntary staff support and input. These programs could generally be classified as either classroom-generated or residential-care-generated, with interest and support remaining fairly exclusive to the area of genesis. That is, the schoolteachers tended to support projects emanating either from their own ingenuity within the classroom or through the Board of Education. Likewise, the counselors and other treatment personnel tended to support projects arising from their own therapeutic network and literature.

Shortly after we began training sessions for the children and staff who were to participate in the running study, the schoolteachers became enthusiastically involved. Since this program had been developed through the treatment staff at the Center rather than the school, I felt this was a clear message that the running was bearing fruit within the classroom—the students were probably becoming more manageable, motivated, and responsive there.

When I questioned the teachers regarding my hunches, they supplied abundant anecdotal support for this idea and continued to sustain energy and interest throughout the study and beyond. The reports usually indicated that disruptive activity diminished among the children who were running, particularly those who had been receiving psychostimulants as behavioral modifiers. "It is as though he (or she) had received extra medication on those days after running." The running students were seen as less distractible and as exhibiting a longer attention span, particularly for two to four hours after the running session itself.

## Case Histories

### Case 1

The patient was eleven years old when he became involved in the running study group. He had come to the Center with a diagnosis of severe anxiety neurosis approximately four months earlier. He had a lifelong history of being difficult to manage and was often out of control at home and at school. He was described as having cried "constantly" as an infant, and he slept only about four hours out of twenty-four until he was five years old. He had always been excessively active and was a "crib rocker." Throughout school reports he was described as possessing an extremely poor self-image and as being very impulsive, with marked difficulty in controlling anger. He distorted reality to avoid failing. He was wary of his environment and viewed the world as violent and explosive. Ritalin had been tried for "hyperactivity" but was discontinued because it was overly sedative, making him "like a zombie."

In terms of positive qualities, he was described as having a good memory and as being observant and imaginative. His social history pointed to a tendency to withdraw when anxious, avoiding peer confrontation and involvement. This boy was in treatment at the Center for nine months and was involved actively in the running program during the last four months of this period. He was not given psychotropic medications at any time during his treatment at the Center.

Comments from his running group leader include the following: When the patient first started running, he had extremely low self-esteem, even when given great encouragement by his peers—until one day when he covered a complete mile. Then he became motivated and went through a period of pushing himself until he developed "stitch" pains. Once past the "stitch" pains, his resistance to running seemed to disappear. He ran four times a week, at least forty minutes at each session, and became enthusiastic about running. Whereas he had been seen as a "loner," afterward he was described as being "outward." He made more friends and was better accepted by his peers. There was an enormous improvement in self-esteem, and he became active in leadership. His mother was greatly encouraged by his physical performance and the changes in his personality. Since his discharge from the program, he has voluntarily telephoned the running group leader several times to report his progress and to share memories about the group.

## Case 2

The patient was an eleven-year-old boy who was enrolled in the day treatment program at the Center for a total of eleven months and was in the running program for three months. He carried diagnoses of oppositional personality and minimal cerebral dysfunction. Admitting symptoms included impulsivity, oppositional behavior, aggressiveness when he was angry, lying, poor peer relations, and an antagonistic attitude toward his sibling. He had been taking Ritalin by prescription, ten milligrams twice a day, for about one year before his admission. He remained off medication throughout his treatment at the Center. When Ritalin had been discontinued previously his behavior had deteriorated, with an increase in aggressive acting out, leading to his removal from a gifted program in public school.

Notes from the running log include the following description and progress notes: The patient complained of "asthma" early in his running. He ran slower than the rest of the group and maintained his identity as a "loner." Gradually he began to push himself to keep up with the group. His complaints about wheezing and "allergies" decreased. Eventually he was able to keep up and even became a group leader. By this time all his physical complaints had disappeared. He became less cocky. Being in the company of the other children seemed to become more important to him than "being the best." His relations with his peers in the group improved greatly. Running seemed to become a strong "plus" for him.

## Case 3

This boy was eight years old when he was admitted to the residential program. He was transferred from a psychiatric hospital, where he had been in intensive treatment for three months with a diagnosis of undersocialized conduct disorder, aggressive type. He was described as an impulsive, distractible, and immature child who displayed regression of cognitive functioning secondary to stress. Earlier psychological testing reported that he had difficulty integrating both visual percepts and verbal information. He was particularly preoccupied with issues of control. Various psychotropic medications had been tried. His medication regimen at the time of his transfer to the Center was Ritalin, twenty-five milligrams twice a day, and mellaril, twenty milligrams a day. He remained in residential treatment about one year. He was regularly engaged in an active running program for the last ten months of that time. The mellaril was discontinued after one month of running; the Ritalin was continued throughout his treatment. Early on, he was seen as having "excellent slow running ability." After three months he was described as having marked success in the running program (including successfully completing a ten-kilometer race with his treatment coordinator). "Running has a calming effect on him, uses up his excess energy, improves his self-image, and provokes admiration from his peers, parents, and staff."

Comments from this boy's treatment coordinator regarding the running give additional information. During and after the running study the patient was running at least forty-five minutes four times a week. He was described as a "quiet back runner in the beginning who stuck with it." Eventually he was able to keep up with children four to five years older. He became markedly calmer, both in cottage life and in school. His self-confidence grew remarkably. His physical complaints decreased, as did his soiling. Peers who had avoided and "scapegoated" him early in his stay at the Center began to admire his running prowess. His parents became extremely accepting and supportive of his running. He was described as having "regressed in all areas of behavior" when his running decreased upon completion of the formal running study.

## Case 4

This was an eleven-year-old boy who had been a patient in several programs within the Residential Treatment Center over a two-year period. He was first admitted to the Day Treatment Program, then transferred to Residential Treatment owing to clinical regression, and finally transferred to a community group home as his clinical status improved. Problem behaviors persisted, with frequent explosive angry outbursts toward peers and staff. Community contact had been restricted because of physical attacks on neighborhood children. He soiled an average of twice a day. He was frequently suspended from school for defiance. At the time the running study began, this boy was on a waiting list for transfer to another residential facility that was to treat him during his growth into adolescence. His diagnosis had been (1) neurotic tension discharge disorder with acting out of conflict and anxiety and (2) special symptom formation (developmental deviation), manifested by uneven academic, integrative, and social development.

His initial reaction to the running program was resistance. He complained, was disruptive, and tired easily. He gradually became more confident in his running. He asked to run at additional times and was soon running three to four miles four times a week. His progress was gradual, but he remained committed to his running and completed his first ten-kilometer competition after two months in the program.

Daily records reflected dramatic changes in his behavior. Peer relations were improving. He began to verbalize anger and was less explosive; his school reports improved; and the encopresis decreased to three to four times a week. After two and a half months of running the patient fractured his toe and was told he could not run for five to six weeks. Within one week the staff observed regression in many areas. A call from the school counselor established that regression had also occurred at school. (The counselor was not aware of the running program.)

Once the injury had healed and he was able to return to running, he resumed positive gains, and he is to be discharged to his home rather than to another institution, as was planned before his running.

*Case 5*

This was an eleven-year-old boy who was admitted to Residential Care with a diagnosis of overanxious disorder of childhood. His medication upon admission was Ritalin, thirty milligrams twice a day. Preadmission behaviors included lying, stealing, destruction of property, rages, and poor relations with other children. He was described as being "counterphobic—meaning that beneath his tough aggressive exterior he is anxious and very fearful."

This boy entered the running study immediately upon admission. After two months of running his medication was reduced to ten milligrams of Ritalin twice a day and was discontinued completely four months into his treatment. He was seen as having a natural ability for running. The record noted that his self-image improved as he continued to run and began to participate in organized races. His acting out decreased. He began teasing other children less and was less argumentive with authority figures. He was able to maintain these improvements and interests without psychotropic medication.

## The Running Study

The original design of the study included a running group and a control group, with the running group participating in slow long-distance running for forty-five minutes four times a week for twelve weeks. This design was modified during the six-week training period before the study began, and we dispensed with the control group. We intended that study participation be enjoyable for the children and not compromise any aspect of their regular programs. We wanted the participation to be voluntary, not restricted in terms of running versus control-group activity. The children who wanted to run did so, and those who did not develop enthusiasm for running were not required to take part.

After eighteen weeks (six weeks of training followed by twelve weeks of the running study), a total of fifty-six children between the ages of six and thirteen were participating in the study. The amount they ran during the study was recorded by the running group leaders. The running groups averaged eight children, with two adult staff members as leaders. Following the six-week training period for staff and children, the groups were encouraged to run a maximum of forty-five minutes, four times a week, for twelve weeks. At the termination of the study, change scores on the tests involved were plotted against total running time. All the participants had been tested before and after the twelve-week study period. Tests involved various measures of sensorimotor perception, integration, and function as well as the standardized behavioral rating scale.

Statistically the changes correlated to some degree with the total running time, suggesting a trend in only three areas of change. Two were related to visual memory and one was classified as auditory memory for unrelated words. The objective findings did not match the enthusiasm and anecdotal information received from staff members during the study. We were puzzled.

Then we retrospectively reviewed the children's clinical records, paying particular attention to medication changes. Participation in the study was found to be significantly related to reduction in psychotropic medication, particularly the psychostimulant treatment of over aggressive, impulse-ridden, and hyperkinetic children. The medications for these children had merely been manipulated "as usual" during the study, disregarding their running participation, since the supervising psychiatrists were not aware of any particular child's level of involvement in the running project.

Further review identified thirty-four children as having received some type of psychotropic medication during the study. When these thirty-four were divided into two groups (the seventeen who ran "more," compared with the seventeen who ran "less"), ten of the twelve children showing "significant reduction" in medication fell into the "ran more" category. The more a child ran, the less psychotropic medication was needed. Eureka![1]

There are some other aspects of the study that I feel are probably more significant than the findings described above. Staff members from different departments worked closely together during the study in an atmosphere of mutual support and cooperation that bridged the usual interdepartmental gaps. Social workers, psychologists, psychiatrists, teachers, clerical personnel, occupational therapists, recreational therapists, child development counselors—all became identified as "running study workers."

Perhaps most impressive were the numbers of instances when parents became positively identified with their children's running. We saw success stories spring out of repeated histories of pessimism, nonaccomplishment, and defeat. The runners wore their T-shirts with pride, and volunteers from the community began to surface to support the study in specialized ways. This was extremely important, because the study was not budgeted or funded within the normal operating funds of the Center, nor was grant money available to support these efforts. Local sports equipment stores contributed supplies. Local runners contributed money. Skilled volunteer services were offered by a sports podiatrist, a pediatrician, a statistician, a professional writer, a track coach, an artist, the director of the local marathon clinic, and many others.

By the time the study was completed, it was obvious that much human potential had been tapped. The running program fostered enormous growth and creativity not only among the participating children, but also among the professional staff and outside community.

## The First Annual Ten Karrot Fun Run

A celebration banquet with awards of gratitude would simply not be sufficient acknowledgment. It became obvious that the San Diego Center for Children should sponsor it's own springtime, pre-Easter "Fun Run."

The occasion was the First Annual Ten Karrot Fun Run. The location was San Diego's serene Mission Bay Park, and the time was Sunday, 5 April 1981, shortly after sunrise on a sparkling clear day. An event that had early on been projected to be a smallish affair for friends, supporters, and participants of the San Diego Center for Children emerged that April morning as a springtime "happening." In the name of supporting running and running studies for children, there occurred a tremendous rallying of community support and imagination, with a timely crescendo during the weeks before the run itself. Local businessmen and corporations donated $3,500 worth of prizes. Volunteers distributed twenty thousand flyers heralding the pleasures of the day. These included several groups of musicians along the route playing extemporaneously for the runners on bagpipes, flutes, and guitars, the Shriner clowns out in force with their calliope, seven-foot dancing rabbits and a large green dragon, brightly outfitted Mexican dancers, refreshments including oranges, yogurt and carrots, specially designed pastel "Runnin' Rabbit" T-shirts, local political figures and sports celebrities, seventeen hundred excited runners and their friends, and a starting line featuring a Volkswagen Rabbit convertible with a six-foot stuffed carrot, dangled over the trunk by an even larger stuffed rabbit, for the runners to chase.

Now such early Sunday morning goings-on may sound rather typical for runners' events, except that all this enthusiasm and cooperation came from within a children's agency whose staff and supporters had no prior interest in, or contact with, recreational running. This enthusiasm and energy developed from and focused on the running study and its effects upon the children, the treatment staff, and their families and friends.

### Conclusion

Slow long-distance running over a period of time generates changes within the runners that overflow into the surrounding community. Running programs seem to be naturally accompanied by enthusiasm, a sense of creativity, and optimism that is unique within organized groups and activities.

Success breeds success, and I see that happening all around me within the world of recreational running. Children, of course, provide an obvious nucleus for such optimism and support. They spontaneously gravitate toward "the action." It seems no wonder that once running groups of children are organized they soon expand to include parents. Running becomes a bridge for understanding between the parents and the therapeutic or educational institution. Parents who may be difficult to corral for sessions within an office can easily find the time for running activites. The changes that occur within the children through running are the foundation for productive sharing between the parents and the institution's staff.

What underlies the changes in adults as well as children who run depends upon the perspective from which the researcher or philosopher is viewing the change. Psychoanalysts speak of ego strength, self-esteem, and sense of mastery. Neurochemists point to possible changes in levels of endorphins and biogenic amines. Other disciplines bring in considerations like conditioning, training effect, runner's high, transcendental states, diffusion of aggressive impulses, reactivation of the runner-hunter identity, and reinforcement of the bonding to mother earth. With all the diversity of opinion on the "causes" (as is characteristic of behavioral sciences), nevertheless there seems to be growing agreement that changes do in fact occur, and that these changes are somehow self-perpetuating and "addictive."

To me the most exciting experiential data to date are the findings that psychotropic medication can be reduced in emotionally disordered children who run. I know of no sensitive clinician who is comfortable using such medications in the ongoing treatment of children. Disturbing and sometimes permanent side effects have made all of us eager for alternatives. Slow long-distance running seems to provide such an option for a significant percentage of children who would otherwise be rendered tolerable in the classroom and at home only through medication. To quote Arnold Mandell (1979, p. 458) regarding psychotropic medications, "Few of us comprehend subjectively the high pitched straitjacket of the tricyclic antidepressants, the flattened topography of fantasy following antipsychotics or Reserpine, the empty joylessness of Lithium and the agitated dysphoria and panic of depersonalization when one's self is changed chemically." The side effects of running seem far more tolerable than those of their neuropharmacologic cousins.

Running and children mix well. They always have; they always will. Here I have attempted to explore possible ways to enhance this interplay so as to promote normal maturation. As a child therapist, I have always believed that the largest single factor working in favor of successful therapy with children is their enormous drive toward growth and individuation. Any activity that adds fuel to that fire is certainly worthy of our closest scrutiny.

## Notes

In addition to the children, staff, financial contributors, volunteers, and Board of Directors of the San Diego Center for Children, I want to thank the following generous professionals for coming and playing with us: Craig Silberman, M.S., Mark Katz, Ph.D., Paul Clopten, M.S., Vince Flaherty, M.S., Jan Hintzman, M.S., Judy Sobel, M.A., Joe Ellis, D.P.M., Austin Gontang, M.A., Lan Barnes, B.A., Richard Woodaman, B.A., Zoame Shipman, Chris Shipman, M.S., and Thaddeus Kostrubala, M.D. 1. Additional work in spring 1982 also demonstrated the positive effects of slow long-distance running on children with behavioral/emotional problems. These studies were carried out at the diagnostic school for neurologically handicapped children, a California state special school in San Francisco. The school's superintendent, Dr. Charles W. Keaster, evaluated a slow long-distance running program with four residential students. The four participants all showed improvement in such areas as peer relations, communication, self-confidence, self-control, determination to succeed, and other behavioral, social, and academic areas. Psychotropic medication was successfully discontinued for two of the boys, who had been medicated for an extended period before participation in the study.

## References

Greist, J. H.; Klein, M. H.; Eischens, R. R.; Faris, J.; Gurman, A. S.; and Morgan, W. P. 1978. Running through your mind. *Journal of Psychosomatic Research* 22:259–94.

Johnson, W. R.; Fretz, B. R.; and Johnson, J. A. 1968. Changes in self-concept during a physical development program. *Research Quarterly* 39:560–65.

Mandell, A. J. 1979. On a mechanism for the mood and personality changes of adult and later life. *Journal of Nervous and Mental Diseases* 167:457–66.

Pearce, J. C. 1977. *Magical child*. New York: E. P. Dutton.

Solomon, E. G., and Bumpus, A. K. 1978. The running meditation response: An adjunct to psychotherapy. *American Journal of Psychotherapy* 32:583–92.

BONNIE G. BERGER

# 9

# Running away from Anxiety and Depression: A Female as Well as Male Race

The need for chapters that focus specifically on women runners reflects basic physiological differences between women and men as well as gender differences in child-rearing, enculturation, and role models in the United States. Despite great strides toward equal rights, the social milieu of women and of women runners in particular differs from that of men. Sport is generally a male-dominated activity that reflects male values such as strength, strategy, and winning. Women who venture into the bastion of male sport find different personal reactions, problems, and benefits than men do. This chapter deals with anxiety and depression, two psychological problems commonly expressed among women, and the use of running to treat them. The material presented here, though directed toward women, is certainly relevant to men as well, since anxiety and depression are common to both sexes.

From a practical viewpoint, running is particularly well suited for women. Many women have not had wide experience with sport and thus have not learned the complex motor skills required in such activities as tennis, swimming, and gymnastics. Since jogging requires little formal instruction, the novice can begin to reap the benefits of exercise with a minimal training period. Another advantage is that running does not require special facilities such as tennis courts, a swimming pool, expensive equipment—or even a partner—so the runner is truly free to participate at her own convenience. And the current popularity of running encourages novice exercisers. From a therapeutic point of view, running is ideally suited to female clients in need of physical activity.

PSYCHOLOGICAL BENEFITS OF RUNNING FOR WOMEN

The experimental literature indicates that running may alleviate psychological problems that are especially prevalent among women. Some possible clinical benefits of running that are particularly important for women include reduction in anxiety and depression and enhancement of self-esteem and self-knowledge.

### Anxiety

Anxiety—a foreboding about some impending disaster that may be real, imaginary, or even unknown—is a serious health hazard in the United States. Anxiety and stress-related diseases afflict women more often than men (Biaggio and Nielsen 1976; Gall 1969; Grove and Tudor 1973; Hodges and Felling 1970; Justice and McBee 1978; Maccoby and Jacklin 1974; Tennenbaum and Milgram 1978). Anxiety is characterized by high levels of activation and somatic complaints such as nausea, tiredness, and headaches. Not only is anxiety costly in terms of increased need for health care and decreased work effectiveness (Mackay and Cox 1974; Petrich and Holmes 1977), it is also a major component in personal unhappiness. A great amount of effort has been expended to define anxiety, delineate it, measure its characteristics, and devise ways of reducing it (Freud 1963; May 1977; Sarason and Spielberger 1976a, b, 1979; Spielberger and Sarason 1975, 1977, 1978).

Separating anxiety into two types, *state anxiety* (A-state) and *trait anxiety* (A-trait) (Cattell and Scheier 1958, 1961; Spielberger 1966), is particularly important in understanding the therapeutic effects of running. State anxiety is a transitory condition associated with autonomic nervous system activity and subjective experiences of apprehension. This form of anxiety is more often affected by habitual aerobic activity. Trait anxiety is a stable, relatively permanent long-range disposition toward anxiety that is hypothesized to be based on parent-child relations centering on punishment (Spielberger 1966). People who score high on A-trait tend to perceive a wide variety of situations as threatening and respond with greater elevations in A-state than those who are low in A-trait (Spielberger 1972). Trait anxiety is less likely to be alleviated by running. Thus, in any study of exercise and mood, it is crucial that a measure of *state* rather than trait anxiety be employed.

Researchers have begun to investigate the relation between anxiety and physical activity, and substantial support has been generated for the hypothesis that vigorous but not exhausting activity lowers state anxiety levels, particularly in people who are highly anxious (Graham 1981; Morgan 1979; Summers and Wolstat 1980 and chap. 5). Graham (1981), a professor of religious studies, noted in his introspective account of why runners run that some compete for better times or distances, others run for health, and a third group, to which he belongs and in whom he is most interested, run as an escape from the pressures of life. "We're the ones for whom the change into ritual clothing, the pain of running, and the shower of cleansing constitute a daily rebaptism into the newness of life" (pp. 149–50). Graham believes that running cannot alleviate the taproot anxiety of death, but that it is a scientifically approved way of extending life: "runners, however, do not so much want to gain an extension as they want to ensure mobility until death comes" (p. 153). Graham illustrated the need for the runner to *run away from anxiety* by noting the agitation many runners experience when they are prevented from running. "But for any runner, a forced lay-off from running is agony: the anxiety of helplessness insistently whispers the message of 'time-is-passing' and 'the-body-is-aging'" (p. 152). Graham's comments are particularly meaningful to women. American society conveys the dual messages that a youthful appearance is more important for women than for men (Rossi 1980) and that women are appreciated more for helplessness than for strength and competence (Kaplan and Bean 1976). Thus women may be especially attracted to running as an escape from the anxieties of aging and helplessness.

Although most experimental studies have employed male subjects, a few investigators who have included both women and men report that both have similar psychological responses to exercise (Wilson, Berger and Bird 1981; Dienstbier et al. 1981; Driscoll 1976; Morgan 1977; Tennenbaum and Milgram 1978; Young 1979). The prevalence of anxiety symptoms in female clients mandates extrapolating results based on male and mixed populations to female clients.

From a practical vantage point, running offers an ideal way for women to reduce their anxiety. The psychological effects can occur in a relatively short period, none of the side effects of drugs are present, and running and therapy together may be more effective than therapy alone (Rueter and Harris 1980). In addition, running is inexpensive and has physiologically healthful effects such as increasing cardiovascular fitness and energy levels and decreasing fat tissue. Key issues for therapists who wish to knowledgeably use exercise to reduce clients' anxiety include (1) delineating the type and amount of exercise that is most beneficial, (2) determining the effects of exercise on both sexes, and (3) developing ways to increase the effectiveness of exercise.

FREQUENCY AND STRENUOUSNESS OF EXERCISE

The strenuousness of the exercise is a major determinant of its success in reducing anxiety. The amount of exercise considered "strenuous" varies from person to person and even differs within the same person depending on how much regular exercise she has had within the previous month. (Refer to chap. 2 for information about exercise prescription.) "Strenuous exercise" is operationally defined in this chapter by three criteria, explained below, and does not reflect exhausting levels. As noted by deVries (1981), exercising to exhaustion may negate the tranquilizing effects of running.

1. *Intensity:* A moderate intensity, as indicated by *sustained heavy breathing,* is the most important requirement for developing a training effect and thus for promoting running ease.

2. *Duration:* A minimum of twenty minutes of activity is required for novices; trained women can maintain twenty to sixty minutes of continuous exertion. Although women runners may run longer than sixty minutes, few if any additional psychological benefits accrue (see chap. 2).

3. *Frequency:* At least *three sessions per week* are required to maintain the training effects of exercise (Pollock 1978; Sharkey 1979).

Not only does the level of exercise that is strenuous differ from person to person, but researchers who have investigated the effect of exercise on psychological well-being do not agree among themselves. Dienstbier et al. (1981) concluded that both "light" and marathon-distance runs significantly decreased anxiety for both women and men as measured by the Mood Adjective Check List (Nowlis and Green 1957). According to the three exercise criteria listed above, these "light" runs, approximately six miles, would constitute a "strenuous" level of exercise for many women. Six-mile runs would require at least forty minutes for most women to complete; would have to be performed at least three times a week so one could run them at the described "easy" pace; and would cause labored breathing. Thus readers must personally define strenuousness according to the three criteria of intensity, duration, and frequency when evaluating the therapeutic effectiveness of running programs reported in the literature.

Although the results of nonsignificant studies (Buffone 1980; Morgan, Roberts, and Feinerman 1971; Sime 1977) are difficult—if not impossible—to interpret, it seems that strenuous forms of exercise such as running and swimming performed at a vigorous pace are more likely to reduce anxiety than are more moderate forms such as walking (Morgan 1979). Undoubtedly some minimum level of intensity, duration, and frequency is required to evoke therapeutic effects. Results of a study comparing the effects of several types of exercise on depression probably are relevant here even though the focus was on depression rather than anxiety (Brown, Ramirez, and Taub 1978). Softball players who participated in intermittent rather than continuous physical activity were similar to the controls who did not exercise and showed no change in depression. Runners who jogged five days a week, compared with those who jogged three days a week and those who participated in the other sports, reported the greatest reduction in depression.

It should be noted, however, that less strenuous forms of exercise sometimes are reported to decrease anxiety. In a study of the effect of ''minimal'' exercise on three chronic psychiatric patients living in a halfway house, two of whom were women, Lion (1978) reported a significant decrease in anxiety as measured by the State-Trait Anxiety Inventory (Spielberger, Gorsuch, and Lushene 1970). He concluded by noting, ''The most important finding is that exercise, *even minimal exercise* for a short duration, alleviated anxiety'' (p. 1217; italics added). This ''minimal'' exercise consisted of alternately running and walking a block for a total distance of one mile, three times a week for two months. For the middle-aged psychiatric patients in Lion's study, this walking and running could have constituted ''strenuous'' exercise as defined here. It is not clear whether the change was in A-state, A-trait, or the two scales together. Lion presented ''state-trait'' scores in his table 1 that were the scores for either A-state or A-trait. In his abstract Lion reported, ''the jogging group showed significantly less post-test trait anxiety'' (p. 1215). However, A-trait, by definition, is a stable personality characteristic and is much less inclined to change than is A-state (Spielberger, Gorsuch, and Lushene 1970). Since Lion does not again mention the reported change in A-trait rather than the more usual change in A-state, the results of the study remain unclear.

Although light exercise per se does not seem to reduce anxiety (Brown, Ramirez, and Taub 1978; Morgan 1979),[1] anxiety reduction may accompany such programs. Byrd (1964) reported that 87 percent of 263 bowlers felt less tense after bowling, light exercise for most people. A variety of mechanisms other than physical activity itself might account for the reduction in anxiety: the social support, the change of pace, or the diversionary nature of the activity. At present, however, it is not clear whether noncontinuous mild exercise decreases anxiety and depression. Since the therapeutic effects of moderate to strenuous exercise are better substantiated, the female client should engage in *intense* activity for at least twenty minutes (*duration*) three times a week or more (*frequency*) to maximize the effectiveness of running in reducing anxiety.

## A CAUSAL OR AN ASSOCIATIVE RELATION

Although the issue of causality versus association has not been resolved, personal reports of feeling "good" after exercise (Berger and Owen, in press; Dienstbier 1978; Harper 1979; Lilliefors 1978; Morgan and Pollock 1978) and empirical evidence (Andrews 1978; Cogan 1976; Dienstbier 1980; Dienstbier et al. 1981) support the possibility that strenuous exercise significantly decreases anxiety. In their review of literature and the conclusion to their study of female and male runners Dienstbier et al. (1981) noted that greater sympathetic nervous system activation and hormonal capacities as developed by running are associated with more positive responses to stressful situations, less emotional upheaval, and less anxiety. Such changes were particularly pronounced in runners who said running was central to their self-concepts. In another article written for runners, Dienstbier (1978, 32) professed, "I believe that a regular exercise program prolongs the ability of the body to tolerate stressors and delays the perception of exhaustion by prolonging the stage of resistance as defined by Selye. . . . Prolonging resistance and delaying exhaustion should allow one to work harder, longer, and in more psychologically demanding circumstances without the perception of stress or exhaustion."

In a subsequent presentation Dienstbier (1980) refined the traditional model of stress in which catecholamines and physiological arousal are accepted as signs of negative emotional states. He proposed that in highly trained runners catecholamines are *less needed* for energy mobilization in stressful situations because of runners' physiological efficiency but are *more available* if required. Thus runners and other highly trained athletes react better and experience less anxiety in stressful situations than the untrained or "normal" population. Dienstbier's model of the effect of strenuous physical activity on emotional stability, particularly on anxiety, directly supports a causal relation. (See Dienstbier, chap. 14.)

If Dienstbier's model of exercise and the sympathetic nervous system is correct, it may partially explain why more women than men tend to be anxious. Women traditionally have been less inclined to participate in vigorous physical activity and thus are likely to have lower levels of catecholamines available in stressful situations.

A major handicap in demonstrating that physiological changes in physical activity cause long-term changes in personality is an inability to overcome difficult control-group problems: (1) the need for similar expectancies for change in both running and control groups; (2) the need to reduce runners' tendencies to change their patterns of eating, sleeping, and drug use or other living habits; and (3) the need to separate personality changes due to a physiological response to strenuous exercise from those accruing from a host of psychological effects such as feelings of competence and enhanced self-concept (Dienstbier et al. 1981). Although the concomitant psychological effects mentioned interfere with the examination of physiological effects of running on personality, they are important psychological effects of jogging. Chapter 10 examines in detail the relation between running, self-concept, self-esteem, and self-awareness.

An early study also supported a causal rather than associative relation between exercise and decreases in anxiety and stress. In an imaginative and systematic investigation, deVries and Adams (1972) compared the effects of single doses of exercise at a heart rate of 100 beats per minute, exercise at 120 beats per minute, 400 milligrams of meprobamate, 400 milligrams of lactose (a placebo), and a control condition on anxiety as measured by the electrical activity in the right elbow flexor groups. The ten elderly subjects received each treatment on three different occasions. Of the four treatments, only the exercise at 100 heartbeats per minute produced a significantly greater effect upon rising muscular tension than did the control condition. (See note 1, for additional comments about this study.)

In another physiological study that supported the causal effects of exercise on stress, Graveling (1980) reported that exercising for approximately thirty minutes immediately following a mentally stressful situation reduced the tendency of mental stress to change the normal pattern of urinary excretion. Suspecting that the beneficial effects of exercise on psychological well-being may result from social and psychological factors associated with sports participation, Graveling controlled the form and intensity of exercise by having the eight male subjects pedal a bicycle ergometer at a workload that represented 60 to 70 percent of their maximum aerobic capacity. The urinary analyses included separate analyses of the 17-oxygenic steroids. Since any deviation from a normal homeostatic pattern can be harmful, Graveling tentatively concluded that one source of stress—exercise—can alleviate the potentially harmful physiological effects of another.

In contrast to the physiological studies, several behavioral investigations support an associative relation between exercise and anxiety reduction (Bahrke and Morgan 1978; Wilson, Berger, and Bird 1981). Bahrke and Morgan compared physical activity at 70 percent of maximum with Benson's relaxation response (Benson et al. 1975), and a control group that rested in a Lazyboy recliner and found that all three groups of subjects reported significant decreases in ongoing levels of A-state as measured on the State-Trait Anxiety

Inventory (STAI). This finding led the investigators to speculate that diversion rather than exercise or meditation was the critical element in reducing A-state. Additional support of the "time-out" or diversionary hypothesis has been provided by Wilson, Morley, and Bird (1980). Each of three activities— running, participating in an organized exercise class, and eating—significantly reduced the female and male participants' postactivity levels of A-state (STAI) compared with their preactivity levels.

In an attempt to preclude the possibility that the observed changes in stress tolerance resulted from the "time-out" or diversionary aspects of running, Dienstbier et al. (1981) tested their runners several hours after their short (six-mile) runs and an average of five hours after their marathon-distance runs. They noted that it seemed unlikely that a brief time away from one's usual activities would retain its effects several hours after return to them. The marathon run provided a longer "time-out" than the shorter run, yet marathon running was not as consistently effective as moderate running in producing positive physiological and psychological changes.

A causal effect certainly argues more strongly for exercise as a therapuetic approach to anxiety reduction than does an association effect (Morgan 1979). Regardless of the underlying mechanisms, however, aerobic conditioning does seem to decrease anxiety. Since inexpensive, convenient, easily conducted anxiety-reduction techniques are greatly needed in today's society, we can legitimately argue for using exercise as a means of anxiety reduction whether the reduction is a direct result of exercise or an accompaniment.

COGNITIVE AND SOMATIC ANXIETY

One reason it is difficult to support a causal relation between exercise and anxiety reduction may be investigators' failure to partition anxiety into two relatively independent types—cognitive and somatic (Barrett 1972; Borkovec 1976; Davidson and Schwartz 1976; Driscoll 1976), or psychic and somatic (Buss 1962; Hamilton 1959; Schalling, Cronholm, and Asberg 1975). Symptoms of cognitive anxiety include worry, inability to concentrate, and insomnia; symptoms of somatic anxiety include regularly occurring nausea, headaches, and rapid pulse.

After delineating different levels of cognitive anxiety (which can be further subdivided into right- versus left-mediated anxiety) and somatic anxiety (which can be divided into skeletal and autonomic), Davidson and Schwartz (1976) related the existing literature to their psychobiological model of anxiety. They stressed the importance of assessing the *type* of anxiety a client has in order to select the most productive *treatment*. Their model was based on psychobiological specificity and on the theory that particular biobehavioral systems have a finite amount of channel space. Thus, if a person has a large amount of somatic anxiety, further somatic activation such as exercise competes for the channel space and causes attenuation of the somatic anxiety (Schwartz 1979).

To test their model, Schwartz, Davidson, and Goleman (1978) observed the influence of two types of anxiety reduction—exercise (a somatic technique) and meditation (a cognitive technique)—in reducing cognitive and somatic anxiety. The practice periods for both anxiety-reduction treatments were approximately six months. Exercisers averaged 3.6 one-hour sessions each week; meditators practiced daily. Since the exercise group (predominantly women) and the meditation group (nearly equal proportions of women and men) did not differ in overall anxiety at the end of the practice period, the researchers could have concluded that the two modes of treating anxiety were equally effective. However, by measuring separately the somatic and cognitive components of anxiety, they observed a significant interaction between the two components and the anxiety reduction. Exercisers reported less somatic and more cognitive anxiety than meditators. The exercisers also were significantly higher in cognitive anxiety than they were in somatic anxiety. Since the anxiety testing was not performed until the end of the treatments, it was not clear whether the two activities attracted people who differed in their patterning of cognitive and somatic anxiety.

Although the issue of cause and effect has not yet been resolved, Schwartz, Davidson, and Goleman (1978) have presented evidence for a causal relation. They noted that their findings were consistent with the initial hypothesis that meditating and exercising may be associated with the differential patterning of somatic and cognitive symptoms of anxiety. The possibility that running is more successful in alleviating somatic symptoms of anxiety than cognitive symptoms seems to be an important consideration in using running as a therapeutic technique.

LEVELS OF ANXIETY AT DIFFERENT TIMES AFTER RUNNING

Runners' anxiety may fluctuate during the interval between exercise sessions. Although the one existing study in this area employed only male subjects, the time concept is important in running therapy, and additional studies employing female joggers are needed. Suspecting that the effect of strenuous exercise upon level of anxiety may not remain constant throughout a twenty-four-hour period, Morgan (1973) measured anxiety at different times and in sessions of different durations. Forty men were tested on the STAI before, immediately after, and twenty to thirty minutes after vigorous workouts that lasted approximately forty-five minutes. Anxiety increased slightly immediately after exercise but decreased significantly below the baseline level twenty to thirty minutes later. Similar results were observed in another study of fifteen men who followed the same protocol but exercised for only fifteen minutes (Morgan 1973).

How long state anxiety is reduced by strenuous exercise is not known. Perhaps the reduction is temporary and the runner "needs" regular bouts of exercise to maintain the lowered A-state (Sime 1979). As reported by Wilson, Berger, and Bird (1981), preactivity anxiety was inversely related to the number of runs per week ($r = -.58$; $p<.01$). This temporary lowering of anxiety after running may partially account for running addiction. As the time between running sessions increases, anxiety may return to its higher level so that the runner desires additional activity to lower it. Dienstbier's (1980; Dienstbier et al. 1981) hypothesis that running results in *long-term* temperament changes that include reduction in anxiety may be more accurate for trained runners, such as those in his marathon preparation class, than for novices. Continual exercising may maintain greater sympathetic nervous system activation and hormonal capabilities and thus enable trained runners to reduce levels of anxiety for long periods. A study in which A-state is monitored several times a day for practiced and novice runners during several months of an exercise program followed by a month of inactivity would provide needed information about the time relation between running and anxiety reduction.

APPLICATION OF LABORATORY STUDIES TO REAL LIFE

Strenuous exercise seems to reduce anxiety in controlled laboratory studies, and these studies provide important information on what aspects of exercise influence the anxiety/exercise relation. However, most people do not exercise in laboratories. An important consideration for the therapeutic use of exercise is how laboratory studies apply to real-life conditions.

A psychologist and a psychiatrist have jointly described their successful use of running therapy outside the laboratory as *one* approach to treating anxious female and male clients. In their presentation at the 1980 American Medical Joggers Association Boston Marathon Medical Symposium, Summers and Wolstat (1980) reported that they viewed a running treatment as supporting a holistic health model. (See Summers and Wolstat, chap. 5.) Improvement in a woman's physical well-being was matched by improvement in her psychological well-being. These clinicians have speculated that the anxious client has an extremely high activation level and that the accompanying feelings are considered to be anxiety: "What is often necessary is to channel or transform that high level of excitement to a positive use. Running can provide this. This is not to say that running is the only physical technique which can be used in the psychotherapy of anxious and depressed people" (Summers and Wolstat 1980, 20).

Mitchum's (1976) field study in which fifteen minutes of racquetball significantly reduced A-state in forty subjects (women and men) supported the previously cited conclusions from laboratory studies. However, in another field investigation Wood (1977) observed a significant decrease in A-state for men, but not for women, after a twelve-minute run. This finding disagrees with the previously mentioned studies in which women as well as men reported lower levels of anxiety after exercising (Dienstbier et al. 1981; Driscoll 1976; Young 1979).

Although Wood's statistical analysis may have contributed to the reported gender differences (Morgan 1979), it is possible that strenuous exercise differentially affected the two sexes. It is unlikely that women and men react differently to the chemical and physiological changes induced by exercise; therefore one explanation for the occasionally reported differential effects of running might be the sex-role conflict experienced by some women athletes (Snyder and Spreitzer 1978). The social and psychological implications of exercise for women who have been highly feminized may counteract its anxiety-reducing benefits. For this select group of women, psychotherapy and other forms of stress reduction may be more helpful than running (Benson et al. 1978). For most women, however, running seems to be socially acceptable. That sex-role conflict of women in sport is lessening has been supported by Joseph and Robbins (1981), who voiced surprise at finding that women runners were not subjected to more complaints from spouses or partners than were men runners.

RUNNING COMPARED WITH OTHER STRESS-REDUCTION
TECHNIQUES

Driscoll (1976) compared the effectiveness of strenuous exercise (running and running plus positive mental imagery) as an anxiety-reducing technique with that of positive mental imagery, taped desensitization, a minimal treatment condition, and an untreated control group. Exercise and positive mental imagery used together produced greater decreases in test anxiety than any of the other treatments except desensitization. However, the desensitization required more time for training subjects. Driscoll's results indicate a need to further investigate the aspects of running that are most conducive to anxiety reduction.

As I noted previously, the separation of anxiety into somatic and cognitive components may account for the conflicting observations concerning the benefits of various techniques in reducing anxiety (Schwartz, Davidson, and Goleman 1978). Comparing the effectiveness of exercise and meditation in reducing the two components of anxiety, Schwartz and his colleagues reported that physical exercise reduced somatic anxiety and that meditation reduced cognitive anxiety. Cognitive, somatic, and even control group activities such as watching television may be differentially effective in reducing the various components of anxiety.

## Conclusion

A considerable body of experimental evidence supports the use of exercise to reduce anxiety, a malady that afflicts a substantially greater proportion of women than men. Although no conclusive evidence has been generated to support a *causal rather than associative effect* of exercise on anxiety reduction, the high incidence of anxiety in women and the resulting psychological pain justify the use of running therapy for this population regardless of the underlying mechanisms.

To maximize the effectiveness of running as a treatment for anxiety, the therapist should ensure that specific conditions are met. For example, the running should be *vigorous,* should occur *at least three times a week,* and should last *at least twenty minutes* for treatment effects to become noticeable. (See Berger, chap. 2, for additional information on the novice woman runner.) Exercise that is frequent and strenuous has been demonstrated to be most effective in reducing anxiety. The anxiety-reducing capabilities of jogging also may be enhanced by directing the runner's thoughts (Driscoll 1976). (See Sachs, chap. 16, for additional information.)

Although running tends to be more successful in reducing the *somatic* aspects of anxiety while cognitive techniques such as meditation work best with the *cognitive* aspects, both have some effect on the multiple physiological systems of anxiety. How long running decreases anxiety may depend on the time interval between exercise and measurement of anxiety, on the number of runs per week, and on the number of months a person has been running. Since maximum decreases may occur about an hour after running, it is likely that the greatest effects of the treatment would be noted at this time. Highly trained, habitual exercisers may reduce their ongoing levels of anxiety for longer than novices. Running may tax the sympathetic nervous system and hormonal systems sufficiently to produce increased capacity or efficiency in responding to stress.

### Depression

"Depression" denotes a heterogeneous group of depressive disorders (Akiskal and McKinney 1975). It is characterized by generalized feelings of hopelessness, despair, sadness, self-hate, and pessimism and has replaced anxiety as the most common psychological complaint (Klerman 1979). Its ultimate behavioral expression is suicide, and the term "melancholia" is employed to designate this extreme level of depression (Akiskal and McKinney 1975). Less severe behavioral manifestations include irritability, social withdrawal, indecisiveness, self-disturbance, loss of appetite, and fatigue (Akiskal and McKinney 1975; Beck et al. 1961; Penfold 1981). Like anxiety, depression affects people of all ages and is especially prevalent in women (Chesler 1973; Justice and McBee 1978; Penfold 1981; Scarf 1979; Weissman and Klerman 1977; Weissman and Paykel 1974). Depending on the figures cited, two to six women are diagnosed as suffering from depression for every man so diagnosed (Penfold 1981). Refer to Akiskal and McKinney (1975) for a thorough integrative review of ten models of depression and a new model that synthesizes findings from different schools. These two psychiatrists have conceptualized depressive illness as the feedback interaction of different variables at chemical, experiential, and behavioral levels, with the diencephalon serving as the field of action.

In her systematic and thought-provoking analysis of women and depression, Penfold (1981) concurred with Akiskal and McKinney that a major problem with current classification systems for depressive disorder is the differential emphasis on such factors as mood, activity level, genetic predisposition, severity, and contact with reality. In addition, examining the depressed person's behavior from endocrine, genetic, psychodynamic, cognitive, social, and behavioral viewpoints further complicates the picture of depression.

Although its nature and causes are unclear, depression is a major source of personal unhappiness and must be treated. As Penfold (1981, 29) concluded: "the need for new models and new understanding is clear." Rather than focusing on the individual's dysfunction and working toward change in her, Penfold emphasizes, therapists need to examine a woman's entire social

environment, consisting of work, husband, children, parents, and other pertinent components. There is often a clear relation between the difficulties a
woman experiences daily and her depression. Rossi's (1980) observation that
family size was strongly and positively correlated with women's use of medication and lowered competence in family roles corroborates the deleterious
effects of environmental stress.

By incorporating a systematic program of physical activity in her life, a
depressed client may be able to alleviate some of her unhappiness and begin to
change her social environment (Jones 1979). Of course the explanation of the
mechanism(s) by which running serves to decrease feelings of depression will
differ according to a therapist's school of thought. In rather simplistic terms, a
therapist who emphasized a cognitive approach might view running as a way
for the client to reduce her negative attitudes toward herself (Beck 1967) and
the way she presented herself to others. For example, she might begin to see
herself as organized, strong, competent, and successful, actively enhancing her
physical health and energy level and improving her appearance by reducing
body fat and toning her muscles. In addition to these psychological effects of
running, the physical benefits such as reduced fatigue and increased endurance,
strength, and ability to sleep would alleviate depression. Behavioral therapists
who view depression as a state of "learned helplessness" (Seligman 1972)
could use running to alter the client's misapprehension that passivity, unre-
sponsiveness, and helplessness are effective ways to deal with environmental
traumas. Should the client be so fortunate as to experience an altered state of
consciousness or "runner's high" (Mandell 1979; Solomon and Bumpus 1978)
while exercising, she would secure at least a temporary respite from depression. (See also Sachs, chap. 15.)

In another review of the literature on women and depression, Scarf (1979)
concluded that, despite Chesler's (1973) claim in *Women and Madness,*
women exhibit gender-appropriate behavior even in psychological dysfunc-
tioning and thus tend to develop the more "passive" syndromes of depression
and schizophrenia. Men exhibit more action-oriented psychological disorders
such as alcoholism, drug addiction, and violent behavior (Justice and McBee
1978; Scarf 1979). Although both women and men may feel the same way, they
behave very differently (Phillips and Segal 1969).

Seeking to determine why a disproportionate number of women are depressed,
Scarf eliminated hormonal differences and focused on the encouragement of
dependency in American women and their consequent strong need for approval.
To counterbalance dependency, one needs an independent sense of self, which is
developed by setting goals and attaining them with reasonable frequency (Scarf

1979). Thus physical fitness and sports skills (two easily attained goals) could be key elements in reducing and preventing depression in women. (See chap. 2 for a detailed discussion of running goals.)

The content of many popular magazine and newspaper articles (Bernstein and Rothman 1978; Hammer 1980; Higdon 1978; *U.S. News and World Report* 1979) leads one to believe that running is a bona fide cure for depression. Bernstein and Rothman (1978, 32) noted that nearly everyone will experience depression at some time and listed tips from the Mental Health Association of Houston for combating simple depression. Several of their suggestions are validated by running research.

1. Concentrate on doing things you do well to increase self-esteem. (With minimal practice, most women can increase the distance, speed, and ease of their running.)
2. Engage in any type of physical activity.
3. Share your feelings with a friend. (Those who run with a companion often have unusually intimate conversations.)
4. Focus your energy on someone who is lonely or ill.
5. Break up your usual routines by taking a different way to work or eating something new for lunch. (Running provides an abrupt change from the sedentary, indoor activities of most women.)
6. List as many of your accomplishments as you can. (The runner can note the number of times a week she runs, the distance covered, the feelings experienced while running, and her speed. She should focus upon her accomplishments rather than upon goals she has not yet met.)
7. Work at making your physical appearance as attractive as possible. (Running tends to reduce body fat and to increase muscle tone and energy levels. Thus, running can easily improve a woman's appearance.) Altshul (1981), a professor of psychiatry at Yale University who described himself as both a runner and a depressive, noted: "This does not mean that running—or psychoanalysis, for that matter—is superior therapy. It does mean that running is a superior blank screen, available for projections. And it does mean that running is likely to be experienced as therapy by those who feel an intense inner need for therapy" (p. 52). Experimental studies on the effects of running on depression fail to offer a clear and consistent connection. To examine systematically the conflicting results of the research that has been done, I will group studies according to their subject populations: (1) athletes compared with nonathletes and with the general population; (2) heart patients; (3) depressed adults who were not characterized as having coronary heart disease; and (4) the "normal" (nondepressed) adult population.

ATHLETES, NONATHLETES, AND THE GENERAL POPULATION

If regular, vigorous physical activity is related to depression, it seems logical that athletes, who exercise far more than the average person, should be below average in depression. Tharp and Schlegelmilch (1977), in one of the few studies of athletes' personalities that has included a measure of depression, produced evidence that habitual exercisers differ from novice exercisers. By comparing trained subjects selected from a YMCA and university population with nontrained subjects, the researchers concluded that the trained subjects were significantly lower in anxiety and depression as measured by the Multiple Affect Adjective Check List (Zuckerman and Lubin 1965) and were more relaxed, emotionally stable, self-assured, and secure (Cattell 1972). Unfortunately, the retrospective nature of the study precluded gaining information about initial personality differences between the trained and untrained exercisers. People who are low in depression may be more inclined to exercise, and thus the habitual and novice exercisers may have differed in depression as a result of self-selection.

In a comprehensive comparison of depression in athletes, Morgan and Pollock (1977) reported that high-level United States wrestlers, rowers, and runners (both world class marathon and middle-distance runners and college middle-distance runners) had similar psychological profiles as measured by the Profile of Mood States (POMS) (McNair, Lorr, and Droppleman 1971). Since sex of the runners was not specified, it probably is safe to assume they were all males. However, there is considerable evidence that outstanding athletes of both sexes are more similar to one another in personality than are athletes and nonathletes of the same sex (Harris 1973). The athletes in Morgan and Pollock's work (1977) scored below the mean reported for college students in depression as well as in tension/anxiety, fatigue, and confusion. Acknowledging that the low levels of depression and anxiety in long-distance runners may be attributable either to initial differences or to the exercise itself, Morgan and Pollock opted for the latter. They reasoned that because their runners and other athletes were similar to the general college population in the relatively stable personality traits of extroversion and neuroticism, it was likely that their low anxiety and depression scores—more unstable measures—were a consequence of the chronic and acute physical activity of running rather than antecedent conditions.

More recently, Morgan (1980, 93) has stated, based on his own research and on that of others in the field, that "One general finding has consistently emerged: successful athletes in all sports possess superior mental and emotional health. They consistently show fewer signs of psychopathology and lower levels of anxiety, neuroticism, and depression than less successful athletes and the general population." The "iceberg" profile that Morgan (1979, 1980; Morgan and Pollock 1977) repeatedly observed in the scores of outstanding athletes on the POMS is presented in figure 1. Elite athletes, including runners, tend to score below the mean or "surface" on the negative psychological constructs of tension, depression, anger, fatigue, and confusion.

The results of Joesting's (1981a) study, which compared the POMS scores of Olympic-hopeful runners (24 females; 106 males) and sailors (8 females; 41 males) differed from Morgan's findings (1979, 1980; Morgan and Pollock 1977). Rather than runners and sailors both reporting enhanced psychological well-being on the six POMS subscales as would be expected from Morgan's

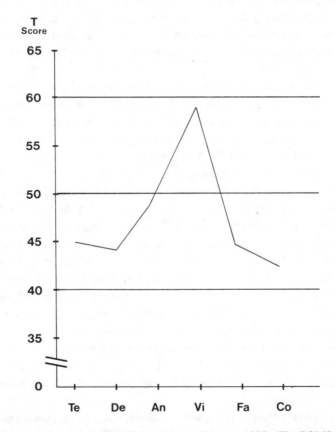

Figure 1. Iceberg mood profile of elite runners (Morgan 1980). The POMS subscales include tension/anxiety (Te), depression (De), anger (An), vigor (Vi), fatigue (Fa), and confusion (Co).

studies, the male runners were significantly less depressed (means = 8.02 and 12.66, $p. < .01$), less anxious (means = 8.04 and 11.98, $p < .01$), and less fatigued (means = 7.02 and 9.39, $p < .05$) than the male sailors. The only other significant difference between groups was that female runners were less fatigued than female sailors (means = 5.83 and 12.75, $p < .01$). Differences in pre- and posttest competition scores on the POMS were not observed for either female or male runners or sailors. Joesting speculated that these findings that favored runners may reflect differences in the two sport environments, such as the sailors' use of equipment and their need to cope with partners during competition. Of course the possibility of a self-selection factor cannot be overlooked.

HEART PATIENTS

Depression is very common in "postcoronary" patients (Kavanagh, Shephard, and Tuck 1975; Kavanagh et al. 1977; Lebovitz et al., 1967). In a five-year prospective study of 1,990 males, Lebovitz et al. (1967) reported that survivors of coronary heart disease (CHD) were significantly more depressed, as measured by the Minnesota Multiphasic Personality Inventory (MMPI), than subjects matched for age and educational status who had no major illness. The nonsurvivors who were tested soon after their attacks were more depressed than CHD patients who survived. It seemed that depressed CHD patients did not have a "will" to live.

In a recent article T. Hackett, a psychiatrist at Massachusetts General Hospital, was quoted as saying that a prescribed program of physical activity strengthens the heart and that for survivors of CHD exercise "is the single most effective way to lift a patient's spirits, to alleviate anxiety, and to restore feelings of potency about all aspects of life" (Brody 1980). When moved from the hospital to home, the recovering heart attack patient tends to falsely attribute fatigue to physiological deterioration and often exhibits "homecoming depression." A prescribed program of exercise can improve cardiovascular functioning and enhance the patient's confidence in her or his physical capabilities. Since the major reasons for depression in heart patients are thought to be the patients' own anxiety, lack of confidence, and fear of sudden death (Fisher 1970), a program of supervised running is likely to reduce depression.

The experimental literature on the effect of regular exercise on heart patients clearly supports an accompanying decrease in depression (Kavanagh et al. 1977; Noble 1976). In a study of forty-four "postcoronary" patients who were very high in depression as indicated by a percentile score of seventy or above on the MMPI, a significant decrease in depression from the initial testing in 1972 to subsequent testing in 1976 was noted after an exercise-based rehabilitation program (Kavanagh et al. 1977) consisting of personally prescribed slow long-distance running over a two- to four-year period. Although the men, as a group, significantly decreased their ongoing levels of depression, the effects were not universal. Of the forty-four depressed men, twenty-seven significantly decreased their depression, ten showed no change, and seven became more depressed. Kavanagh et al. noted that a variety of contaminating factors could have affected the decrease, but it seemed that compliance, as indicated by attending at least 60 percent of the running sessions, influenced the decrease in depression. The compliance group reduced their depression scores from 29.2 ± 3.6 to 25.3 ± 5.5. The noncompliance group's level of depression remained the same (27.1 ± 4.5 to 27.1 ± 2.3).

The results of this field study were complicated because some subjects were taking mood-elevating drugs (diazepam and chlorpromazine) and propranolol, a drug that supresses angina but has a depressant effect. It was not surprising that the two patients who decreased their depression the most were taking mood-elevating drugs, even though such drugs tend to provoke dysrhythmia and sudden death. The propranolol, though a depressant, suppresses angina and dysrhythmia and may have allowed for greater participation in the exercise program.

Exercise seems to be a very effective means of reducing depression in postcoronary patients, but, generalizations based on this population are exceedingly speculative. The unique characteristics of heart patients are emphasized by Noble (1976), who concluded a review of the psychological characteristics of myocardial infarction patients (MI) with the observation that such patients are psychologically different from normal subjects and even from coronary-prone subjects before a cardiac episode. Since depression has been proposed as a psychological precursor of MI, exercise programs for people who have had one or more heart attacks are particularly important. The physiological effects of exercise alone would justify the program. In addition, it is likely that exercise would decrease their depression.

EFECT OF RUNNING ON NONDEPRESSED ADULTS
WHO HAVE NO FORM OF CORONARY HEART DISEASE

In early study of the psychological effects of physical activity, Morgan et al. (1970) sought to elucidate the ''feeling better'' sensation that results from regular strenuous exercise. The study was conducted in two phases. In the first part, a variety of physiological measures were correlated with depression scores (Zung 1965) of sixty-seven male college professors. None of the correlations were significant; no evidence was produced that depression was related to age, height, weight, percentage of body fat, physical working capacity, or grip strength.

In the second portion, thirty-four male professors were added to the study ($N = 101$). All 101 men were tested on the depression scale (Zung 1965), and received both resting and exercise electrocardiograms. The professors chose one of four vigorous activities (circuit training, jogging, swimming, and laboratory exercises of treadmill running or bicycle ergometry) and participated in the program three days a week for six weeks. A control group was composed of those who could not arrange an activity to fit their schedules ($n = 16$). As in many studies of nondepressed populations, no significant change in depression was observed between the pre- and postexercise depression scores. Morgan et al. (1970) speculated that the lack of change may have been because the training program was not of sufficient intensity (85 percent predicted maximum) or duration (six weeks), or because decreases in depression may not occur among people who are already in the normal range.

Since 11 of the 101 professors had earned raw scores of 50 or above on Zung's scale, a unique opportunity was available for comparing pre- and postexercise depression scores of the *clinically depressed*. Indeed, the depressed group in contrast to the nondepressed men did lower their depression scores, dropping from the initial mean of 51.45 to 44.45 ($p \leq .01$). The results of this study indicate that decreases in depression in response to an exercise program are more obvious in a depressed than in a normal population.

In a two-part study that included both nondepressed or "normal" and depressed high-school and college students, Brown, Ramirez, and Taub (1978) investigated the psychological correlates of a ten-week exercise program. No subjects were receiving treatment of any kind for emotional problems. In the first part, nondepressed women ($n = 96$) and men ($n = 71$), except for six control subjects, selected a physical activity in which they participated for an average of thirty minutes a day three times a week: jogging, softball, tennis, wrestling, or a varied program. Contact between subjects and investigators was limited to the pre- and postactivity testing sessions that included measures of resting pulse rates, the Zung Depression Scale (Zung 1965), and the Eysenck Personality Inventory (Eysenck and Eysenck 1968). All subjects except the softball players and controls significantly decreased in depression.

The second phase of the study separated those who were depressed from those who were not and included 561 university students: clinically depressed students who jogged ($n = 91$), depressed subjects who served as nonjogging controls ($n = 10$), nondepressed subjects who jogged ($n = 406$), and non-depressed subjects who served as a nonexercising control group ($n = 54$) (Brown, Ramirez, and Taub 1978). Each subject chose whether to jog three times a week, five times a week, or not at all. The two jogging groups gradually increased their exercise to a minimum of thirty minutes a session. Although *both* the depressed and the nondepressed groups of joggers significantly decreased their levels of depression, the changes were much larger for the depressed populations. Decreases in depression were attributed to jogging because no changes were observed for the depressed and "normal" groups who did not jog. Based on their two-part study, the experimenters concluded that the antidepressant effect of exercise seemed to depend on the intensity, duration, and frequency of exercise. Softball players who did not participate in aerobic (continuous) exercise were similar to the nonexercising control group in showing no change in depression; tennis players had significant but slight reductions in depression; and joggers who ran five days a week evidenced the largest decreases.

Wilson, Morley, and Bird (1980) compared the depression levels of "marathoners" who ran between six and twenty miles six to seven days a week ($n = 10$) with those of "joggers" who averaged one to two miles three to five days a week ($n = 10$) and of nonexercisers who had participated in no regular physical activity during the previous year ($n = 10$). The study included only males and thus awaits replication employing female subjects. However, the results are impressive for a normal, nondepressed population. Marathoners and joggers were significantly lower in depression as measured on the POMS (McNair, Lorr, and Droppleman 1971) than nonexercisers. Marathoners also were significantly lower in depression than joggers. The retrospective nature of the study precluded the establishment of a causal effect. Thus, it was unclear whether the observed differences in depression were related to the distance run, the type of individual attracted to running, an expectation of positive benefits from running, or a host of other influences.

In another study of runners' levels of depression, Joesting (1981b) compared the depression scores of female ($n = 21$) and male ($n = 79$) runners who were competing in a Florida race with the nonpsychiatric norms for the Depression Adjective Check List (Lubin 1967). Both the female and the male runners were significantly ($p \leq .01$) less depressed than the normative population. As in all studies in which subjects are not randomly assigned to treatment groups and in which no control groups are employed, the cause(s) of the low depression scores could not be specified. In all these studies, though, runners—members of a nonclinical population—are consistently low in depression.

In a recent study of the relation between physical fitness and personality, Jasnoski and Holmes (1981) produced evidence that, among 103 college women enrolled in aerobics training classes, the women who *initially* were higher in aerobic capacity were significantly less depressed. This finding is particularly interesting because the investigators employed the same depression scale (Zung 1965) used by Brown, Ramirez, and Taub (1978) and Morgan et al. (1970). Aerobic capacity—the maximum amount of oxygen the body can process during a specified amount of time (Cooper 1968), estimated by the women's performance on a twelve-minute walk/run test—was employed to measure physical fitness levels.

Since aerobic capacity is heavily influenced by running, Jasnoski and Holmes's results supported the conclusion that nondepressed women who run are lower in depression than those who are less fit. Like Morgan et al. (1970), Jasnoski and Holmes produced no evidence that the fifteen weeks of exercise classes further reduced the women's initial levels of depression.

An explanation for failure to observe changes as a result of exercise among people within a "normal" range of depression may be that the measures are not sensitive to *small* changes or whatever makes chronic exercisers report that exercise makes them "feel better." Supporting a need for more discriminating tests of depression, Morgan and Pollock (1978) noted that fifty-five men in a running program for twenty weeks at the Institute for Aerobic Research in Texas also did not change their levels of depression as measured by the Profile of Mood States (McNair, Lorr, and Droppleman 1971). Although these men reported normal levels of depression and thus may have been less likely to decrease their ongoing levels, their own opinions were that they were less depressed. That 77 percent of those who ran one day a week and 76 percent of those who ran five days a week reported decreases compared with only 22 percent of the recreational group who participated in less vigorous physical activity leads to the conclusion that aerobic exercise decreases depression (Morgan and Pollock 1978). Of course, this could reflect the men's expectations of "feeling better" from their exercise programs.

Harris (1981) reported results similar to those of Morgan and Pollock in her study of runners' ($N = 411$) perceptions of the benefits of running. The runners differed in sex (132 women, 277 men), age (10–71 years), running ability (1–120 miles per week), occupation, and ethnicity and thus seemed to represent a cross section of runners for the Albuquerque, New Mexico, area. Although

Harris administered no indexes of personality or mood, it seems likely that these runners were within the normal range in such psychological characteristics as depression and mood. Their major reasons for participating were to feel better physically (92.5 percent), to feel better psychologically (87.3 percent), to control their weight (54.8 percent), and to relax (55.5 percent). An important question that needs further study is whether runners who attain their goals continue running more often than runners who do not. The more serious runners—those who had run for more years, run faster, or run longer distances—were more addicted to running and became more depressed when they stopped running than the less serious runners, so it might be concluded from Harris's study that running did provide psychological benefits. She specifically noted that those who began running in hopes of feeling less depressed tended to report sleeping better. That the runners who reported the greatest improvement in nutrition were most likely to report feeling better both psychologically and physically supported the possibility that the physical and psychological effects of running interact to influence runners' feelings of psychological well-being (Engle 1977; Pelletier 1979; Sheehan 1980).

### EFFECT OF RUNNING ON CLINICALLY DEPRESSED ADULTS WHO HAVE NO FORM OF CORONARY HEART DISEASE

Supporting repeated observations of a decrease in depression resulting from a running program among a moderately depressed population, Greist and his colleagues concluded that a supervised running program was at least as effective as ten-session time-limited and time-unlimited psychotherapy programs (Greist et al. 1978, 1979). Thirteen men and fifteen women who sought treatment for neurotic or reactive depression were assigned randomly to running or to one of two forms of psychotherapy. The eight patients who remained in the running therapy treatment were encouraged to run individually with or without a running leader at least three times a week for an hour each time. The purpose of the running leader was to ensure that patients ran or walked at a comfortable pace, using their ability to converse while running as a guide.

Interspersing running with walking helped patients avoid pain and fatigue. In contrast to the attrition rate of 30 to 70 percent observed in running groups in the general population (Morgan 1977; Pollock et al. 1977), the attrition rate in this study was only 11 percent, probably because of the graduated, gentle approach to running (Greist et al. 1978). The topic of depression was avoided during the sessions and conversations focused on the running itself. By teaching the correct approach to running, the leaders hoped to encourage patients to continue treatment by themselves after the ten-week study. Most attrition in running programs occurs in the first six weeks (Morgan 1977; Pollock et al. 1977).

Two women in the running treatment showed little decrease in depression. One had a scheduling problem and found running difficult because of her low level of fitness. However, she did initiate a regular walking program during the sixth week of treatment and "had a dramatic remission of symptoms during the sixth week of the follow-up period" (Greist et al. 1979, 46). Another woman who did not significantly reduce her depression while running stated that she thought running never "could be treatment" (Greist et al. 1978, 276), thus illustrating that running therapy is not always effective in treating moderate depression. Her disbelief in running as therapy and the accompanying lack of change in her depression level highlight the great need to compare the effects of a jogging program with those of any control activity for which subjects have similar expectations of change, perhaps acting as a self-fulfilling prophecy. An interesting sidelight is that this second woman seemed to have an underlying problem of attachment to and separation from significant males. When a male friend who had been away returned to town, her depression promptly subsided (Greist et al. 1978, p. 46).

Greist and his colleagues (1978, 1979) reported that the running therapy was at least as effective in alleviating depressive symptoms as were the two forms of psychotherapy. They suggested that the underlying mechanisms that alleviated depression in the running program included:

1. sense of mastery or success
2. awareness of a capacity for change as illustrated by improved health, appearance, and body image
3. generalized effects of a new positive self-image
4. relief of anger and anxiety as well as depression, and pleasure in the act of running that becomes a justification to continue
5. consciousness alteration
6. biochemical changes.

In an exploratory study of moderately to severely depressed patients, Buffone (1980) investigated the effects of an eight-week therapy program that combined a cognitive-behavioral approach with an aerobic running program on a variety of psychological parameters. The five subjects (four females, one male) who participated in the entire treatment process significantly reduced their ongoing levels of depression as measured by the Beck Depression Inventory (Beck et al. 1961) and the "Mini-Mult" form of the Minnesota Multiphasic Personality Inventory (MMPI) (Hathaway and McKinley 1967).

Buffone noted that the failure to find changes in a second psychological characteristic, anxiety, may in part have been a result of the measuring instrument employed (MMPI). The lack of change in body image as measured by a modified version of Secord and Jourard's (1953) scale was thought to have been related to the subjects' low fitness levels and their tendency to be overweight. Buffone speculated that the *intensity* (walking and jogging), *duration* (thirty minutes), *frequency* (once a week as part of a group and independently two or three times a week), and *length* of the exercise program (eight weeks) were insufficient to produce any major physical changes that might have influenced the subjects' body images. Since no subjects continued to jog two months after the formal termination of the study and since subjects reported a recurrence of depression, information on factors that promote exercise adherence is crucial to the success of this therapeutic approach. (See Buffone, Sachs, and Dowd, chap. 11.)

Supporting the effectiveness of running therapy for both women ($n = 18$) and men ($n = 4$) who were clinically depressed, Rueter and Harris (1980) concluded that, after a ten-week treatment period, running combined with counseling produced significantly greater decreases in depression than did counseling alone. The volunteers, who had sought university-sponsored psychological services and who initially were moderately depressed as measured on the Beck Depression Inventory (Beck et al. 1961), were assigned randomly to one of two treatment conditions: to counseling only or to counseling plus running. The prospective nature of the study, the random assignment of clients to treatment conditions, and the significant decreases in depression observed for the running and counseling group during the ten weeks of therapy strongly supported the causative rather than associative effects of running in reducing depression.

Adding to the accumulating evidence that running is effective in reducing depression among those who are "moderately" depressed, Blue (1979) reported two case studies of former inpatients who were hospitalized because of their depression. After their release from a psychiatric hospital, both the female client and the male client failed to improve as a result of antidepressant medication, empathy, and cognitive-behavioral therapy in the ensuing eight to ten weeks. Each patient then was encouraged to begin jogging two or three times a week. After only three weeks of jogging, the woman reduced her scores on the Zung Depression Scale by fifteen points and the man reduced his by eighteen points (Zung 1965). Both changed from the "moderately depressed" category to either "mildly" or "minimally" depressed. Although it is difficult to maintain strict experimental control in case studies, the failure of these two patients to respond to traditional types of treatment followed by a rapid response to running is impressive.

## Conclusions and Suggestions for Conducting Running Therapy Programs

It is impossible to conclude that regular strenuous exercise alleviates depression in *all* people. What is fairly certain is that *athletes* tend to score lower in depression than their less physically active peers. *Heart patients* who are deeply depressed report significant decreases in depression when they participate in rehabilitation programs that include physical activity. After a heart attack, patients often worry that any kind of physical exertion may precipitate another attack. A program of supervised physical activity can reduce their fears of impotency, decrease their feelings of helplessness, and renew their confidence in their physical capacities.

The implications of research on running and depression for the *nondepressed* portion of the population, however, are not clear. Nonetheless, so many runners attest to the depression-reducing qualities of exercise that the attribution is hard to refute. For *clinically depressed* persons, many of whom are women with no history of CHD, running seems an ideal way to reduce depression. The treatment is relatively inexpensive, requires little supervision after a brief instruction period, and needs no scheduling.

In contrast to these attractive characteristics of running therapy, other treatments for depression have negative consequences. Drug therapy is not always effective (Akiskal and McKinney 1975) and can result in drug dependence and a host of other undesirable side effects. The unpredictable effects of electroshock therapy and the lack of knowledge concerning its underlying mechanisms make both therapists and patients reluctant to use it. Psychotherapy can be an expensive and lengthy process. Running therapy, in contrast to the more conventional approaches to treating depression, tends to be effective and has the desirable side effects of increasing cardiovascular fitness, leg strength, and calorie expenditure. For many persons running is enjoyable as well as therapeutic. It differs from one's daily tasks and provides opportunities to be outdoors and commune with nature, to test one's ability, and to see concrete signs of progress. However, in spite of the evidence that supports the therapeutic use of running to reduce moderate levels of depression, Greist et al. (1978, 287) have sounded a note of caution: "In our opinion, running as treatment for depression remains experimental, in need of replication by additional controlled studies and potentially dangerous to depressed individuals.''

Possible problems in using running as therapy for depressed persons include: (1) risk of cardiovascular misadventure, which can be minimized by requiring exercise stress tests before therapy; (2) lack of evidence that jogging is helpful in managing severe rather than moderate depression; and (3) incorrect running prescription and the resulting problem of poor adherence (Greist et al. 1978). Therapists should take care to individualize running programs according to clients' capabilities and fitness levels. Results of an investigation of factors that affect both initial recruitment and continued participation in industrial fitness programs (Shephard and Cox 1980) are particularly applicable to running therapy programs. Of primary importance are (1) matching activity to body build, since obese women will have greater difficulty running than thin ones; (2) providing gradual progressions in running to avoid discouragement; (3) paying attention to the individual's goals, such as decrease in stress anxiety, release of tension, improved appearance, or sense of accomplishment; and (4) helping clients resolve time conflicts that might limit the participation of ''type A'' individuals.

As noted in a multitude of articles in popular running magazines, many novices expect and demand more running of themselves than they can produce. Women who exceed their capabilities find running exhausting, painful, and unpleasant, so they stop. In encountering another failure, women who already are depressed could become even more so. As Greist et al. (1978, 289) concluded, it is likely that running is most effective in reducing depression for individuals ''who run within the 'therapeutic window' of their adaptive capacity.'' Running more or less than this critical amount will detract from the treatment effectiveness and may even cause further problems.

## Notes

I wish to thank Drs. Mary Duquin, Vietta Wilson, and Jerome Winter for their constructive comments and suggestions on an earlier draft of this chapter.

1. DeVries and Adams (1972; deVries 1981) observed a significant decrease in muscular tension in ten elderly volunteers who considered themselves to have anxiety-tension problems and who exercised (walked) and maintained a heart rate of 100 beats per minute. (I consider exercising at a heart rate of 100 beats per minute *very mild* in intensity.) In contrast to those who maintained exercise heart rates of 100 beats per minute, the elderly subjects who exercised at 120 beats per minute approached but did not reach a significant decrease in muscular tension. No evidence was produced to

indicate that the subjects receiving meprobamate or the placebo differed from the controls. Since no other investigators have demonstrated changes in anxiety at this intensity of exercise, the results are exceeding difficult to interpret and await additional investigation.

### References

Akiskal, H. S., and McKinney, W. T. 1975. Overview of recent research in depression. *Archives of General Psychiatry* 285–305.

Altshul, V. A. 1981. Should we advise our depressed patients to run? In *Psychology of running,* ed. M. H. Sacks and M. L. Sachs. Champaign, Ill.: Human Kinetics Publishers.

Andrews, V. 1978. *The psychic power of running.* New York: Ballantine Books.

Bahrke, M. S., and Morgan, W. P. 1978. Anxiety reduction following exercise and meditation. *Cognitive Therapy and Research* 2:323–34.

Barrett, E. S. 1972. Anxiety and impulsiveness: Toward a neuropsychological model. In *Anxiety: Current trends in theory and research,* vol. 1, ed. C. Spielberger. New York: Academic Press.

Beck, A. T. 1967. *Depression: Clinical, experimental and theortical aspects.* London: Staples Press.

Beck, A. T.; Ward, C. H.; Mendelson, M.; Mock, J.; and Erbaugh, J. 1961. An inventory for measuring depression *Archives of General Psychiatry* 4:561–71.

Benson, H.; Frankel, F. H.; Apfel, R.; Daniels, M. S.; Schniewind, H. E.; Nemiah, J. C.; Sifneos, P. E.; Crassweller, K. D.; Greenwood, M. M.; Kotch, J. B.; Arns, P. A.; and Rosner, B. 1978. Treatment of anxiety: A comparison of the usefulness of self-hypnosis and a meditational relaxation technique. *Psychotherapy and Psychosomatics* 30:229–42.

Benson, H., and Klipper, M. Z. 1975. *The relaxation response.* New York: Avon.

Berger, B. G., and Owen, D. R. 1983. The mood enhancing effects of swimming: Swimmers really do "feel better." *Psychosomatic Medicine,* in press.

Bernstein, T., and Rothman, S. 1978. One of seven Americans can expect to suffer depression. *National Enquirer,* 26 September, 32–33.

Biaggio, M. K., and Nielsen, E. C. 1976. Anxiety correlates of sex-role identity. *Journal of Clinical Psychology* 32:619–23.

Blue, F. R. 1979. Aerobic running as treatment for moderate depression. *Perceptual and Motor Skills* 48:228.

Borkovec, T. D. 1976. Physiological and cognitive processes in the regulation of anxiety. In *Consciousness and self-regulation: Advances in research,* vol. 1, ed. G. E. Schwartz and D. Shapiro. New York: Plenum Press.

Brody, J. E. 1980. Personal health. *New York Times,* 30 April, C–14.

Brown, R. S.; Ramirez, D. E.; and Taub, J. M. 1978. The prescription of exercise for depression. *Physician and Sportsmedicine* 6(12):34–37, 40–41, 44–45.

Buffone, G. W. 1980. Psychological changes associated with cognitive-behavioral therapy and an aerobic running program in the treatment of depression. Ph.D. diss., Florida State University.

Buss, A. H. 1962. Two anxiety factors in psychiatric patients. *Journal of Abnormal and Social Psychology* 65:426–27.

Byrd, O. E. 1964. Viewpoints of bowlers in respect to the relief of tension. *Physical Educator* 21:119–20.

Cattell, R. B. 1972. *Manual for sixteen personality factor questionnaire*. Champaign, Ill.: Institute for Personality and Ability Testing.

Cattell, R. B., and Scheier, I. H. 1958. The nature of anxiety: A review of thirteen multivariate analyses comprising 814 variables. *Psychological Reports* 4:351–88.

———. 1961. *The meaning and measurement of neuroticism and anxiety*. New York: Ronald Press.

Chesler, P. 1973. *Women and madness*. New York: Avon Books.

Cogan, M. 1976. The possible role of physical activity in adaptation to psychological stress. In *Tension control: Proceedings of the second meeting of the American Association for the Advancement of Tension Control*, ed. F. J. McGuigan. Blacksburg, Va.: University Publications.

Cooper, K. H. 1968. A means of assessing maximal oxygen uptake. *Journal of the American Medical Association* 203:201–4.

Davidson, F. J., and Schwartz, G. E. 1976. The psychobiology of relaxation and related states: A multi-process theory. In *Behavior control and modification of physiological activity*, ed. D. I. Mostofsky. Englewood Cliffs, N.J.: Prentice-Hall.

deVries, H. A. 1981. Tranquilizer effects of exercise: A critical review. *Physician and Sportsmedicine* 9(11):46–49, 52–53, 55.

deVries, H. A., and Adams, G. M. 1972. Electromyographic comparison of single doses of exercise and meprobamate as to effect on muscular relaxation. *American Journal of Physical Medicine* 51:130–41.

Dienstbier, R. A. 1978. Running and personality change. *Today's Jogger* 2(1): 30–33, 48–49.

———. 1980. Exercise, catecholamines, and personality. Paper presented at the Third Annual Psychology of Running Seminar, Cornell University Medical College, New York City, 24 October.

Dienstbier, R. A.; Crabbe, J.; Johnson, G. D.; Thorland, W.; Jorgensen, J. A.; Sadar, M. M.; and LaVelle, D. C. 1981. Exercise and stress tolerance. In *Psychology of running*, ed. M. H. Sacks and M. L. Sachs. Champaign, Ill.: Human Kinetics Publishers.

Driscoll, R. 1976. Anxiety reduction using physical exertion and positive images. *Psychological Record* 26:87–94.

Engle, G. L. 1977. The need for a new medical model: A challenge for biomedicine. *Science* 196(4286):129–36.

Eysenck, H. J., and Eysenck, S. B. 1968. *Eysenck personality manual*. San Diego: Educational and Industrial Testing Service.

Fisher, S. 1970. International survey on the psychological aspects of cardiac rehabilitation. *Scandinavian Journal of Rehabilitative Medicine* 2–3:71–77.

Freud, S. 1963. *The problem of anxiety*. New York: Psychoanalytic Quarterly Press.

Gall, M. D. 1969. The relationship between masculinity-femininity and manifest anxiety. *Journal of Clinical Psychology* 25:294–95.

Graham, W. F. 1981. The anxiety of the runner: Terminal helplessness. In *Psychology of running*, ed. M. H. Sacks and M. L. Sachs. Champaign, Ill.: Human Kinetics Publishers.

Graveling, R. A. 1980. The modification of the hormonal and metabolic effects of mental stress by physical exercise. In *Stress and tension control*, ed. F. J. McGuigan, W. E. Sime, and J. M. Wallace. New York: Plenum Press.

Greist, J. H.; Klein, M. H.; Eischens, R. R.; Faris, J.; Gurman, A. S.; and Morgan, W. P. 1978. Running through your mind. *Journal of Psychosomatic Research* 22: 259–94.

———. 1979. Running as treatment for depression. *Comprehensive Psychiatry* 20: 41–54.

Grove, W. R., and Tudor, J. F. 1973. Adult sex roles and mental illness. In *Changing women in a changing society*, ed. J. Huber. Chicago: University of Chicago Press.

Hamilton, M. 1959. The assessment of anxiety states by rating. *British Journal of Medical Psychology* 32:50–55.

Hammer, S. 1980. How boredom can rev up your life. *Mademoiselle* 86:132–33.

Harper, F. D. 1979. *Jogotherapy: Jogging as a therapeutic strategy*. Alexandria, Va.: Douglass.

Harris, D. V. 1973. Self-concept: Does physical activity affect it? In *Involvement in sport: A somatopsychic rationale for physical activity*. Philadelphia: Lea and Febiger.

Harris, M. B. 1981. Runners perceptions of the benefits of running. *Perceptual and Motor Skills* 52:153–54.

Hathaway, S. R., and McKinley, M. D. 1967. *Minnesota multiphasic personality inventory*. New York: Psychological Corporation.

Higdon, H. 1978. Can running cure mental illness? *Runner's World,* 13:36–43.

Hodges, W. F., and Felling, J. P. 1970. Types of stressful situations and their relationship to trait anxiety and sex. *Journal of Consulting and Clinical Psychology* 34:333–37.

Jasnoski, M. L., and Holmes, D. S. 1981. Influence of initial aerobic fitness, aerobic training and changes in aerobic fitness on personality functioning. *Journal of Psychosomatic Research* 25:553–56.

Joesting, J. 1981a. Comparison of personalities of athletes who sail with those who run. *Perceptual and Motor Skills* 52:514.

————. 1981b. Running and depression. *Perceptual and Motor Skills,* 52:442.

Jones, A. 1979. Running madness. *Running Psychologist* 2(2):17–18.

Joseph, P., and Robbins, J. M. 1981. Worker or runner? The impact of commitment to running and working on self-identification. In *Psychology of running,* ed. M. H. Sacks and M. L. Sachs. Champaign, Ill.: Human Kinetics Publishers.

Justice, B., and McBee, G. W. 1978. Sex differences in psychological distress and social functioning. *Psychological Reports* 43:659–62.

Kaplan, A. G., and Bean, J. P., eds. 1976. *Beyond sex-role stereotypes: Readings toward a psychology of androgyny.* Boston: Little, Brown.

Kavanagh, T.; Shephard, R. J.; and Tuck, J. A. 1975. Depression after myocardial infarction. *Canadian Medical Association Journal* 113:23–27.

Kavanagh, T.; Shephard, R. J.; Tuck, J. A.; and Qureshi, S. 1977. Depression following myocardial infarction: The effects of distance running. *Annals of the New York Academy of Sciences* 301:1029–38.

Klerman, G. L. 1979. The age of melancholy. *Psychology Today* 12:36–42, 88.

Lebovitz, B. Z.; Shekelle, R. B.; Ostfeld, A. M.; and Paul, O. 1967. Prospective and retrospective psychological studies of coronary heart disease. *Psychosomatic Medicine* 29:265–72.

Lilliefors, J. 1978. *The running mind.* Mountain View, Calif.: World Publications.

Lion, L. S. 1978. Psychological effects of jogging: A preliminary study. *Perceptual and Motor Skills* 47:1215–18.

Lubin, B. 1967. *Manual for the depression adjective check lists.* San Diego: Educational and Industrial Testing Service.

Maccoby, E. E., and Jacklin, C. N. 1974. *The psychology of sex differences.* Stanford, Calif.: Stanford University Press.

Mackay, C., and Cox, T. 1974. Stress at work. In *Stress,* ed. T. Cox. Baltimore: University Park Press.

McNair, D. M.; Lorr, M.; and Droppleman, L. F. 1971. *Profile of mood states manual.* San Diego: Educational and Industrial Testing Service.

Mandell, A. J. 1979. The second second wind. *Psychiatric Annals* 9:57–69.

May, R. 1977. *The meaning of anxiety.* Rev. ed. New York: W. W. Norton.

Mitchum, M. L. 1976. The effect of participation in a physically exerting leisure activity on state anxiety level. Master's thesis, Florida State University.

Morgan, W. P. 1973. Influence of acute physical activity on state anxiety. Proceedings, National College Physical Education Association for Men, Seventy-sixth Annual Meeting.

————. 1977. Involvement in vigorous physical activity with special reference to adherence. In *Proceedings of the 1977 National Association of Physical Education for College Women and National College Physical Education Association for Men joint conference,* ed. L. Gedvilas and M. Kneer. Chicago: University of Illinois at Chicago Circle.

————. 1979. Anxiety reduction following acute physical activity. *Psychiatric Annals* 9:141–47.

————. 1980. Test of champions: The iceberg profile. *Psychology Today* 14:92–99, 101, 108.

Morgan, W. P., and Pollock, M. L. 1977. Psychologic characterization of the elite distance runner. *Annals of the New York Academy of Sciences* 301:382–403.

————. 1978. Physical activity and cardiovascular health: Psychological aspects. In *Physical activity and human well-being,* ed. F. Landry and W. A. Orban. Miami, Fla.: Symposia Specialists.

Morgan, W. P.; Roberts, J. A.; Brand, F. R.; and Feinerman, A. D. 1970. Psychological effect of chronic physical activity. *Medicine and Science in Sports* 2:213–17.

Morgan, W. P.; Roberts, J. A.; and Feinerman, A. D. 1971. Psychologic effect of acute physical activity. *Archives of Physical Medicine and Rehabilitation* 52:422–25.

Noble, B. J. 1976. Cardiac rehabilitation: Psychological implications. In *American Alliance for Health, Physical Education, and Recreation Symposia Proceedings.* Washington, D.C.: American Alliance for Health, Physical Education, and Recreation.

Nowlis, V., and Green, R. F. 1957. The experimental analyses of mood. Technical report, Office of Naval Research, contract number Nonr-668.

Pelletier, K. R. 1979. *Holistic medicine.* New York: Delacorte Press.

Penfold, S. 1981. General papers: Women and depression. *Canadian Journal of Psychiatry* 26:24–31.

Petrich, J., and Holmes, T. H. 1977. Life changes and onset of illness. *Medical Clinics of North America* 61:825–38.

Phillips, D. L., and Segal, B. E. 1969. Sexual status and psychiatric symptoms. *American Sociological Review* 34:58–72.

Pollock, M. L. 1978. American College of Sports Medicine position statement on the recommended quantity and quality of exercise for developing and maintaining fitness in healthy adults. *Sports Medicine Bulletin* 13(3):1, 3–4.

Pollock, M. L.; Gettman, L. R.; Milesis, C. A.; Bah, M. D.; Durstine, L.; and Johnson, R. B. 1977. Effects of frequency and duration of training on attrition and incidence of injury. *Medicine and Science in Sports* 9:31–36.

Rossi, A. S. 1980. Life-span theories and women's lives. *Journal of Women in Culture Society* 6:4–32.

Rueter, M. A., and Harris, D. V. 1980. The effects of running on individuals who are clinically depressed. Paper presented at the annual meeting of the American Psychological Association, Montreal.

Sarason, I. G., and Spielberger, C. D. 1976a. *Stress and anxiety.* Vol. 2. New York: John Wiley.

————. 1976b. *Stress and anxiety.* Vol. 3. New York: John Wiley.

————. 1979. *Stress and anxiety.* Vol. 6. New York: John Wiley.

Scarf, M. 1979. The more sorrowful sex. *Psychology Today* 12:45–52, 89–90.

Schalling, D.; Cronholm, B.; and Asberg, M. 1975. Components of state and trait anxiety as related to personality and arousal. In *Emotions: Their parameters and measurement,* ed. L. Levi. New York: Raven Press.

Schwartz, G. E. 1979. Relaxation is not relaxation is not relaxation: Cognitive and somatic patterning in meditation versus exercise. *Tension control: Proceedings of the fifth annual meeting of the American Association for the Advancement of Tension Control,* ed. F. J. McGuigan. Louisville: American Association for the Advancement of Tension Control.

Schwartz, G. E.; Davidson, R. J.; and Goleman, D. J. 1978. Patterning of cognitive and somatic processes in the self-regulation of anxiety: Effects of meditation versus exercise. *Psychosomatic Medicine* 40:321–28.

Secord, P. F., and Jourard, S. M. 1953. The appraisal of body-cathexis: Body-cathexis and the self. *Journal of Consulting Psychology* 17:343–47.

Seligman, M. E. P. 1972. Learned helplessness. *Annual Review of Medicine* 23:407.

Sharkey, B. J. 1979. *Physiology of fitness.* Champaign, Ill.: Human Kinetics Publishers.

Sheehan, G. 1980. Body and soul. *Physician and Sportsmedicine* 8(2):43.

Shephard, R. J., and Cox, M. 1980. Some characteristics of participants in an industrial fitness programme. *Canadian Journal of Applied Sport Sciences* 5:69–78.

Sime, W. E. 1977. A comparison of exercise and meditation in reducing physiological response to stress. *Medicine and Science in Sports* 9:55.

———. 1979. Psychological concomitants of running. In *American Alliance for Health, Physical Education, and Recreation research consortium symposium papers,* vol. 2, book 2, ed. R. Cox. Washington, D.C.: American Alliance for Health, Physical Education, and Recreation.

Snyder, E. E., and Spreitzer, E. 1978. *Social aspects of sport.* Englewood Cliffs, N.J.: Prentice-Hall.

Solomon, E. G., and Bumpus, A. K. 1978. The running meditation response: An adjunct to psychotherapy. *American Journal of Psychotherapy* 32:583–92.

Spielberger, C. D. 1966. Theory and research on anxiety. In *Anxiety and behavior,* ed. C. D. Spielberger. New York: Academic Press.

———. 1972. Current trends in research and theory on anxiety. In *Anxiety: Current trends in theory and research,* vol. 1, ed. C. D. Spielberger. New York: Academic Press.

Spielberger, C. D.; Gorsuch, R. L.; and Lushene, R. 1970. *State-trait anxiety inventory manual.* Palo Alto, Calif.: Consulting Psychologists Press.

Spielberger, C. D., and Sarason, I. G. 1975. *Stress and anxiety.* Vol. 1. New York: John Wiley.

———. 1977. *Stress and anxiety.* Vol. 4. New York: John Wiley.

———. 1978. *Stress and anxiety.* Vol. 5. New York: John Wiley.

Summers, J., and Wolstat, H. 1980. Creative running. *American Medical Joggers Association Newsletter,* November, 20–22.

Tennenbaum, G., and Milgram, R. M. 1978. Trait and state anxiety in Israeli student athletes. *Journal of Clinical Psychology* 34:691–93.

Tharp, G. D., and Schlegelmilch, R. P. 1977. Personality characteristics of trained versus nontrained individuals. *Medicine and Science in Sports* 9:55.

*U.S. News and World Report.* 1979. Is jogging really good for you? Pro and Con, 19 March.

Weissman, M. M., and Klerman, G. L. 1977. Sex differences and epidemiology of depression. *Archives of General Psychiatry* 34:98–111.

Weissman, M. M., and Paykel, E. S. 1974. *The depressed woman: A study of social relationships.* Chicago: University of Chicago Press.

Wilson, V. E.; Berger, B. G.; and Bird, E. I. 1981. Effects of running and of an exercise class on anxiety. *Perceptual and Motor Skills* 53:472–74.

Wilson, V. E.; Morley, N. C.; and Bird, E. I. 1980. Mood profiles of marathon runners, joggers, and non-exercisers. *Perceptual and Motor Skills* 50:117–18.

Wood, D. 1977. The relationship between state anxiety and acute physical activity. *American Corrective Therapy Journal* 31:67–69.

Young, R. J. 1979. The effect of regular exercise on cognitive functioning and personality. *British Journal of Sports Medicine* 13:110–17.

Zuckerman, M., and Lubin, B. 1965. *Manual for the multiple affect adjective check list.* San Diego: Educational and Industrial Testing Service.

Zung, W. W. K. 1965. A self-rating depression scale. *Archives of General Psychiatry* 11:63–70.

# 10

---

# Running toward Psychological Well-being: Special Considerations for the Female Client

As psychologists become more interested in enhancing psychological well-being, exercise therapy is likely to become more prevalent. Running has been found to positively influence self-concept, body awareness, and self-esteem (Andrews 1978; Joesting and Clance 1979; Kurtz and Hirt 1970; Rossi and Zoccolotti 1979; Snyder and Kivlin 1975). By emphasizing traditionally masculine personality characteristics such as vigor and physical competence, running may enable women to become psychologically more androgynous (Harris and Jennings 1977) and thus more capable of responding appropriately in a variety of situations (Bem 1974, 1976, 1979; Spence and Helmreich 1978, 1979). Jogging also gives a woman a wonderful opportunity to increase her conscious awareness of feelings, values, and their underlying psychodynamics. Not only is the woman jogger free to explore her stream of consciousness as she runs, she also can begin to question whether she really wishes to run farther or faster, and even why she chooses to run (Berger 1979; Berger and Mackenzie 1980; Besson 1978, 1979; Schofield and Abbuhl 1975).

In the recent past, only the few women who dared to be athletes could report on the feelings of personal confidence, physical power, and competence gained from developing motor skills and attaining high levels of proficiency (Andrews 1978; Huey 1976; Price 1970). Now the upsurge in women's participation in sports is opening the door for many women to begin exercising or to increase their physical activity. The potential of physical activity, especially running, for improving a woman's self-concept, self-esteem, and body concept is exciting. I shall present current information on each of these concepts to help therapists select the most appropriate strategies for their clients.

## Self-Concept

Traditionally, the self-concept has been described as a collection of tentative hypotheses about the self, primarily learned from other people's responses to the individual (Diggens and Huber 1976; Gergen 1971). As Diggens and Huber noted (1976, 204), self-concept refers not to the person herself, but to what she sees when she stands back from herself. One's self-concept is composed of statements by which one relates oneself to one's environment (Washburn 1962). Since the self-concept is a primary determinant of behavior (Diggens and Huber 1976, 204), its enhancement is an important part of psychotherapy.

### SELF-THEORY

The importance of the self-concept to overall psychological well-being is emphasized by Epstein (1976), who enlarges the definition of self-concept to include nearly all aspects of behavior. Epstein reclassified this broader conceptualization as "self-theory." Like most theories, one's self-theory is a hierarchy of major and minor postulates. Invalidating or changing minor postulates of one's self-theory requires only minimal adjustments and poses no great threat to the theory's stability. But invalidating a major postulate may subject the entire theory to collapse, as in cases of schizophrenic disorganization. The most important function of the self-theory is to maintain a favorable pleasure/pain balance, but it also assimilates the data of significant experiences and helps one maintain self-esteem (Epstein 1976).

A running therapy program that positively influences all three functions of the self-system is more likely to improve a woman's self-concept than other types of running programs. In general, running should result in more overall pleasure than pain, provide new data about the self that influence minor rather than major postulates, and enhance the runner's self-esteem. Running programs that influence major self-theory postulates can also enhance a woman's self-concept, but they require close therapeutic supervision so the resulting disorganization can provide opportunities for adaptation, assimilation, and reorganization.

To the extent that a woman's implicit self-theory can fulfill the three enumerated functions, the theory is stable. She has a sense of well-being, and she is motivated to extend her range of experience. Primarily pleasant emotions result from a stable self-theory and are related to specific response tendencies: attraction to stimulation and social interaction, self-acceptance and acceptance by others, and increased achievement motivation. Dysphoric emotions tend to evoke the opposite responses and result in problem solving or defensiveness (Epstein 1976).

## VERSIONS OF SELF

One woman's concept of self will differ greatly from another's, and each woman has several versions of her self: a *real self,* a *perceived self,* an *ideal self,* and a *self observed by other people* (Gergen 1971; Gough, Lazzari, and Fioravanti 1978; Harris 1973; White 1972). In addition to these four versions of self, people also differ in the number of selves they employ (Snyder 1980). Women who constantly monitor their own behavior and adapt their "real" selves to particular situations have been designated "high self-monitors" (Snyder 1974, 1979, 1980). High self-monitors tend to view their "real" selves as whomever they appear to be at any particular time (Snyder 1980). Although it is not clear what high self-monitors are responding to, they seem to be especially good at anticipating, understanding, and following role prescriptions in particular situations rather than responding to persons around them (Dabbs et al. 1980). High self-monitors have been compared to onions; they have many layers of roles and facades, but no inner core (Campbell and Smith 1976). In contrast to these multiselves, impression managers, or "low self-monitors," have a firmer, more single-minded idea of their "true" selves (Snyder 1974, 1979, 1980). The high self-monitor can be considered either more flexible or more superficial than the low self-monitor.

The desirability of a primary self versus multiple selves and of agreement between real and ideal selves is not clear (Diggens and Huber 1976; Gough, Lazzari, and Fioravanti 1978; Miskimins et al. 1971; Snyder 1980). The multiple selves of high self-monitors allow such women to act appropriately in a variety of social situations and thus evoke positive reactions from others. In fact, an inability to change masks has been observed to reflect severe emotional stress, rigidity, or maladaption (Gergen 1971; Snyder 1980). Despite the benefits of high self-monitoring, a problem may arise because such people communicate very little of their private attitudes and feelings. Jourard (1971) has stated that it is primarily through self-disclosure that a person achieves self-discovery and self-knowledge. Moderate self-monitoring thus seems most desirable.

Women vary widely in the degree of discrepancy between their real and ideal selves. This discrepancy has been labeled both "self-esteem" and "self-image disparity." Psychologists who favor psychodynamic interpretations believe such discrepancies indicate maladjustment; cognitive-developmentalists consider the discrepancies a natural concomitant of normal growth and development (Phillips and Zigler 1980). Since we need to clarify the meaning of real/ideal disparities, it seems safe to conclude that both high and low discrepancies may be related to neuroticism (Diggens and Huber 1976). Self-dissatisfied people (high-discrepancy) tend to be hypochondriacal, depressed, and even psychotic. Self-satisfied (low-discrepancy) individuals tend to be overcontrolling and constricted, to lack candor, and to deny problems. People characterized by moderate amounts of discrepancy are inclined to be reasonable, to accept their self-appraisals, and not to deny their problems (Block and Thomas 1955). Indeed, moderate disparity between real and ideal selves may promote striving for personal improvement and social effectiveness (Gough, Lazzari, and Fioravanti 1978).

GENDER DIFFERENCES

According to observed differences in self-concept between woman and men, women describe both their actual and their ideal selves as more tender, submissive, and socially competent than do men (Bledsoe 1973; Carlson 1965; Maccoby and Jacklin 1974; Moffett 1975; Stoner and Kaiser 1978). However, high self-esteem, indicated by little discrepancy between a person's ideal self and actual self, is significantly and positively related to a man's masculinity score, but not to a woman's femininity score (Sappenfield and Harris 1975). The researchers speculated on the absence of a relation between self-esteem and femininity by noting that masculinity, which connotes assertiveness, competence, and self-reliance, is becoming a desirable characteristic for women as well as for men.

Now more than ever women are recognizing that the traditional feminine gender role, defined by such characteristics as warm, gentle, and eager to soothe hurt feelings, does not enhance one's self-concept. The underlying processes responsible for gender differences in self-concept are illustrated in a promotional flier for *Ms*. magazine. The brochure addresses the woman who wants to scream every time she hears remarks like "May I speak to your husband? It's important" and "You know men don't like girls who are too smart" and encourages women who are offended by such daily assaults upon their self-concepts to buy the magazine. The magazine's success supports the observation that women need and desire to change their self-concepts.

## EFFECT OF RUNNING ON WOMEN'S SELF-CONCEPTS

Linda Huey, a national collegiate record holder, demonstrated the positive relation between her self-concept and running when she remarked, "I yell 'Track!' to a jogger plodding along and whiz by on the inside lane. Again, at last, *I am powerful and in control*. After the workout, I can feel that *the way I carry myself has changed drastically*. I look at my shadow again. *My head is up* and *I'm walking with real sureness and physical pride. 'This is what I've needed.'* I say to myself. 'This is what I've missed' " (Huey 1976, 18; italics added).

Investigating the apparent relation between participation in physical activity and self-concept, researchers have observed a positive and significant correlation between sport participation and the self-concepts of male rehabilitation clients (Collingwood 1972), obese male teenagers (Collingwood and Willett 1971), emotionally disturbed and retarded females and males (Johnson, Fretz, and Johnson 1968), elementary school children of both sexes (Kraft 1978; Martinek, Cheffers, and Zaichkowsky 1978; Zaichkowsky, Zaichkowsky, and Martinek 1978), and seventh-grade boys who were low in self-concept (McGowan, Jarman, and Pedersen 1974). As happens in many areas of psychological research, other investigators have failed to find a significant relation (Darden 1972; Leonardson and Gargiulo 1978).

In one of the few studies focusing specifically on the effectiveness of running in elevating students' self-concepts, Hilyer and Mitchell (1979) compared three types of college physical education classes. (1) running and stretching; (2) running and stretching plus personalized counseling; and (3) a control class of "basic physical education." The forty-three women and seventy-seven men were randomly assigned to the various treatments and exercised one hour three times a week for ten weeks. Unfortunately the experimenters made no attempt to examine a possible gender influence when investigating the effects of exercise on self-concept. The counseling group met with the experimenters for an additional hour each week, during which students expressed their feelings about the activity, learned facts about the value of exercise, were taught techniques for dealing with the occasional unpleasantness inherent in exercise, and were assisted in setting their own exercise goals in a supportive, accepting atmosphere.

As in most field studies, a host of contaminating factors precluded definitive conclusions. The two experimenters together taught the running and counseling groups; someone else taught the regular physical education group. No attempt was made to control for a halo effect or for the increased attention and faculty-student interaction in the counseling group. Time alone—four hours rather than three hours a week during the ten weeks—may have accounted for the enhanced effectiveness of the counseling group. Despite such practical methodological problems, the systematic changes in overall self-concept scores for students who were below the mean in the pretest were impressive. The low-self-concept students in the running-plus-counseling group showed the greatest changes in both overall and subscale measures. Students in the running group that had no counseling also significantly improved their overall self-concept scores as measured before and after the ten-week program. In support of their initial hypotheses, Hilyer and Mitchell found no evidence that the regular physical education students changed in self-concept. No change was reported by students who were above the mean in self-concept; thus it seems these students had already learned they were adequate and capable.

Hilyer and Mitchell (1979) speculated that the running program influenced self-concept through generalized increases in efficiency and physical functioning and through a sense of mastery or control over self and the environment. Not only did the counseling program help students overcome the difficulties and resistance common in the beginning programs, but it was viewed as reinforcing the natural benefits of running. Exercise counseling, in addition to the actual exercise program, may shorten the time necessary for normally occurring changes in self-concept. Future studies are needed to determine the relative durability of the changes in self-concept resulting from running alone and from running plus counseling and also to establish whether and how long one must continue to exercise to maintain the changes in self-concept.

Additional support for a positive relation between exercise and self-concept has been provided by Sharp and Reilley (1975), who reported that aerobic fitness scores were related to favorable responses about self on the MMPI, and by Leonardson (1977), who observed a positive relation between perceived rather than actual physical fitness and the self-concepts of high-school students. It seems likely that physical activity improves a woman's image of her body (Joesting and Clance 1979; Kurtz and Hirt 1970; Snyder and Kivlin 1975) and her feelings of competence (Roberts, Duda, and Kleiber 1980), which in turn are related to her self-concept (Mahoney 1978; Rosen and Ross 1968; Weinberg 1960).

Of particular importance when examining the influence of running on women's self-concepts is the possibility that running might create gender-role conflicts for particularly "feminine" women (Corbin and Nix 1979; Wark and Wittig 1979). Traditionally, the "athlete" and "woman" roles have been dissonant. Marty Liquori, a world-class runner, commented on this conflict; "They can take two young girls of equal talent and ability, one being great looking and the other being ugly and the great looking one won't stand a chance of making it in the athletic world. She'll have too many alternatives presented to her, too many social pressures put on her. But the ugly girl will probably stay with athletics as her one form of outlet for success and recognition" (Huey 1976, 10). Huey emphasized the poignancy of Liquori's observation by concluding, "I didn't realize then that reconciling the female-athlete dichotomy would take me through a series of identity crises. I thought of myself as an exception, but I was wrong" (Huey 1976, 11).

Because sports participation may be unacceptable to a woman who is highly sex-typed, it is not surprising that the results of some studies examining the relation between women's self-concepts and physical activity are ambiguous. Because of differences in methodology, in the sports included, and in the scales used to measure self-concept, as well as the changing role models of women, interstudy comparisons are unproductive. In spite of the problems, however, there is an emerging body of evidence for a positive relation between a woman's self-concept and participation in certain types of physical activity (Cochran et al. 1977; McElroy and Willis 1979; Snyder and Kivlin 1975; Snyder, Kivlin, and Spreitzer 1976; Van der Merwe 1982; Vincent 1976). As Snyder, Kivlin, and Spreitzer (1976) concluded, the expected negative associations between female sports participation and self-concept often are not observed.

Jorgenson and Jorgenson (1979) examined the relation between habitual running and the perception of self and others. Female and male runners who had averaged about twenty-two miles a week during the preceding three years completed a questionnaire that focused on their perceptions of change produced by the running. No significant differences were observed between females' and males' perceptions, and thus there was no evidence of a gender-role conflict for the women runners. An extremely high proportion (92 percent) of the runners perceived increased emotional well-being as a result of running; 73 percent reported an increase in the number of their friendships; 68 percent indicated they felt more critical of those who seemed out of shape physically. Further evidence of enhanced self-concept was that 74 percent of those who lived with their families perceived an increase in their families' appreciation of their physical appearance. The retrospective nature of the study precluded comparison of the perceived changes with actual changes in self-concept.

### Self-Esteem

Self-esteem is one's conception of the relation between one's real and ideal selves (Christian 1978; Rogers and Dymond 1954) and defines one's perception of one's own worth (Ziller et al. 1969). As I said earlier, unusually large and unusually small difference scores tend to indicate poor mental health. A person with low self-esteem feels there is a huge gap between who she is and who she wants to be. Conversely, someone with exceedingly high self-esteem may feel she is "perfect."

## ANDROGYNY

Androgyny, the possession of both feminine and masculine personality characteristics, enables a person to respond appropriately and competently without being constricted by stereotyped ideas about gender-appropriate behavior (Bem 1974, 1976, 1979; Locksley and Colten 1979; Pedhazur and Tetenbaum 1979; Spence and Helmreich 1978, 1979; Spence, Helmreich, and Stapp 1974). In her reflective review of the literature on androgyny, Gilbert (1981) indicated that the generally accepted stereotypes of masculine and feminine personality traits are consistent with Parson and Bales's (1955) description of *instrumental* qualities in men and *expressive* qualities in women and also with Bakan's (1966) concept of *agency,* or sense of self, as a masculine principle and *communion,* or sense of selflessness, as a feminine principle. The reconception of masculinity and femininity as coexisting within the same person has led to the hypothesis that androgynous rather than gender-typed individuals enjoy better mental health and are personally more effective (Deutsch and Gilbert 1976; Gilbert 1981; Jones, Chernovetz, and Hansson 1978).

The importance of androgyny for women's psychological health has been noted by Kaschak (1976), who reported that it was *impossible* to be a healthy adult woman and at the same time a healthy human being defined by male psychological traits. Successful women, who should have high self-esteem, tend to view themselves as "imposters" who have fooled others into thinking they are intelligent (Clance and Imes 1978). Emphasizing the importance of androgyny for both women and men, Bem (1979, 1053) concluded:

If there is a moral to the concept of psychological androgyny, it is that behavior should have no gender. But there is an irony here, for the concept of androgyny contains an inner contradiction and hence the seeds of its own destruction. . . . But to the extent that the androgynous message is absorbed by the culture, the concepts of femininity and masculinity will cease to have such content and the distinctions to which they refer will blur into invisibility. Thus, when androgyny becomes a reality, the *concept* of androgyny will have been transcended.

According to the traditional concepts of femininity and masculinity, the terms represent opposite ends of a single continuum. The greater one's femininity, the lower must be one's masculinity and vice versa. The more recent formulations of gender roles (Bakan 1966; Bem 1974, 1976, 1979; Constantinople 1973; Spence and Helmreich 1978; Spence, Helmreich, and Stapp 1974) depict the coexistence of femininity and masculinity in the same person. Anyone can be assigned to one of four groups according to the interrelation of their masculine and feminine scores on the Personal Attributes Questionnaire (PAQ) (Spence, Helmreich, and Stapp 1974);

1. *feminine,* this person's femininity score is much higher than their masculinity score,
2. *masculine,* this person's masculinity score is much higher than their femininity score,
3. *androgynous,* this person has high scores on both scales, and
4. *undifferentiated,* this person has low scores on both scales. (Helmreich and Spence 1977).

Bem (1977), the author of another commonly employed test of psychological androgyny, also noted a need to distinguish between individuals who are high in both femininity and masculinity, or "androgynous," and those who are low in both characteristics, or "undifferentiated." Undifferentiated individuals of both sexes repeatedly have been observed to be lowest of the four groups in self-esteem as measured on the Texas Social Behavior Inventory (Bem 1977; Helmreich and Spence 1977; Helmreich and Stapp 1974; Helmreich, Stapp, and Ervin 1974; Spence, Helmreich, and Stapp 1974). Feminine individuals were the next lowest in self-esteem. Psychologically masculine and androgynous individuals, regardless of sex, were highest in self-esteem. These results differ slightly from those of Jones, Chernovetz, and Hansson (1978), who observed that masculine rather than androgynous individuals of both sexes had the highest self-esteem scores.

Women athletes and scientists in the Helmreich and Spence (1977) study were preponderantly classified as "androgynous" or "masculine." This was strikingly different from the classification of female college students, who were predominantly in the "feminine" category (Helmreich and Spence 1977). Helmreich and Spence concluded:

> Thus, it appears that, following our conceptual and empirical analyses, those women who have outwardly specifiable, agentic concerns also score higher on our measure of masculinity. The joint distribution also suggests that those women (both athletes and scientists) who succeed in those areas of endeavor defined as stereotypically masculine do not do this at the expense of their

femininity. Indeed, these data suggest that rather than suffering a deficiency of femininity, *high achieving women . . . are more likely than their male counterparts to possess both masculine and feminine attributes*. At the least, these data suggest that *our stereotypic conceptions of masculinity and femininity in relation to achieving women may have been overly simplistic*. (p. 42; italics added)

Comparing the androgyny characteristics of female and male physical education majors and athletes, Duquin (1977) found that both the women majors and the women athletes were more androgynous than the men and more androgynous than Bem's sample at Stanford. Whether participating in the physical activity actually influenced the women's androgyny or whether the physical education majors and athletes were different from the beginning could not be determined because of the retrospective design of the study.

Rather than being negative characteristics for women, both androgyny and masculinity have been found to be related to desirable behaviors, social competence, mental health, and high self-esteem (Deutsch and Gilbert 1976; Flaherty and Dusek 1980; Gilbert 1981; Harris and Jennings 1977; O'Connor, Mann, and Bardwick 1978). Since women who participate in individual sports tend to have more positive self-concepts than women who play team sports and than those who do not participate in any physical activity (Cochran et al. 1977), running may be a particularly successful therapeutic approach to improving a woman's self-esteem. An article by a woman who had just completed her first marathon supports the experimental literature (Karetsky 1978). She described her development as a runner as follows: "At first the effort was exhausting. Sometimes I felt discouraged and lonely. Then, after six weeks, I sensed a change. My body was growing stronger. I was developing as an athlete. But something more was happening. I was developing as a woman too. I felt different about myself. *Brave. And strong. And beautiful*. (p. 9; italics added)

In their study of the self-perceptions of women distance runners, Harris and Jennings (1977) reported that both scholastic runners who ranged between fourteen and twenty-three years of age and club runners between twenty-six and fifty-nine tended to be either androgynous or masculine as measured by the PAQ. These results are in direct agreement with those of Duquin (1977) mentioned previously. Again the retrospective nature of the study precluded obtaining information about cause or effect.

Balazs and Nickerson (1976) also produced evidence that women athletes tend to demonstrate personality characteristics traditionally considered masculine. As indicated by their scores on the Edwards Personal Preference Schedule, national-class women athletes scored in the seventieth percentile on the *autonomy* scale and in the seventy-fourth percentile on *achievement*, indicating that they were considerably higher than the normative population in these characteristics. These women athletes liked to make their own decisions, to accomplish tasks that required effort and skill, to do their best, and to be unconventional and nonconforming. They also scored lower than the "average" woman (whose scores fall between the fortieth and sixtieth percentiles) on affiliation (thirty-eighth percentile) and on intraception (thirty-fifth percentile). They had little need to do things with others, had little concern for what others thought of them, and tended not to analyze their own actions. Since otherwise the women's personality scores resembled those of the normative female population, these women athletes who possessed both masculine and feminine characteristics can be considered androgynous.

Del Rey and Sheppard (1981) have produced additional evidence that, among women athletes, those who were androgynous (PAQ) were significantly higher in self-esteem as measured by the Texas Social Behavior Inventory (Helmreich, Stapp, and Ervin 1974) than those who were either feminine or undifferentiated. No attempt was made to separate the 119 women athletes, who attended three large universities in different parts of the country, according to type of sport. Since the androgynous women athletes were significantly higher in self-esteem, Del Ray and Sheppard reported that stereotypically feminine women were operating with an impoverished model in regard to self-esteem. They concluded that competitive sports may provide ideal training environments for women who wish to become more androgynous and thus raise their self-esteem.

## RAISING SELF-ESTEEM

Although low self-esteem seems to seriously impair psychological well-being and achievement, little information is available on what can be done to raise self-esteem (Baron, Bass, and Vietze 1971; Parrott and Hewitt 1978). Noting that psychotherapy (Rogers and Dymond 1954), experience in sensitivity training groups (Gibb 1971), and learning to swim (Kocher 1971) have had positive effects, Parrott and Hewitt (1978) investigated the effects of three programs on self-esteem. The program of major interest, a goal-attainment program, required subjects to maintain a daily checklist stating degree of compliance in meeting ten specific goals thought by the experimenters to raise self-esteem. Two of the ten goals could be satisfied or promoted by running: ten minutes of exercise, and ideal weight achievement. In a second program, the participants were instructed to enjoy themselves rather than to work on goal attainment—thus it was the opposite of the goal-attainment condition. Since an

Table 1. Sample Checklist for Use in Developing
Achievable, Important Running Goals

| DAILY RUNNING GOALS | Date _____ | | | | | | |
|---|---|---|---|---|---|---|---|
| | Days That Goals Are Successfully Completed | | | | | | |
| | S | M | Tu | W | Th | F | S |
| 1. Today's run maintains a pattern of running every other day. (Runners can take one day a week off to maintain a schedule of running three times a week.) | | | | | | | |
| 2. Today I completed my personal goal of running/walking continuously for twenty minutes. | | | | | | | |
| 3. I did at least five minutes of stretching exercises. | | | | | | | |
| 4. I ran/walked two miles. | | | | | | | |
| 5. (If underweight) I ate three meals today, regardless of how much I ate at one meal. | | | | | | | |
| or | | | | | | | |
| (If overweight) I eliminated a dessert at a meal and ate less starch than usual. | | | | | | | |

increase in self-esteem was observed only in the goal-attainment program, compliance with important goals seems to enhance self-esteem, especially in people who are low initially. Parrott and Hewitt cautioned that they did not ascertain whether their ten goals were important personal goals for the subjects.

Based on Parrott and Hewitt's observations that those with low self-esteem who were in the goal-attainment condition significantly increased in self-esteem, therapist and client together might set reachable running-related goals that are important to the client. By using a daily checklist to indicate degree of compliance, the client receives immediate reinforcement for the desired behavior and is reminded of her goals. Table 1 suggests client-related running goals. After the first weeks of running, the client and therapist may alter the goals as needed.

Although those with low self-esteem significantly increased their self-esteem by participating in Parrott and Hewitt's goal-attainment condition, they rated the procedure low in terms of being enjoyable and worthwhile. Apparently they preferred to indulge themselves or to talk about their problems to others rather than actively pursue activities meant to raise their self-concepts. The therapist who expects such responses can be prepared to offer weekly encouragement, to reinforce the importance of the program, to reevaluate particular items on the checklist, and to support the client's continuation. (Refer to chap. 2 for additional information about initial compliance and adherence.)

In an investigation of the influence of praise on both task performance and self-esteem, Baron, Bass, and Vietze (1971) noted that a low frequency of praise (25 percent) was significantly more effective in enhancing women's self-images than a higher (75 percent) frequency. They explained that low-frequency praise was more effective for enhancing women's self-image because it was more consistent with the women's past experience and thus more creditable, so it had greater persuasive influence. Although the subjects in this study were black women of relatively low socioeconomic status, the general observation that the therapist's praise should be consistent with the client's previous experience as well as with task accomplishment probably can be generalized to most women.

Analyses of sex differences in the components of self-esteem indicate that women's self-esteem, in contrast to men's, is contingent on their certainty that other people like them (Berger 1968). The results of the previously mentioned study by Baron, Bass, and Vietze (1971) support the importance of the social element in women's self-esteem. Praise of the *person* rather than praise of *task* performance significantly enhanced women's self-concepts as measured by several subscales of the Tennessee Self-Concept Scale (Fitts 1965). It seems that a client's social concerns are important considerations in encouraging her to participate in a running program. Novice women runners tend to be particularly sensitive to the reactions of others. Concerns about what to wear, where to run, running form, and what others will think if she runs slowly should be acknowledged and explored during therapy.

### Body Concept

Closely allied to self-concept and self-esteem is body concept, a broad, rather vague term that includes a host of components. Some of these components are (1) *body cathexis,* the degree of acceptance and rejection of various body parts or processes such as hair, complexion, appetite, and height (Secord and Jourard 1953); (2) *body image* and *body boundaries* as indicated by barrier and penetration scores (Fisher 1963; Fisher and Cleveland 1958); and (3) *body awareness,* which is reflected in a person's awareness of different zones or parts of the body (Fisher 1970; Fisher and Cleveland 1958).

BODY CATHEXIS

Secord and Jourard (1953) theorized that body cathexis is integral to the self-concept. As stated by Fisher (1973, ix), "all that you perceive, think, and believe occurs in the context of your body experiences." Testing the Body Cathexis-Self-Concept Scale, Secord and Jourard (1953) produced evidence that (1) feelings about the body are commensurate with feelings about one's self; (2) low body cathexis is associated with anxiety; and (3) low body cathexis is associated with insecurity. As noted in Fisher's first two studies (1964), women were less inclined than men to be satisfied (body cathexis) with their legs (Bennett 1960; Calden, Lundy, and Schlafer 1959; Wittreich and Grace 1955). Fisher (1964) attributed this gender difference in body cathexis to two independent factors. Women, more than men, are judged in appearance according to their legs. And men enjoy greater mobility and movement in space, primarily accomplished by the use of their legs. Assuming the accuracy of this second explanation, increasing a woman's mobility by encouraging her to run would enhance her satisfaction with her legs.

In a comparison of the body cathexes of nationally ranked women athletes (basketball players and gymnasts) and women nonathletes, Snyder and Kivlin (1975) reported significant differences between the athletes and nonathletes on twenty-five of the twenty-nine items in the modified Secord and Jourard scale (1953). These findings were particularly impressive because each of the differences favored the athletes. The athletes clearly had more positive feelings toward their legs, hips, faces, arms, busts, and so forth than the nonathletes. In addition to their positve body cathexes, the athletes were significantly higher than nonathletes on three measures of psychological well-being.

In one of the few studies of runners and body cathexis, Joesting and Clance (1979) observed that male runners who participated in local races were significantly more positive than nonrunners on the Body-Cathexis and Self-Cathexis scales (Secord and Jourard 1953). The differences between women runners and nonrunners were in the direction hypothesized but were not significant. The failure to find a difference between women runners and nonrunners in a single study is difficult to interpret. Running may not affect women's body cathexes, or the effect simply may not have been evident in this particular study. A question that arises from the work of Joesting and Clance is whether the body cathexis of women runners who do not compete in races is more positive than those of nonrunners.

## BODY IMAGE AND BODY BOUNDARIES

Substantial evidence has been produced that body image and body definiteness are highly related to psychophysiological patterns of reactivity, adjustment to physical disability, ego integration, and communicative skills in small groups (Fisher 1963, 1970, 1973). More recently, interest in this area has focused on the relation of body awareness to personality (Bruchon-Schweitzer 1979; Fisher 1970; Vinck 1979) and on the relation between body boundaries and the aging process (Phillips 1979).

Harris (1974) reviewed the literature on body image and related it to participation in physical activity. Harris made the important observation that body image undoubtedly influences choice of and participation in sports. It is difficult to speculate about the body image conducive to a woman's becoming a runner; however, a high barrier score and a low penetration score would tend to permit her greater freedom to begin this activity. Since women's body cathexis has been shown to change as a result of an awareness-training class (Clance, Matthews, and Joesting 1979), and since men, who tend to be more physically active than women, judged their bodies to be significantly more potent and active than did women (Kurtz 1969), it seems logical that successful participation in a running therapy program would positively affect a woman's body cathexis, body image, and body awareness.

## BODY AWARENESS

Contrary to much psychological theory that postulates that women are less satisfied with their bodies than men and less able to arrive at an articulated, realistic body concept (body awareness), Fisher (1964) presented several converging lines of evidence showing that women have more definite, stable body concepts than men. Subsequent studies have supported women's more accurate body concepts (Kurtz 1969). One interpretation of women's superior body awareness is that a woman's body is more closely related to her "principal" life goals of being attractive to men, marrying, and bearing children. Regardless of the underlying dynamics, the results are encouraging because refined body boundaries and perception are thought to be directly related to a clear definition of self and to body security (Bruchon-Schweitzer 1979; Fisher 1963; Fisher and Cleveland 1958; Mahoney 1974).

Although a woman's body awareness may be more differentiated and accurate than a man's, physical activity in the form of running probably would heighten it. Indeed, in a study of the body perception of male athletes and nonathletes, Rossi and Zoccolotti (1979) found that the athletes were significantly more accurate in judging body dimensions in comparison to objects than were the nonathletes. One might surmise that the same results would be observed for women runners and nonrunners.

### Self-Awareness and Insight

Running provides a woman with an outstanding opportunity to increase awareness of her feelings and behavior and encourages her to examine the underlying psychodynamics (Berger 1979; Berger and Mackenzie 1980; Besson 1978, 1979; Henning 1978; Schofield and Abbuhl 1975). In an attempt to understand why running is meaningful to so many women, Berger and Mackenzie (1980) conducted a case study of a woman runner in her mid-thirties and investigated her stream of consciousness while she was running. The data analyzed included the runner's recordings of her thought processes during thirty-three running sessions over a four-month period and material from three recorded psychiatric interview seesions of approximately fifty minutes, conducted during the final weeks of the study. The following hypotheses reflect broad areas of the woman's thoughts and illustrate the potential of running for increasing self-awareness. They were intended as guides for analyzing data collected from this one individual and are not necessarily applicable to everyone, but they do seem to demonstrate some of the therapeutic effects of jogging.

*Hypothesis 1: "Participation in sports involves experiencing a wide spectrum of emotions ranging from agony to ecstasy"* (Berger and Mackenzie 1980, 7)

As Berger (1979) noted, running provides an opportunity to experience emotions in a relatively nonthreatening environment and thus is particularly important as a therapeutic technique for the woman who is unaware of and cut off from many emotions. Examples of the emotions reported by the woman runner included *competence,* "When I started out, I really felt strong. Went fast and felt great. Seem to recover quickly (p. 7); *control,* "I was watching the lights. Timing everything. I was dodging traffic and I felt like cars couldn't hurt me. . . . I feel great, energetic, alive, the master of my fate" (p. 8); and *guilt,*

"I steal time from things that I should be doing to jog. . . . What else do I have to do? Dinner has to be on the table at 5:30. . . . It's taking time from him [her son]" (p. 8).

*Hypothesis 2: "Sports such as jogging are conducive to introspection as well as to thinking in general"* (Berger and Mackenzie 1980, 8)

Supporting the introspective nature of running, the woman reported, "When I'm running, it seems like I'm dreaming and a lot of thoughts go through my mind very, very quickly" (p. 8). The following personal description of the meaning of running by a psychologist supports the tendency for introspection to occur while running (Shainberg 1977, 1003):

> I am aware that my brain is seeking a kind of order when my memories appear, . . . thought sequences that have *nothing to do with the present run.* . . . Despite the fact that there are an infinite number of details to face every minute, *my brain persists in this habit of going over old situations.* In a way, the brain operates during the run as *it does in dreams,* where the *incomplete events of the day are reworked.* On the run, *puzzles from other parts of life tend to appear.* The past *invades the present,* and attention to the run is shifted to what has been. (Italics added)

Kostrubala (1976) also noted experiencing a dreamlike state while running (see also Kostrubala, chap. 7, on running and therapy):

> In this new therapeutic role, I was doing something markedly different. I was directly participating in the action with the patient—we were both running. And we experienced similar phenomena. . . . If I compare this technique of therapy with *dream analysis, it's like dreaming the same dream as the patient at the same time.* The therapy was immediate. The nuances were immediately available and *my own unconscious was more visible to me and to my patients.* At times, it seemed as if the *archetypes within us rose up to consciousness and lived and talked as we ran along.* (p. 131; italics added)

Noting the introspective opportunities in running, Andrews (1978), in *The Psychic Power of Running,* elaborated on the possibility that running unravels the mysteries of the unconscious.

Experimental evidence for this hypothesis is provided by Hartung and Farge (1977), Ismail and Trachtman (1973), and Simono, Dawson, and Murphy (1979), who reported high imagination scores, as measured by factor M on Cattell's Sixteen Personality Factor Questionnaire, for middle-aged men who participated in supervised fitness or running programs. According to the definition of factor M, high scorers not only tend to have imagination but also are inner-directed, creative, and self-directed (Cattell, Eber, and Tatsuoka 1970). Speculating on the underlying basis for the relationship between factor M and running, Simono, Dawson, and Murphy (1979) noted a strong relation between imagination, physical energy, and health.

*Hypothesis 3: "Engagement in sport satisfies inner psychodynamic needs"* (Berger and Mackenzie 1980, 9)

This hypothesis is particularly important for choosing running as a therapeutic technique. If running does satisfy the inner psychodynamic needs of the participant as Berger and Mackenzie report and as is supported in numerous anecdotal accounts (Anderson 1978; Libby 1978; Shainberg 1977), then jogging may not be compatible with the personality dynamics of all women. Clients who do not like jogging for a variety of reasons may really be saying that running is not the right physical activity for them. The therapist will become adept at distinguishing those women who are simply unfamiliar with exercise procedures and thus are exploring the unknown from those whose personalities are not suitable for running. Some of the physical responses to running that all inexperienced runners will encounter, accept, and perhaps at times enjoy include sensations described by Shainberg (1977, 1004):

> Some days when it is very humid (or cold, or raining), I develop a certain weakness in my knees and legs. I feel that I can't go on; I feel the weather is weighing me down, I am sweating more than usual, and *my legs feel they will not hold me enough to get up this next incline*. There is a sensation of a *big hole at* the bottom of my stomach and my brain *does not bring me the air I need* in this hole. *I am complaining* about running today and *I feel afraid. Finally I stop. I walk.* Suddenly *I realize a silence.* The connection of all these parts is not clear, but when I stop, the *anxious grabbing* is no longer there. (Italics added)

For women who truly dislike the solitary nature of running, its lack of competitive strategy, or its repetitiveness, other psychotherapeutic approaches would be more productive.

*Hypothesis 4: "Awareness of private phenomenological experiences associated with sport can be useful for gaining self-understanding"* (Berger and Mackenzie 1980, 14)

This last hypothesis is highly dependent on a person's openness to personal feelings, her willingness to explore them, and the assistance of the therapist. An example of the woman runner's quest for self-knowledge in the study by Berger and Mackenzie is reflected in her own analysis of her competitive behavior and her dislike of running an unmeasured distance. "I just won't know how far I've gone. . . . Being in great competition with myself, I find that greatly distracting. Why do I get caught up in this race with myself? Can I tolerate not knowing how far I've gone?'' (p. 14). As Berger and Mackenzie noted, having a client run immediately before or even during a therapy session seems to be a particularly productive technique (Kostrubala 1976, 126–61). Kostrubala stated emphatically the powers of running in enhancing the quest for self-knowledge. ''It [running] fostered analysis. It helped the individual discover new depths within himself. . . . It stimulates the unconscious and is a powerful catalyst to the individual psyche'' (p. 133). A psychologist also illustrated the opportunities for self-understanding in his article describing the meditative qualities of running (Shainberg 1977). Such open and introspective reflections would be particularly useful in a therapy session during or immediately after a run while the client still remembers the material.

> Sometimes I cannot help myself, but there is some problem which will have its way. This problem is completely absorbing. I find, for example, that I am thinking of *my early life, my relationship with my mother* when I was an infant, *my fears* in that relationship. It is best when *I watch all of these different, flashing thoughts*. . . . During such runs, *I have discovered patterns in my relationship to my brother, my father, my children, my wife, and my mother*. The *whole panorama goes by* and I *often feel a deeper acceptance* after having been able to run and be *with the whole movement without judgment or choice*. I simply recognize all of this is what makes up my being for the day. (Shainberg 1977, 1004; italics added)

Additional evidence that physical activity is useful in stimulating insight was presented in an experimental study by Schofield and Abbuhl (1975). A significant difference in responsiveness on a projective test was observed between high-school women who had done five minutes of warmup exercises before testing and a control group of nonexercising participants. Although the underlying reasons for the differences remained unclear, Schofield and Abbuhl speculated that either the specific physical activity itself lowered the women's defenses and inhibitions for both experiencing and expressing thoughts and feelings, or that body movement in general stimulated cognitive functioning and thus permitted greater insight and self-awareness.

### Note

Although directed toward female clients, the information contained here is certainly relevant for males as well. I wish to thank Dr. Jerome Winter for his constructive comments on this chapter.

# References

Anderson, B. 1978. Philosophy, part 1: The running movement. *On the Run,* 20 April, 1.

Andrews, V. 1978. *The psychic power of running.* New York: Ballantine Books.

Bakan, D. 1966. *The duality of human existence.* Chicago: Rand McNally.

Balazs, E., and Nickerson, E. 1976. A personality needs profile of some outstanding female athletes. *Journal of Clinical Psychology* 32:45–49.

Baron, R. M.; Bass, A. R.; and Vietze, P. M. 1971. Type and frequency of praise as determinants of favorability of self-image: An experiment in a field setting. *Journal of Personality* 39:492–511.

Bem, S. L. 1974. The measurement of psychological androgyny. *Journal of Consulting and Clinical Psychology* 42:155–62.

———. 1976. Probing the promise of androgyny. In *Beyond sex-role stereotypes: Readings toward a psychology of androgyny,* ed. A. G. Kaplan and J. P. Bean. Boston: Little, Brown.

———. 1977. On the utility of alternative procedures for assessing psychological androgyny. *Journal of Consulting and Clinical Psychology* 45:196–205.

———. 1979. Theory and measurement of androgyny: A reply to the Pedhazur-Tetenbaum and Locksley-Colten critiques. *Journal of Personality and Social Psychology* 37:1047–54.

Bennett, D. H. 1960. The body concept. *Journal of Mental Science* 105:56–57.

Berger, B. G. 1979. The meaning of regular jogging: A phenomenological approach. *American Alliance for Health, Physical Education, and Recreation research consortium symposium papers,* vol. 2, book 2, ed. R. Cox. Washington, D.C.: American Alliance for Health, Physical Education, and Recreation.

Berger, B. G., and Mackenzie, M. M. 1980. A case study of a woman jogger: A psychodynamic analysis. *Journal of Sport Behavior* 3:3–16.

Berger, C. R. 1968. Sex differences related to self esteem factor structure. *Journal of Consulting and Clinical Psychology* 32:442–46.

Besson, G. 1978. *The complete woman runner.* Mountain View, Calif.: World Publications.

———. 1979. Inner workings of the woman runner. *Runner's World,* January, 62–68.

Bledsoe, J. C. 1973. Sex differences in self-concept: Fact or artifact? *Psychological Reports* 32:1252–54.

Block, J., and Thomas, H. 1955. Is satisfaction with self a measure of adjustment? *Journal of Abnormal and Social Psychology* 51:254–59.

Bruchon-Schweitzer, M. 1979. Dimensionality of body perception and personality. *Perceptual and Motor Skills* 48:840–42.

Calden, G.; Lundy, R. M.; and Schlafer, R. J. 1959. Sex differences in body concepts. *Journal of Consulting Psychology* 23:378.

Campbell, C., and Smith, M. B. 1976. Our many versions of the self. *Psychology Today* 9 (February): 74–79.

Carlson, R. 1965. Stability and change in the adolescent image. *Child Development* 37:13–16.

Cattell, R. B.; Eber, H. W.; and Tatsuoka, M. M. 1970. *Handbook for the 16PF.* Champaign, Ill.: Institute for Personality and Ability Testing.

Christian, K. W. 1978. Aspects of the self-concept related to level of self esteem. *Journal of Consulting and Clinical Psychology* 46:1151–52.

Clance, P. R., and Imes, S. A. 1978. The imposter phenomenon in high achieving women: Dynamics and therapeutic intervention. *Psychotherapy: Theory, Research, and Practice* 15:241–47.

Clance, P. R.; Matthews, T. V.; and Joesting, J. 1979. Body-cathexis and self-cathexis in an interactional, awareness training class. *Perceptual and Motor Skills* 48:221–22.

Cochran, T.; Aiken, G.; Hartman, K.; and Young, I. 1977. A comparative study of the self-image and body-image of female and male college team and individual athletes and nonathletes. In *Human performance and behavior: Proceedings of the Ninth Canadian Psychomotor Learning and Sport Psychology Symposium,* ed B. Kerr, Banff, Alberta. Calgary, Alberta: University of Calgary.

Collingwood, T. R. 1972. The effects of physical training upon behavior and self attitudes. *Journal of Clinical Psychology* 28:583–85.

Collingwood, T. R., and Willett, L. 1971. The effects of physical training upon self-concept and body attitude. *Journal of Clinical Psychology* 27:411–12.

Constantinople, A. 1973. Masculinity-femininity: An exception to the famous dictum. *Psychological Bulletin* 80:389–407.

Corbin, C. B., and Nix, C. 1979. Sex-typing of physical activities and success predictions of children before and after cross-sex competition. *Journal of Sport Psychology* 1:43–52.

Dabbs, J. J.; Evans, M. S.; Hopper, C. H.; and Purvis, J. A. 1980. Self-monitors in conversation: What do they monitor? *Journal of Personality and Social Psychology* 39:278–84.

Darden, E. 1972. A comparison of body image and self-concept variables among various sport groups. *Research Quarterly* 43:7–15.

Del Rey, P., and Sheppard, S. 1981. Relationship of psychological androgyny in female athletes to self-esteem. *International Journal of Sport Psychology* 12:165–75.

Deutsch, C. J., and Gilbert, L. A. 1976. Sex role stereotypes: Effect on perceptions of self and others and on personal adjustment. *Journal of Counseling Psychology* 23:373–79.

Diggens, D., and Huber, J. 1976. Self: How are you affected by the way you see yourself? In *The human personality,* ed. D. Diggens and J. Huber. Boston: Little, Brown.

Duquin, M. E. 1977. Perception and sport: A study in sexual attraction. In *Psychology of motor behavior and sport,* vol. 2, ed. R. W. Christina and D. M. Landers. Champaign, Ill.: Human Kinetics Publishers.

Epstein, S. 1976. Anxiety, arousal, and the self-concept. In *Stress and anxiety* vol. 3, ed. I. G. Sarason and C. D. Spielberger. New York: John Wiley.

Fisher, S. 1963. A further appraisal of the body boundary concept. *Journal of Consulting Psychology* 27:62–74.

———. 1964. Sex differences in body perception. *Psychological Monographs: General and Applied* 78:1–22.

———. 1970. *Body experience in fantasy and behavior*. New York: Appleton-Century-Crofts.

———. 1973. *Body consciousness: You are what you feel*. Englewood Cliffs, N.J.: Prentice-Hall.

Fisher, S., and Cleveland, S. E. 1958. *Body image and personality*. Princeton, N.J.: Van Nostrand.

Fitts, W. H. 1965. *Tennessee Self-Concept Scale*. Nashville: Counselor Recordings Tests.

Flaherty, J. F., and Dusek, J. B. 1980. An investigation of the relationship between psychological androgyny and components of self-concept. *Journal of Personality and Social Psychology* 38:984–92.

Gergen, K. J. 1971. *The concept of self*. New York: Holt, Rinehart, and Winston.

Gibb, J. R. 1971. The effects of human relations training. In *Handbook of psychotherapy and behavior change,* ed. A. E. Bergin and S. L. Garfield. New York: John Wiley.

Gilbert, L. A. 1981. Toward mental health: the benefits of psychological androgyny. *Professional Psychology* 12:29–38.

Gough, H. G.; Lazzari, R.; and Fioravanti, M. 1978. Self versus ideal self: A comparison of five adjective check list indices. *Journal of Consulting and Clinical Psychology* 46:1085–91.

Harris, D. V. 1973. Self-concept: Does physical activity affect it? In *Involvement in sport: A somatopsychic rationale for physical activity*. Philadelphia: Lea and Febiger.

———. 1974. Exploration of body image in physical activity involvement. In *Psychology of motor behavior and sport,* ed. M. Wade and R. Martens. Champaign, Ill.: Human Kinetics Publishers.

Harris, D. V., and Jennings, S. E. 1977. Self-perceptions of female distance runners. *Annals of the New York Academy of Sciences* 301:808–15.

Hartung, G. H., and Farge, E. J. 1977. Personality and physiological traits in middle-aged runners and joggers. *Journal of Gerontology* 32:541–48.

Helmreich, R., and Spence, J. T. 1977. Sex roles and achievement. In *Psychology of motor behavior and sport,* vol. 2, ed. R. W. Christina and D. M. Landers. Champaign, Ill.: Human Kinetics Publishers.

Helmreich, R., and Stapp, J. 1974. Short forms of the Texas Social Behavior Inventory (TSBI): An objective measure of self esteem. *Bulletin of the Psychonomic Society,* 4:473–75.

Helmreich, R.; Stapp, J.; and Ervin, C. 1974. The Texas Social Behavior Inventory (TSBI). *JSAS Catalogue of Selected Documents in Psychology* 4:79 (Ms. no. 681).

Henning, J. 1978. *Holistic running: Beyond the threshold of fitness*. New York: Signet.

Hilyer, J. C., and Mitchell, W. 1979. Effect of systematic physical fitness training combined with counseling on the self-concept of college students. *Journal of Counseling Psychology* 26:427–36.

Huey, L. 1976. *A running start: An athlete, a woman*. New York: Quadrangle Books.

Ismail, A. H., and Trachtman, L. E. 1973. Jogging the imagination. *Psychology Today* 6:78–82.

Joesting, J., and Clance, P. R. 1979. Comparison of runners and nonrunners on the body-cathexis and self-cathexis scales. *Perceptual and Motor Skills* 48:1046.

Johnson, W. R.; Fretz, B. R.; and Johnson, J. A. 1968. Changes in self-concepts during a physical development program. *Research Quarterly* 39:560–65.

Jones, W. H.; Chernovetz, M. E.; and Hansson, R. C. 1978. The enigma of androgyny: Differential implications for males and females? *Journal of Consulting and Clinical Psychology* 46:298–313.

Jorgenson, C. B., and Jorgenson, D. E. 1979. Effect of running on perception of self and others. *Perceptual and Motor Skills* 48:242.

Jourard, S. M. 1971. *The transparent self*. New York: Van Nostrand.

Karetsky, C. 1978. Running free: One woman's story from a race of thousands. *Marathon* 1:7–13.

Kaschak, E. 1976. Sociotherapy: An ecological model for therapy with women. *Psychotherapy: Theory, Research, and Practice* 12:61–63.

Koocher, G. 1971. Swimming, competence, and personality change. *Journal of Personality and Social Psychology* 18:275–78.

Kostrubala, T. 1976. *The joy of running*. Philadelphia: J. B. Lippincott.

Kraft, R. E. 1978. Can the movement specialist really influence self-concept? *Physical Educator* 35:20–21.

Kurtz, R. M. 1969. Sex differences and variations in body attitudes. *Journal of Consulting and Clinical Psychology* 33:625–29.

Kurtz, R. M., and Hirt, M. 1970. Body attitude and physical health. *Journal of Clinical Psychology* 26:149–51.

Leonardson, G. R. 1977. Relationship between self-concept and perceived physical fitness. *Perceptual and Motor Skills* 44:62.

Leonardson, G. R., and Gargiulo, R. M. 1978. Self-perception and physical fitness. *Perceptual and Motor Skills* 46:338.

Libby, B. 1978. From actor Bruce Dern: "Running saved my life." *New American Runner*. December, 19–34.

Locksley, A., and Colten, M. E. 1979. Psychological androgyny: A case of mistaken identity? *Journal of Personality and Social Psychology* 37:1010–31.

Maccoby, E. E., and Jacklin, C. N. 1974. *The psychology of sex differences*. Stanford, Calif.: Stanford University Press.

McElroy, M. A., and Willis, J. E. 1979. Women and the achievement conflict in sport: A preliminary study. *Journal of Sport Psychology* 1:241–47.

McGowan, R. W.; Jarman, B. O.; and Pedersen, D. M. 1974. Effects of competitive endurance training program on self-concept and peer approval. *Journal of Psychology* 86:57–60.

Mahoney, E. R. 1974. Body cathexis and self-esteem: The importance of subjective importance. *Journal of Psychology* 98:27–30.

————. 1978. Subjective physical attractiveness and self-other orientations. *Psychological Reports* 43:277–78.

Martinek, T. J.; Cheffers, J. T. F.; and Zaichkowsky, L. D. 1978. Physical activity, motor development and self-concept: Race and age differences. *Perceptual and Motor Skills* 46:147–54.

Miskimins, R. W.; Wilson, L. T.; Braucht, G. N.; and Berry, K. L. 1971. Self-concept and psychiatric symptomatology. *Journal of Clinical Psychology* 27:185–87.

Moffett, L. A. 1975. Sex differences in self-concept. *Psychological Reports* 37:74.

O'Connor, K.; Mann, D. W.; and Bardwick, J. M. 1978. Androgyny and self-esteem in the upper-middle class: A replication of Spence. *Journal of Consulting and Clinical Psychology* 56:1168–69.

Parrott, R., and Hewitt, J. 1978. Increasing self-esteem through participation in a goal-attainment program. *Journal of Clinical Psychology* 34:955–57.

Parson, R., and Bales, R. F. 1955. *Family, socialization and interaction process*. New York: Free Press of Glencoe.

Pedhazur, E. J., and Tetenbaum, T. J. 1979. Bem sex role inventory: A theoretical and methodological critique. *Journal of Personality and Social Psychology* 37:996–1016.

Phillips, D. A., and Zigler, E. 1980. Children's self-image disparity: Effects of age, socioeconomic status, and gender. *Journal of Personality and Social Psychology* 39:689–700.

Phillips, J. R. 1979. An exploration of perception of body boundary, personal space, and body size in elderly persons. *Perceptual and Motor Skills* 48:299–308.

Price, L. F. E. 1970. *The wonder of motion: A sense of life for woman*. Grand Forks: University of North Dakota Press.

Roberts, G.; Duda, J.; and Kleiber, D. 1980. Children in sport: Dimensions of motivation and competence in male and female participants. Paper presented at the annual conference of the North American Society for the Psychology of Sport and Physical Activity, Boulder, Colorado, May.

Rogers, C. R., and Dymond, R. F., eds. 1954. *Psychotherapy and personality change*. Chicago: University of Chicago Press.

Rosen, G. M., and Ross, A. O. 1968. Relationship of body image to self-concept. *Journal of Consulting and Clinical Psychology* 32:100.

Rossi, B., and Zoccolotti, P. 1979. Body perception in athletes and non-athletes. *Perceptual and Motor Skills* 49:723–26.

Sappenfield, B. R., and Harris, C. L. 1975. Self-reported masculinity-femininity as related to self-esteem. *Psychological Reports* 37:669–70.

Schofield, L. J., and Abbuhl, S. 1975. The stimulation of insight and self awareness through body-movement exercise. *Journal of Clinical Psychology* 31:745–46.

Secord, P. F., and Jourard, S. M. 1953. The appraisal of body-cathexis: Body-cathexis and the self. *Journal of Consulting Psychology* 17:343–47.

Shainberg, D. 1977. Long distance running as meditation. *Annals of the New York Academy of Sciences* 301:1002–9.

Sharp, M. W., and Reilley, R. R. 1975. The relationship of aerobic physical fitness to selected personality traits. *Journal of Clinical Psychology* 31:428–30.

Simono, R. B.; Dawson, G.; and Murphy, H. 1979. Factor M as a correlate of physical fitness or just more energy? *Journal of Clinical Psychology* 35:309–11.

Snyder, E. E., and Kivlin, J. E. 1975. Women athletes and aspects of psychological well-being and body image. *Research Quarterly* 56:191–99.

Snyder, E. E.; Kivlin, J. E.; and Spreitzer, E. 1976. The female athlete: An analysis of objective and subjective role conflict. In *Psychology of sport and motor behavior II*, ed. D. M. Landers. University Park: Pennsylvania State University.

Snyder, M. 1974. The self-monitoring of expressive behavior. *Journal of Personality and Social Psychology* 30:526–37.

———. 1979. Self-monitoring process. In *Advances in experimental social psychology*, vol. 12, ed. L. Berkowitz. New York: Academic Press.

———. 1980. The many me's of the self-monitor. *Psychology Today* 13:33–40, 92.

Spence, J. T., and Helmreich, R. L. 1978. *Masculinity and femininity: Their psychological dimensions, correlates and antecedents*. Austin: University of Texas Press.

———. 1979. The many faces of androgyny: A reply to Locksley and Colten. *Journal of Personality and Social Psychology* 37:1032–46.

Spence, J. T.; Helmreich, R. L.; and Stapp, J. 1974. The Personal Attributes Questionnaire: A measure of sex-role stereotypes and masculinity-femininity. *JSAS Catalogue of Selected Documents in Psychology* 4:43 (Ms. no. 617).

Stoner, S., and Kaiser, L. 1978. Sex differences in self-concepts of adolescents. *Psychological Reports* 43:305–6.

Van der Merwe, M. S. 1982. The relationship between physical fitness and the health status of selected Canadian college women. Ph.D. diss., Ohio State University, 1981. *Dissertation Abstracts International* 42(7): 3024-A (University Microfilms no. 8121866, 180).

Vincent, M. F. 1976. Comparison of self-concepts of college women: Athletes and physical education majors. *Research Quarterly* 47:218–25.

Vinck, J. 1979. Body awareness and personality. *Psychotherapy and Psychosomatics* 32:170–79.

Wark, K. A., and Wittig, A. F. 1979. Sex role and sport competition anxiety. *Journal of Sport Psychology* 1:248–50.

Washburn, W. C. 1962. The effects of physique and intrafamily tension on self-concepts in adolescent males. *Journal of Consulting Psychology* 5:460–66.

Weinberg, J. R. 1960. A further investigation of body-cathexis and the self. *Journal of Consulting Psychology* 24:277.

White, R. W. 1972. *The enterprise of living: Growth and organization in personality.* New York: Holt, Rinehart, and Winston.

Wittreich, W. J., and Grace, M. 1955. Body image and development. *Technical Reports,* 29 March. Princeton University, Contract N6 ONR 270(14), Office of Naval Research.

Zaichkowsky, L. D.; Zaichkowsky, L. B.; and Martinek, T. J. 1978. Physical activity, motor development and self-concept: Age and sex differences. In *Physical activity and human well-being: Motor learning, sport psychology, pedagogy, and didactics of physical activity,* ed. F. Landry and W. A. R. Orban. Miami: Symposia Specialists.

Ziller, R. C.; Hagey, J.; Smith, M. D.; and Long, B. H. 1969. Self-esteem: A self-social construct. *Journal of Consulting and Clinical Psychology* 33:84–95.

GARY W. BUFFONE, MICHAEL L. SACHS,
AND E. THOMAS DOWD

# 11

# Cognitive-Behavioral Strategies for Promoting Adherence to Exercise

Exercise prescriptions appear to offer considerable promise for use in clinical practice, but adherence to the prescribed regimen is crucial to its effectiveness. A most important, but neglected, aspect of behavior change programs is the maintenance of established patterns of behavior *after* the original controlling conditions have been discontinued. For example, Turner, Pooly, and Sherman (1976) presented a behavioral approach to individualized exercise programs. They discuss in detail the acquisition of new exercise behaviors but spend little time on their maintenance. The persistence of behavior change, in this case exercise behaviors, may be promoted by a variety of methods.

Interest in the use of exercise in physical and psychological therapy has brought up two critical questions. First, what general factors affecting adherence to physical activity programs should be considered in designing exercise regimens for clients? Second, what specific technique or combination of techniques will enhance adherence to exercise?

## Adherence Factors

Therapists should be aware of factors affecting adherence when they decide to prescribe exercise as an adjunct therapy. The dropout rate in exercise programs varies widely, from 1.2 percent to 95 percent (Danielson and Wanzel 1978), with most dropout rates ranging from 30 percent to 70 percent of the participants in a program (Morgan 1977). It should be noted, however, that these figures do not reflect percentages for those who begin (and perhaps stop) exercising on their own, without the associated benefits or drawbacks of an organized exercise program.

Numerous factors have been suggested as significantly related to adherence to exercise (Dishman 1980), including attitudes toward physical activity, self-perceptions of exercise ability, and feelings of responsibility for health. These factors have *not* been shown, however, to significantly *predict* adherence, though their role in determining *initial involvement* in physical activity may be important.

The extent to which participants remain free of injuries (Massie and Shephard 1971; Pollock, Gettman, and Milesis 1975) has also been cited in the literature. Clearly, it is difficult for the participant to reap any benefits if injuries make it impossible to continue the activity.

Another factor is the support of significant others. Participants whose spouses had favorable attitudes toward their physical activity displayed considerably better adherence patterns than those whose spouses were neutral or negative (Heinzelmann and Bagley 1970; Jones and Jones 1977).

Where the exercising is done can also be important. Participants in one study had campus offices significantly closer to the testing/exercise areas than non-participants (Hanson 1976). Similarly, Teraslinna et al. (1970) found that those willing to participate in an exercise program lived nearer to the exercise area than those who were unwilling. Particularly in the beginning stages, readily accessible locations will increase the likelihood that participants will continue the activity.

An additional factor is attainment of exercise objectives. Danielson and Wanzel (1978) found that those who failed to attain their objectives dropped out of the exercise program much faster than those who succeeded. Setting reasonable, attainable goals in most situations will increase satisfaction and enhance the likelihood of continuing.

Another potential factor is that individuals have either predominantly fast-twitch or predominantly slow-twitch muscle fibers. Roughly, those with mostly fast-twitch muscle fibers find sprinting "easier," while those with mostly slow-twitch muscle fibers find long-distance running easier. D. L. Costill (personal communication) notes a number of anecdotal and intuitive reports of what one of his colleagues calls the "fast twitch personality." (See Dienstbier, chap. 14, for a discussion of the effect of exercise on personality.) Of particular relevance here is Ingjer and Dahl's (1979) report of a Finnish study indicating a higher dropout rate for exercise program participants with predominantly fast-twitch as opposed to slow-twitch muscle fibers. Perhaps particular attention needs to be given to those with predominantly fast-twitch muscle fibers.

Dishman (1981) has shown that the health of participants is related to adherence. Patients with a disability associated with disease, such as cardiovascular problems, were more inclined to adhere to a training program.

As noted above, however, though the factors cited may be *associated* with adherence, they have not been shown to be useful in *predicting* adherence. In considering whether to prescribe exercise for a given client, it would be particularly valuable to know how likely that person is to drop out.

Dishman, Ickes, and Morgan (1980) have drawn upon the psychobiological perspective adopted by Alexander and Selesnick (1966) and further developed by Morgan (1973a) in sport psychology. Dishman, Ickes, and Morgan found that body weight, percentage of body fat, and self-motivation could be used to diagnose dropout proneness at the outset of involvement with roughly 80 percent accuracy. Specifically, those who were heavier, had a higher percentage of body fat, and lacked self-motivation had a higher probability of dropping out of an exercise program. Of particular interest to the researchers was that "self-motivation proved to be the best discriminator between exercise adherers and dropouts among the psychological variables employed and was strongly related to program adherence" (1980, 115).

Striking similarities have been observed between dropout rates for physical activity and relapse rates for smoking, alcoholism, and heroin addiction (Morgan 1977). Hunt and Bespalec (1974) evaluated current studies on modifying smoking behavior and found that a wide range of treatments have been successful. The variable of motivation, however, underlies the selection of subjects in these studies. All subjects who participate want to quit smoking, though many drop out before completing the program. Hunt and Bespalec suggest that the specific treatment is of minor importance once the smoker is attracted to the program and is motivated to change. Morgan (1977, 244) suggests that exercise adherence can be viewed in the same manner: "The challenge then becomes one of developing, first, attraction strategies that will be successful in enticing sedentary people to become active, and programmatic strategies that will facilitate adherence." Certainly, motivation for participation underlies initial involvement in, as well as adherence to, a program of regular physical activity.

We can therefore cite a number of general strategies for promoting adherence: use of groups, accessible exercise locations, support of significant others, limited intensity to avoid injury, and attainment of training objectives. It would be valuable to initially assess the client's likelihood of dropping out, perhaps using the model proposed by Dishman, Ickes, and Morgan (1980) or personality profiles of dropouts (D. L. Costill, personal communication; Thirer 1980).

Determining what features of the exercise setting might influence given individuals would allow one to manipulate these situational factors so as to enhance clients' likelihood of adherence.

## Measurement of Adherence

The accurate assessment of adherence to a prescribed exercise regimen allows the clinician to determine the efficacy of the client's prescription and detect errors the client might be making in following the regimen.

In their report on adherence to diet and drug regimens, Dunbar and Stunkard (1979) state that one of the most effective methods of measurement is daily self-reports. Clinical interviews, though useful, do not detect specific problems the client encounters in following the regimen. Also, poor adherence may be underreported in interviews.

Self-report techniques have been used successfully in studies on weight control (Leon 1976; Stunkard 1975) and appear to be of considerable value in improving exercise adherence. The positive therapeutic implications of self-monitoring have been presented by Kazdin (1974) and Mahoney (1974). The daily self-report can provide continuous data on the client's exercise behaviors that will help the therapist detect and identify potential problems with the prescribed exercise regimen. The clinician may then, with the assistance of the client, make the necessary adjustments to ensure continued participation. However, record keeping has a reactive effect and will vary under different conditions, which should be considered by therapists who use this technique. A major problem with this method, as in interview methods, is that clients may misrepresent their actual participation and underreport poor adherence. This might be corrected with the assistance of significant others, who could collect information as a reliability check for the client's self-report data.

In one study (Wysocki et al. 1979), subjects contracted to observe and record the exercise of other subjects and to perform independent reliability observations each week demonstrated high levels of interobserver reliability. Thus training inexperienced observers seems to offer promise as an accurate and efficient method for assessing exercise participation.

Self-recording can focus on different aspects of exercise behavior. In running, for example, differential emphasis may be placed on duration, frequency, and intensity. (See Berger, chap. 2, for a more detailed discussion of these factors.) Duration can easily be assessed if the runner checks a clock before and after the run or carries a watch. Frequency is, of course, the number of times the client runs each week.

Intensity may be more difficult to assess. The ideal measure would be percentage of maximum oxygen uptake during the run, but this cannot be measured accurately without sophisticated laboratory equipment. Heart rate, on the other hand, offers a fairly effective measure of the percentage of maximum heart rate being utilized—60 to 70 percent for twenty minutes or more, three times a week, is suggested for maximum benefit (American College of Sports Medicine 1978). However, few runners care to stop in the middle of a run to record heart rate. Assessment of recovery time by measuring heart rate at the conclusion of the run and several minutes afterward can indicate the effort expended and the runner's recovery efficiency.

Detailed diaries, such as the running diary developed by Osman and Johnson (1979), are available for the runner interested in maintaining a record of activity and may enhance adherence. Some may find it more reinforcing to develop their own recording instruments.

As the research indicates, there is no completely reliable measure of adherence to prescribed regimens. Obviously, adherence measurement is at a relatively low level of sophistication and requires further research. The therapist who wants accurate information on adherence might best obtain data from a number of sources, particularly the clinical interview, self-report, and reports from significant others in the client's environment.

## Interventions

A number of interventions may be useful in reducing the 30 to 70 percent dropout rate reported in the literature (Morgan 1977). These techniques can be classified as cognitive, behavioral, and social-facilitative.

### COGNITIVE MAINTENANCE STRATEGIES

Cognitive strategies have recently come to be viewed as playing a major role in maintaining and generalizing behavior change (Franks and Wilson 1978). In particular, recent formulations have recognized that clients' appraisals of the meaning of their own actions affect the durability of the effects produced by a wide variety of change-inducing treatments (e.g., Bandura 1977). Several cognitive strategies with important maintenance implications have been isolated.

*Self-Statements*

Meichenbaum (1977) pointed out the importance of positive and negative self-statements in regulating behavior. In a similar vein, Beck (1976) discussed the effects that positive and negative automatic thoughts have on moods and consequent emotional life. Both are saying that we give ourselves internal messages, or talk to ourselves, and that the content of these self-statements is an important determinant of our actions and moods.

It has repeatedly been demonstrated that maintenance of therapeutic gain, in this case exercise, can be enhanced by programming specific coping self-statements and by eliminating maladaptive self-statements. Clients, for example, can be taught to eliminate maladaptive self-statements, such as self-blame ("I knew I could never stick to my exercise program") or self-pity ("Why am I such a weak person?") and focus instead on more adaptive self-statements ("Just because I have a relapse doesn't mean I can't succeed").

The therapist can help clients reduce self-statements that decrease the likelihood of exercising, perhaps by first teaching them to recognize those statements through self-monitoring and then to extinguish these statements by pairing them with an aversive stimulus (a rubber-band pop on the wrist, for example). These negative self-statements, once they are brought to conscious awareness, may also be modified with the help of the therapist so that they are more realistic and adaptive and will not inhibit the patient's motivation to exercise. The therapist can work in much the same way to increase the patient's positive self-statements ("I like the changes exercise causes," "Exercise makes me feel good").

Both Beck and Meichenbaum, however, emphasize that client self-statements are often virtually automatic, below the level of conscious awareness. Therapists should therefore also pay particular attention to their clients' underlying belief systems.

*Cognitive Rehearsal*

A second cognitive strategy that may enhance exercise adherence is cognitive rehearsal. McFall and his colleagues (McFall and Lillesand 1971; McFall and Twentyman 1973) demonstrated that covert and overt behavior rehearsal were helpful in assertion training, contributing to both maintenance and generalization of change. Moreover, they found that covert response rehearsal was as effective as overt rehearsal. Clients can be asked to imagine themselves responding appropriately in a problematic situation, or they can be asked to cognitively rehearse certain elements and expected outcomes of a treatment program. For example, clients might cognitively rehearse the reasons they began their exercise programs and the outcomes they expect or imagine—how healthy, strong, or attractive they will feel if they continue. They can also, via imagery, picture themselves as, for example, slim and healthy. This cognitive rehearsal might easily be prompted by exercise-related cues in the environment (running magazines, decals, shorts).

Recently more attention has been paid to the *meaning* of relapse (nonmaintenance of behavior) to the individual (Marlatt 1978; Wilson 1978). Clients who do not maintain their exercise programs, for example, may interpret it to mean that they will never be able to maintain a program, that they lack control over themselves, or that they are basically weak. On the other hand, they may interpret a relapse to mean they should redouble their efforts. The particular meaning assigned to a relapse in exercise behavior may be all-important in determining whether a client persists in an exercise program. In this connection, Marlatt (1978) suggested a "programmed relapse" as a laboratory exercise to help a client control any negative reactions while the counselor is still available. The therapist would discuss with patients the possibility of an exercise relapse and then help them define such a relapse as a temporary setback that can easily be overcome. Patients should be prevented from interpreting a break in their exercise routine as more than what it is—a brief break in a regular, continued schedule of exercise.

### Self-Efficacy

A third cognitive variable that may affect continuation of an exercise program is expectation of results. Bandura (1977) argued that maintenance of treatment effects depends on increasing the client's self-efficacy—one's sense that one can achieve a favorable outcome. Likewise, Schlegel and Kunetsky (1977) obtained evidence that clients' expectation of a positive outcome is important in maintaining a reduction in smoking. This suggests that maintenance of exercise behavior will be enhanced if clients believe that a program of that nature *can* be maintained, and that they have the ability to do it. It is therefore crucial that relapses be interpreted as expected occurrences in a progression toward an achievable goal rather than as a sign that the cause is hopeless. The therapist must instill, through encouragement and example, the positive expectation (hope?) that clients can maintain an exercise program.

*Attribution*

There has been increasing recognition that attribution plays a major role in counseling outcomes, indeed that counseling itself could be thought of as a reattributing process (Strong 1978). Abramson, Seligman, and Teasdale (1978) argued that those who have "learned helplessness" tend to make internal attributions for failure (blame themselves) and external attributions for success (believe something or someone else was responsible). Likewise, Franks and Wilson (1978) summarized data indicating that self-attribution of behavior change (clients' belief that they, rather than the therapist were responsible for treatment success) may in part account for maintenance of treatment effects.

Thus the therapist should help clients attribute successes in the exercise program (including maintenance) to their own efforts and abilities. In this sense the therapist must "give" them the power of their own behavior change. Likewise, the therapist should help clients avoid attributing failure to their own defects or weaknesses. Failure should be presented as normal and expected, not as reflecting badly on the individual. If clients are encouraged to maintain a problem-solving set, coping strategies can be devised to overcome these adherence failures.

## BEHAVIORAL MAINTENANCE STRATEGIES

A number of behavioral techniques can also be applied to the maintenance of exercise behavior.

*Shaping*

The first behavioral strategy is shaping—the process of reinforcing gradual, successive approximations toward a terminal response rather than reinforcing only the terminal response. Clients are guided through progressively more complex behaviors to the desired goal, allowing them to master each component of the exercise regimen and providing checks on potential mistakes or problems that may require attention before adherence is impeded. This intervention is related to the tailoring of the exercise regimen in that both gradually increase the reinforcing value of the exercise behavior by assigning accomplishable tasks compatible with the client's level of functioning.

Crucial to the shaping process is beginning the initial exercise task at the client's current level of performance. This may require breaking down the prescribed exercise into small, manageable parts that the client can handle, thus increasing the probability of continued participation. For example, initially assigning obese or cardiac patients to a rigorous running program not only will impede their adherence but could also result in a serious mishap. Establishing realistic, attainable goals is important if clients are to improve and not be discouraged by unrealistic expectations. They must experience reinforcement throughout the exercise experience. The importance of prescribing an appropriate regimen has also been discussed by Dunbar and Stunkard (1979).

Greist et al. (1978) used a graduated running program with depressed clients, who typically have difficulty participating in any physical activity. The running program, based on small increments, produced an attrition rate of only 11 percent compared with the 30 to 70 percent found in most programs (Morgan 1977).

The exercise regimen should be tailored to fit as conveniently as possible into the client's daily routine, to reduce interference and increase adherence. An inappropriately designed training regimen may lead to injuries, nonattainment of goals and objectives, disillusionment, and dropping out.

### Stimulus Control

A behavioral technique frequently used in behavior weight control programs is stimulus control (Bandura 1969), generally to decrease the frequency of eating. One can also rearrange antecedent environmental stimuli to change the occurrence of other specific behaviors such as exercise. For example, one might have patients schedule their exercise sessions, change into exercise clothing whenever possible, or associate with people who exercise regularly. The goal is to increase the number of environmental cues that might encourage exercise. A creative therapist can help patients engineer their environments to increase their tendency to exercise regularly.

A more systematic analysis of the antecedent conditions of exercise may lead to new techniques for promoting exercise adherence. Prompts associated with exercise may enhance the likelihood of the behavior and the client can eventually use them to maintain participation.

### Modeling

A third strategy for influencing exercise participation involves the therapist's own lifestyle. Modeling is an important method of enhancing adherence and is apt to be particularly successful when a person has developed a strong positive tie to a prestigious model (Bandura and Huston 1961), a condition emphasized in psychotherapy. The clinician who runs or participates in physical activity can be a valuable role model, but the overweight, out-of-shape, chain-smoking therapist may find clients skeptical of his or her espousal of the benefits of physical activity.

Studies of modeling effects show that a person tends to perform the model's behavior in the model's abence (Bandura, Ross, and Ross 1963), suggesting that once the therapist's attitudes and behaviors have been adopted, they continue to influence and indirectly control the client's actions though the clinician is not physically present. Differential reinforcement is a necessary component of observational learning or modeling, and the modeling/reinforcement approach merits serious consideration in the development of exercise adherence strategies.

### Reinforcement

Reinforcement is probably the most potent technique available for promoting exercise, and reinforcement strategies are part of virtually all behavior therapy. Positive reinforcement has been used extensively in most behavioral weight control programs, for example, and a number of studies (Agras et al. 1974; Mahoney, Moura, and Wade 1973) have shown it to be the single most effective element in treatment.

Reinforcement may range from praise and the social rewards of recognition to tangible rewards for walking or jogging a designated time or distance each day. Although the initial reinforcement may be administered by the therapist, reinforcement control should gradually be shifted to clients themselves (Mahoney 1975; Stuart and Davis 1972) or to significant others in their environment. This fading from therapist-prompted to naturally occurring or environmentally programmed reinforcers is a necessary step in encouraging the patient to continue exercise after the formal treatment ends.

Exercise behaviors can also be supported by their intrinsic sensory consequences. Artificial incentives and a great deal of initial encouragement may be required to induce the client to exercise, but once proficiency is achieved, physical activity is likely to be continued for its own physiological and psychological benefits.

This is a critical point. The problems of reinforcing exercise behaviors are similar to those encountered in weight control programs. Reinforcement immediately following the target behavior is most effective in initially modifying behavior. Once the behavior is established, delayed or intermittent reinforcement may effectively maintain it. In exercise programs, especially those not carefully planned and supervised, the initial outcomes (which are frequently punishing—pain or injury) may deter future exercise. The positive health outcomes the novice is looking for will not materialize for weeks or months. Unfortunately many, if not most, will drop out before their outcomes are realized. Therefore, though improved health may be a sustaining factor for long-term exercisers, a more immediate form of reinforcement must be made available for most beginners.

This might be accomplished through a group format, with posted attendance and running records, public recognition for accomplishing goals (e.g., certificates, tangible rewards), and the pairing of exercise mates to actively encourage and reinforce each other. The personal attention of the instructor or therapist is also important, and clinicians should recognize the reinforcement value of their time and attention. The client's therapy time might be contracted as a reward for adhering to the exercise prescription. There is evidence that the amount of time the clinician spends with the client is related to adherence (Jeffrey, Wing, and Stunkard 1978).

### Contracting

Another method that has proved useful with a number of behavior problems is contingency contracting. Dunbar and Stunkard (1979) have reviewed several advantages of this method in adherence programs. First, contracts provide a written, readily available outline of treatment goals. Second, in developing a contract clients can discuss possible problems or solutions, involving them in decisions about their regimens. Third, the contract itself acts as an incentive by establishing rewards from self or others for accomplishing treatment goals. Last, the contract requires an explicit commitment to the remediation program. As Kanfer et al. (1974) suggested, the promise and intentions outlined in the contract may themselves foster self-control.

Although several studies have supported the use of behavioral contracts in encouraging physical exercise (Turner, Pooly, and Sherman 1976; Vance 1976; Wysocki et al. 1979), few have specifically discussed contracting in promoting exercise adherence. The study by Wysocki et al. (1979) has demonstrated the effectiveness of contracting in modifying and maintaining exercise behavior, and this area deserves further attention in both research and practice.

SOCIAL-FACILITATION STRATEGIES

In addition to cognitive and behavioral techniques, social supports have been suggested as a key to increasing the likelihood that a client will follow the therapeutic regimen (Dunbar and Stunkard 1979). This strongly supports a commonsense approach in treatment prescription that may prove one of the most promising routes to an effective adherence program. The cooperation of significant others can be important in the systematic application of behavioral contingencies and can greatly increase the effectiveness of strategies for behavior change.

Although the literature is not clear on whether "serious" running has positive or negative effects on family relations (Jones and Jones 1977; Jorgenson and Jorgenson 1978; Joseph and Robbins 1981), it is certain that if one or more members run regularly there are important effects on family life. As noted earlier, participants whose spouses had favorable attitudes toward programs of physical activity displayed considerably better adherence patterns than those whose spouses were neutral or negative (Heinzelmann and Bagley 1970; Jones and Jones 1977). Wankel (1979, 41) notes that families should be included in exercise programs wherever possible or should "at least be consulted and informed about the program so that they can plan to best accommodate it into the family life-style."

Although the family has received some attention as an important support system in adherence strategies, the occupational setting has largely been neglected. On-the-job treatment has been demonstrated effectively in one study (Alderman 1976) involving hypertensive patients. This research was dramatically successful and strongly suggests that work has great significance in the treatment of a variety of clinical problems. The dramatic growth of the American Association for Fitness Directors in Business and Industry (AAFDBI) suggests that fitness programs in industry are now being seen as important in maintaining workers' physical and psychological health. Wanzel and Danielson (1977a,b,c) provide a detailed study of dropouts from the employee fitness program of a large Canadian firm and suggest ways to improve adherence to fitness programs in general. They discuss crowding, distance of the exercise area from home or work, social support, and the role of instructors.

Other social-facilitation settings that might be programmed into treatment are clubs and organizations. Individuals appear to affiliate with others who share behavioral norms and reinforce the standards they have adopted (Bandura 1969). Membership and participation in these social systems (e.g., running and swimming clubs) should be encouraged in the early stages of treatment and may support the client during and after the formal treatment contract ends, providing reinforcement from natural environmental contingencies.

Group involvement directly motivates participation in the fitness group (Brawley 1979; Wankel 1979). Such motivation develops over time, and the leader can play an important role in developing fitness-group solidarity. Enhancing identification with the group (perhaps by T-shirts bearing the group name), engaging in friendly competition with other groups (such as age-group handicap relays), and interdependent action can all be used. General social psychological principles are helpful in understanding the role the fitness group and its members play in individual achievement and success. The social environment—including car pools where appropriate, a clean exercise setting, direct and well-planned leadership, knowledge of results and verbal praise, and role models—can be a great aid in enhancing adherence.

## Conclusions

Physical exercise is gaining attention as an adjunct to more traditional psychotherapeutic practices. As with other behaviors, maintaining adherence to exercise after the termination of formal programming is a problem.

A number of cognitive-behavioral strategies can help the clinician promote development and maintenance of exercise behavior. Experience clearly indicates, however, that the best strategies are ineffective if the client is not motivated to participate.

Dishman, Ickes, and Morgan (1980) offer a first step in diagnosing those who are least likely to adhere to an exercise program, citing psychobiologic factors related to dropout proneness. Other factors most likely will also be found to relate to adherence. For example, O'Halloran et al. (1979) noted that dropouts from an antihypertensive drug regimen were significantly more suspicious than adherers, as measured by Cattell's Sixteen Personality Factor Inventory.

Much has been written about noncompliance in health care as well as drug and diet regimens (see particularly Dunbar and Stunkard 1979; Haynes, Taylor, and Sackett 1979). Clinicians can easily familiarize themselves with this research. Problems of exercise adherence are now being explored (Dishman 1980, 1981; Dishman, Ickes, and Morgan 1980). We cannot overemphasize the importance of considering adherence in planning programs of exercise. By discussing with clients whether to prescribe an exercise program, then working with them on its development and initiation, the clinician can greatly increase the probability of adherence.

## References

Abramson, L. Y.; Seligman, M. E. P.; and Teasdale, J. D. 1978. Learned helplessness in humans: Critique and reformulation. *Journal of Abnormal Psychology* 87: 49–74.
Agras, W. S.; Barlow, D. H.; Chapin, H. N.; Abel, G. G.; and Leitenberg, H. 1974.

Behavior modification of anorexia nervosa. *Archives of General Psychiatry* 30: 279–86.

Alderman, M. H. 1976. Organization for long-term management of hypertension. *Bulletin of the New York Academy of Medicine* 52:697–717.

Alexander, F. G., and Selesnick, S. T. 1966. *The history of psychiatry.* New York: Harper and Row.

American College of Sports Medicine. 1978. Position statement on the recommended quantity and quality of exercise for developing and maintaining fitness in healthy adults. *Sports Medicine Bulletin* 13(3):1, 3–4.

Bandura, A. 1969. *Principles of behavior modification.* New York: Holt, Rinehart and Winston.

————. 1977. Self-efficacy: Toward a unifying theory of behavior change. *Psychological Review* 84:191–215.

Bandura, A., and Huston, A. C. 1961. Identification as a process of incidental learning. *Journal of Abnormal and Social Psychology* 63:311–18.

Bandura, A.; Ross, D.; and Ross, S. A. 1963. Imitation of film-mediated aggressive models. *Journal of Abnormal and Social Psychology* 66:3–11.

Beck, A. T. 1976. *Cognitive therapy and the emotional disorders.* New York: International Universities Press.

Brawley, L. R. 1979. Motivating participation in the fitness group. *Recreation Research Review* 6(4):35–39.

Buffone, G. W. 1980. Exercise as therapy: A closer look. *Journal of Counseling and Psychotherapy* 3:101–15.

Costill, D. L. 1981. Responses and adaptations to anaerobic muscular effort. Paper presented at the annual meeting of the New England chapter of the American College of Sports Medicine, Boxboro, Massachusetts, November.

Danielson, R. R., and Wanzel, R. S. 1978. Exercise objectives of fitness program dropouts. In *Psychology of motor behavior and sport, 1977,* ed. D. M. Landers and R. W. Christina. Champaign, Ill.: Human Kinetics Publishers.

Dishman, R. K. 1980. Prediction of adherence to habitual physical activity. In *Exercise in health and disease,* ed. H. J. Montoye and F. J. Nagle. Springfield, Ill.: Charles C. Thomas.

————. 1981. Biologic influences on exercise adherence. *Research Quarterly for Exercise and Sport* 52:143–59.

Dishman, R. K.; Ickes, W. J.; and Morgan, W. P. 1980. Self-motivation and adherence to habitual physical activity. *Journal of Applied Social Psychology* 10:115–31.

Driscoll, R. 1976. Anxiety reduction using physical exertion and positive images. *Psychological Record* 26:87–94.

Dunbar, J. M., and Stunkard, J. A. 1979. Adherence to diet and drug regimen. In *Nutrition, lipids, and coronary heart disease,* ed. R. Levy, B. Rifkind, B. Dennis, and N. Ernst. New York: Raven Press.

Franks, C. M., and Wilson, G. T. 1978. *Annual review of behavior therapy: Theory and practice.* New York: Brunner/Mazel.

Greist, J. H.; Klein, M. H.; Eischens, R. R.; Faris, J.; Gurman, A. S.; and Morgan, W. P. 1978. Running through your mind. *Journal of Psychosomatic Research* 22:259–94.

Hanson, M. G. 1976. Coronary heart disease, exercise, and motivation in middle-aged males. Ph.D. diss., University of Wisconsin.

Haynes, R. B.; Taylor, D. W.; and Sackett, D. L., eds. 1979. *Compliance in health care*. Baltimore: Johns Hopkins University Press.

Heinzelmann, R., and Bagley, R. W. 1970. Response to physical activity programs and their effects on health behavior. *Public Health Reports* 85:905–11.

Hunt, W. A., and Bespalec, D. A. 1974. An evaluation of current methods of modifying smoking behavior. *Journal of Clinical Psychology* 30:431–38.

Ingjer, F., and Dahl, H. A. 1979. Dropouts from an endurance training program. *Scandinavian Journal of Sports Sciences* 1:20–22.

Jeffrey, R. W.; Wing, R. R.; and Stunkard, A. J. 1978. Behavioral treatment of obesity: The state of the art—1976. *Behavior Therapy* 9:189–99.

Jones, S. B., and Jones, D. C. 1977. Serious jogging and family life: Marathon and sub-marathon running. Paper presented at the annual meeting of the American Sociological Association, Chicago, 5–9 September.

Jorgenson, D. E., and Jorgenson, C. B. 1978. Perceived changes in intrafamilial relations: A study of runners/joggers. Paper presented at the annual conference of the Western Social Science Association.

Joseph, P., and Robbins, J. M. 1981. Worker or runner? The impact of commitment to running and work on self-identification. In *Psychology of running*, ed. M. H. Sacks and M. L. Sachs. Champaign, Ill.: Human Kinetics Publishers.

Kanfer, F., II; Cox, L. E.; Gruner, J. M.; and Karoly, P. 1974. Contracts, demand characteristics, and self-control. *Journal of Personality and Social Psychology* 30:605–19.

Kazdin, A. E. 1974. Self-monitoring and behavior change. In *Self-control, power to the person*, ed. M. J. Mahoney and C. E. Thoresen. Monterey: Brooks/Cole.

Layman, E. M. 1973. Physical activity as a psychiatric adjunct. In *Science and medicine of exercise and sports*, ed. W. R. Johnson. New York: Harper and Row.

Leon, G. R. 1976. Current directions in the treatment of obesity. *Psychological Bulletin* 83:557–78.

McFall, R. M., and Lillesand, D. B. 1971. Behavior rehearsal with modeling and coaching in assertion training. *Journal of Abnormal Psychology* 77:313–23.

McFall, R. M., and Twentyman, C. T. 1973. Four experiments on the relative contributions of rehearsal, modeling, and coaching to assertion training. *Journal of Abnormal Psychology* 81:199–218.

Mahoney, M. J. 1974. Self-reward and self-monitoring techniques for weight control. *Behavior Therapy* 5:48–57.

———. 1975. The behavioral treatment of obesity. In *Applying behavioral science to cardiovascular risk*, ed. A. J. Enelow and J. B. Henderson. Dallas: Heart Association.

Mahoney, M. J.; Moura, N. G. M.; and Wade, T. C. 1973. The relative efficacy of self-rewards, self-punishment and self-monitoring techniques for weight loss. *Journal of Consulting and Clinical Psychology* 40:404–7.

Marlatt, G. A. 1978. Craving for alcohol, loss of control and relapse: A cognitive-behavioral analysis. In *Alcoholism: New directions in behavioral research and treatment,* ed. P. E. Nathan and G. A. Marlatt. New York: Plenum.

Massie, J., and Shephard, R. 1971. Physiological and psychological effects of training. *Medicine and Science in Sports* 3:110–17.

Meichenbaum, D. 1977. *Cognitive-behavior modification.* New York: Plenum.

Morgan, W. P. 1973a. Efficacy of psychobiologic inquiry in the exercise and sport sciences. *Quest* 20:39–47.

————. 1973b. Influence of acute physical activity on state anxiety. *Proceedings, National College Physical Education Association for Men,* Seventy-sixth Annual Meeting. Chicago: University of Illinois at Chicago Circle, Office of Publications Services.

————. 1977. Involvement in vigorous physical activity with special reference to adherence. *Proceedings of the NCPEAM/NAPECW National Conference.*

O'Halloran, M. W.; Zacest, R.; Barrow, G. G.; and Wilson, L. L. 1979. Suspiciousness trait: A factor in antihypertensive drug trials? Letter to the editor, *Lancet II,* 1298.

Osman, J. D., and Johnson, M. F. 1979. *AMJA runner's daily diary.* North Hollywood, Calif.: American Medical Joggers Association.

Pollock, M. L.; Gettman, L. R.; and Milesis, C. A. 1975. *Physical fitness manual for correctional institutions.* Report no. 1AR-1975-0017. Dallas: Institute for Aerobics Research.

Schlegel, R. P., and Kunetsky, M. 1977. Immediate and delayed effects of the "five day plan to stop smoking" including factors affecting recidivism. *Preventive Medicine* 6:454–61.

Strong, S. R. 1978. Social psychological approach to psychotherapy research. In *Handbook of psychotherapy and behavior change,* ed. S. L. Garfield and A. E. Bergin. New York: John Wiley.

Stuart, R. B., and Davis, B. 1972. *Slim chance in a fat world: Behavioral control of obesity.* Champaign, Ill.: Research Press.

Stunkard, A. J. 1975. From explanation to action in psychosomatic medicine: The case of obesity. *Psychosomatic Medicine* 37:195–236.

Teraslinna, P.; Partanen, T.; Oja, P.; and Koskela, A. 1970. Some social characteristics and living habits associated with willingness to participate in a physical activity intervention study. *Journal of Sports Medicine and Physical Fitness* 10:138–44.

Thirer, J. 1980. Distinguishing the successful runner from the running drop-out. Paper presented at the Third Annual Psychology of Running Seminar, Cornell University Medical College, New York City, 24 October.

Turner, R. D.; Pooly, S.; and Sherman, A. R. 1976. A behavioral approach to individualized exercise programming. In *Counseling methods,* ed. J. D. Krumboltz and C. E. Thoresen. New York: Holt, Rinehart and Winston.

Vance, B. 1976. Using contracts to control weight and to improve cardiovascular physical fitness. In *Counseling methods,* ed. J. D. Krumboltz and C. E. Thoresen. New York: Holt, Rinehart and Winston.

Wankel, L. M. 1979. Motivating involvement in adult physical activity programs. *Recreation Research Review* 6(4):40–43.

Wanzel, R. S., and Danielson, R. R. 1977a. Improve adherence to your fitness program: Part I. *Recreation Management* 20(5):16–19.

———. 1977b. Improve adherence to your fitness program: Part II. *Recreation Management* 20(6):38–41.

———. 1977c. Improve adherence to your fitness program: Part III. *Recreation Management* 20(7):34–37.

Wilson, G. T. 1978. Booze, beliefs and behavior: Cognitive processes in alcohol use and abuse. In *Alcoholism: New directions in behavioral research and treatment,* ed. P. E. Nathan and G. A. Marlatt. New York: Plenum.

Wysocki, T.; Hall, G.; Iwata, B.; and Riordan, M. 1979. Behavioral management of exercise: Contracting for aerobic points. *Journal of Applied Behavior Analysis* 12:55–64.

# 12

# Future Directions:
# The Potential for
# Exercise as Therapy

A new field of inquiry, knowledge, and practice has developed within the areas of physical exercise and mental health (Folkins and Sime 1981; Sacks and Sachs 1981). The field of running or exercise therapy is one manifestation of interest in the mind/body perspective. This related holistic view, closely aligned with behavioral medicine and health psychology, is also undergoing enormous expansion. Recent developments in the behavior-health fields include the formation of professional societies (e.g., Society of Behavioral Medicine, 1978), the planning and publication of books and journals (Davidson and Davidson 1980; *Journal of Health Psychology),* and a new division within the American Psychological Association (Division 38, Health Psychology).

Regardless of the increased enthusiasm for exercise as a form of psychotherapy, there appears to be limited understanding of the method. The refinement and application of exercise therapy remain in the earliest stages, and skeptics will continue to find sufficient grounds to question this approach. At this point considerable skepticism seems warranted.

There are basically two kinds of skeptics, uninformed and informed. The uninformed know little of the method and question the use of any treatment that appears to depend more on the clients' own effort than those of the therapist.

Informed skeptics in this area, who are likely to be exercisers, demand of themselves and their professional colleagues the highest standards of proof of efficacy. They are not content with the numerous anecdotal and research accounts that reflect favorably on the use of exercise as therapy. They want to know if the studies were designed to rule out extraneous factors in apparent successes. They want to know, as definitively as possible, whether exercise can produce specific psychological improvements and how these can be made to occur. It is these concerns that I address.

Before running or other exercise can be widely accepted by professionals as a viable treatment alternative, a number of issues must be clarified: the current state of research and theory; limitations on the use of this method; specific clinical concerns about assessment and treatment; and application to special populations.

## Research

One of the major obstacles to the widespread use of running therapy is the lack of *definitive* research on the method. There is voluminous anecdotal material but few well-controlled studies supporting the use of physical exercise as therapy. Although one may argue that all research on the outcome of psychotherapy is questionable, research in the use of running as therapy must still be significantly improved, with more soundly controlled studies. A critical review of the research is essential if we are to separate fact from fiction.

To date, most studies on the psychological effects of physical exercise have been poorly designed and inconclusive. A number of design problems threaten both internal and external validity (e.g., history, test-taking effects, maturation, instrumentation) (Campbell and Stanley 1963).

Aside from design problems, variations in exercise prescriptions make the results of these studies difficult to interpret. In many cases the intensity of exercise has been insufficient to achieve a training effect. Experimenters must carefully document subjects' cardiovascular output after exercise (heart or pulse rate) to standardize the training effects achieved.

Specific research plans are discussed in chapter 17 by Silva and Shultz. Dienstbier (chap. 14) also presents a number of issues important to researchers interested in investigating this complex phenomenon. We would do well to heed their guidelines for future research.

To improve the quality of the research, we need to rule out, as far as possible, extraneous variables that may be producing or affecting the reported successful outcomes. I must counsel a conservative attitude, especially to those among us who, because of our own position and exercise experiences, have become evangelical. As with any new treatment approach (recall the introduction of behavior therapy in the 1960s), we should not make claims that cannot be substantiated by research. The problems are much more complex than they may appear, and simplistic solutions are not feasible. At this point the "exercise evangelist" stands to do more harm than good by extolling the unsubstantiated benefits of exercise. Many of the original questions have yet to be answered by sound, well-controlled, quality research.

As research goes, so goes theory. Most of the research to date has been atheoretical or mechanistic. There is need for unifying theory that can explain the psychological effects of exercise. Harris (1973) proposed that a "somato-psychic" perspective might serve as a conceptual framework to generate causal hypotheses on the effects of exercise. Harris states: "The somatopsychic rationale for man's involvement in physical activity and sport, in brief, is the theory that bodily activity and function influence his behavior" (p. 240). But this "somatopsychic" theory does not address the question of "how" these changes in physical fitness influence psychological factors.

There have been a number of theories, physiologically based (Michael 1957; Morgan 1974; Schwartz, Davidson, and Goleman 1978; Stein and Belluzzi 1978) and psychologically based (Bahrke and Morgan 1978; Hollandsworth 1979; Morgan 1979; Solomon and Bumpus 1978), that have attempted to explain the psychological effects of physical exertion. Lazarus (1975) presented one of the best-integrated theoretical models for biofeedback. This model places research and practice within the broad context of a cognitive theory of emotion and adaptation. This is perhaps the first theoretical offering that could effectively combine the various claims for cause and effect in the area of physical exercise and mental health. Research in this area seems greatly inhibited by the lack of an integrated theoretical model that can explain the reported changes.

### Limitations

As with any treatment, there are problems with running therapy. First, there have been claims that a running or exercise treatment is effective with anorexia nervosa, "lifestyle changes," poor self-esteem, alcoholism, psychosis, and drug addiction (Dodson and Mullens 1969; Gary and Guthrie 1972; Kostrubala 1976). There is considerable question whether running alone can produce significant improvements in these problems. Exercise as a psychological treatment is similar to any other treatment—it will work only with certain people with certain types of problems under certain therapeutic conditions. This is a considerable qualification of a treatment that some have offered as a panacea.

Like other somatic therapies, running therapy must be carefully prescribed. It is interesting to note several similarities between running and exercise treatments and companion somatic therapies such as medication. (*a*) Running, like medication, must be administered at a particular dosage (duration, frequency, intensity) to produce a therapeutic effect. As with medication, this dosage will vary depending on a number of important variables, including type of problem prescribed for, physical condition of client, motivation and likelihood of compliance, and availability of significant others for support. (*b*) Running appears to produce biochemical changes that correspond with psychological changes. (*c*) There is a latency period, after the patient initiates the exercise program, before a therapeutic effect is achieved. (*d*) Running, like medication, must be done regularly to be effective. The runner "needs" regular doses of exercise to maintain the therapeutic effect (Sime 1977). Similarly, compliance to the exercise regimen is vital in order to first produce and then maintain a successful outcome. See chapter 11 by Buffone, Sachs, and Dowd for more information on compliance. (*e*) The psychological improvement associated with running subsides after the patient discontinues the regimen. (*f*) Last, a running treatment, like medication, seems to be most effective when used in conjunction with supportive and other psychotherapies. The use of running as a therapeutic treatment is fraught with special problems, some common to other somatic treatments, and like medication it should be carefully prescribed and monitored.

It is naive to expect running therapy to be any more of a panacea than primal therapy was several years ago. In fact it may follow the same route as primal and other "popular" therapies that were not soundly based, empirically or theoretically, and hence never found their way into the mainstream of psychotherapy. It behooves us to heed the lesson of these therapies that have "come and gone" and devote our research to determining what problems and clients are most amenable to such an approach. There are also a number of contraindications for this method of treatment, discussed in chapter 1.

### Assessment and Treatment

One area that has received limited attention is the assessment of potential participants in exercise therapy. Consistent clinical efficacy demands careful client-specific assessment—clinicians must pay attention to individual differences that reflect significant variations in ability to benefit psychologically from an exercise prescription. Some factors that require early assessment are patients' values, expectations for treatment, belief systems, cognitive and affective sets, and coping repertoires. Applying any therapeutic intervention such as running indiscriminately to broadly defined problems like depression almost guarantees failure. Are we treating reactive or endogenous depression, unipolar or bipolar?

The treatment, regardless of its nature, must be tailored to the patient. The clinician may be "oversold" on particular methods, in this case running, by researchers working with preselected populations and reporting averaged data. Different treatments need to be prescribed for different clinical problems. For example, physical exercise may be beneficial for patients experiencing anxiety at the somatic level, while meditation may prove a better strategy for those overburdened by cognitive anxiety (Schwartz, Davidson, and Goleman 1978).

Why is it so vital to conduct a comprehensive assessment of the patient? Primarily because of the complexity of the presenting problems, which dictates multilevel intervention. The patient who presents a primary problem of anxiety may manifest this anxiety in one specific response channel or several channels. Research evidence suggests that the cognitive (e.g., subjective distress), motoric (e.g., avoidance behavior), and physiological response channels are not necessarily highly intercorrelated. There is increasing evidence that cognitive techniques are most effective in reducing subjective distress (Wein, Nelson, and Odum 1975) and that in vivo procedures are differentially effective in modifying avoidance behavior (Leitenberg et al. 1971), and there is some suggestion that systematic desensitization might be differentially effective in reducing conditioned autonomic responses (Bellack and Hersen 1977).

The complexity of the clinical problems that have been treated by running has been largely ignored, as happened in the early introduction of other therapeutic strategies. Despite the promise held out by initial behaviorists, more recent evidence catalogs only moderate success in maintaining and generalizing treatment effects. These somewhat disappointing results can generally be traced to the naive assumption that the respective disorders involve identical symptoms or causes that will respond to unitary treatments. On the contrary, recent emphasis on systematic assessment has demonstrated the complexity of these problems and shown that multiple interventions are often necessary.

This again stresses the importance of not only a thorough pretreatment assessment, but also continual reassessments throughout treatment. This is necessary to identify false starts or trouble spots that may hamper the effects of an exercise treatment or require supplementary methods.

One last question on the assessment stage of exercise therapy is, What are some of the practical issues? Besides the necessary demographic, historical, and clinical (mental status) information, what other information would prove useful? It seems that general guidelines for additional assessment data would include past physical exercise (frequency, intensity, duration), attitudes toward exercise, physical condition (possible contraindications such as weight or cardiovascular risk), motivation to initiate and maintain an exercise program, and potential support from family, work, and environment. Compliance with an exercise regimen is vital to its continued success. As with all treatments, compliance outside the therapist's office is a problem. A number of factors and strategies (see Buffone, Sachs, and Dowd, chap. 11; Dunbar and Stunkard 1979) may be used in designing an exercise program so the patient can become positively addicted (see also Sachs and Pargman, chap. 13.)

What about the actual use of running or other exercise as a therapeutic technique? At this point clinicians are left pretty much to their own devices. Although there are several guides for conducting such a program (see prior chapters on application by Berger, Eischens, and Greist), some do not provide specific guidelines for implementation. Several issues require consideration. First, are the client and the problem amenable to such an approach? This can be answered only by a careful analysis of the client and by study of the literature reporting on the use of exercise with the particular problem. Second, if this intervention does appear appropriate, then the patient must be "sold" on the procedure and be willing to participate. It is at this point that the clinician may either lose patients or decide on an alternative treatment, since many clients expect to passively receive a "cure" in therapy. They may be extremely uncomfortable at discovering that they are expected to actively—in fact strenuously—participate in treatment. They also discover that their treatment outcome depends greatly upon their own efforts. In this model the therapist is likely to act more as a consultant who assists clients in improving their emotional condition.

If the client clears this obstacle, the exercise dosage or prescription is set. The dosage must be tailored to the client's physical condition (regarding weight, exercise history, cardiovascular fitness) so it will produce the desired therapeutic effect. With patients in extremely poor physical condition (e.g., obese chain smokers), lifestyle changes may have to be included, such as weight loss, cessation of smoking, or involvement in other programs designed to alter lifestyle.

Generally it seems that thirty minutes of walking/jogging three or four times a week is appropriate for the beginner. See Berger (chap. 2) and Eischens and Greist (chap. 3) for more specific suggestions on exercise prescriptions and beginning an exercise program.

Clients must be closely supervised in the early weeks to detect any difficulties and correct any problems that may impede adherence. They must also, as is sometimes true with medication, be told that visible effects may take several weeks so they will not be discouraged if they gain no immediate symptomatic relief. The latency period for improvement may vary from several days to several weeks depending on a variety of factors (e.g., particular problem, client's expectancies, or physical condition). Many patients become discouraged because results are not "instant" in the true American sense of the word. One real advantage of this method is that much of the running can be assigned, after minimal instruction, as homework, so most of the session is available for other interventions.

As mentioned in chapter 1, running functions best as an adjunct to verbally oriented therapies. Thus far running has been used in combination with psychoanalysis, cognitive-behavior therapy, hypnosis, guided imagery, "counseling," and less well specified treatment methods. It is likely that it may be combined with yet other methods in the future.

### Special Populations

Running and exercise have already been used to improve the psychological functioning of a number of analogue and clinical populations (Folkins and Sime 1981). Improvements have been reported with children (see Shipman, chap. 8), adolescents, and geriatric populations, drug- and alcohol-addicted patients, anxious, phobic, and depressed individuals, and persons experiencing insomnia or poor self-concept. Since these applications have been presented in the chapters by Eischens and Greist, Berger, and others, I will focus on other special groups.

One such group is the developmentally disabled. Miller (1981) has used an aerobic running program with the developmentally handicapped and has developed a training manual for clinicians.

Adolescents, whose problems are not particularly amenable to traditional forms of verbal psychotherapy, may also respond to an organized running program. The limited research conducted with this population (Holden 1962; Howard, Heaps, and Thorstenson 1972; Johnson 1962) offers at least tentative support for this suggestion. Shipman (chap. 8) further discusses the potential for such an approach with children and adolescents with emotional disorders.

Women seem to benefit greatly from physical exercise. Berger (see chaps. 2, 9, 10) and Oglesby (1981) present excellent discussions of running and exercise as tools to decrease psychological dysfunction and improve the status and well-being of women.

A fourth special population that merits attention is the elderly. Considering the high incidence of depression in this age group, aerobic activity may be an efficient and effective alternative for improving psychological functioning. It appears certain from the available literature that exercise particularly benefits the aged (see, for example, Bennett, Carmack, and Gardner 1982). A number of studies have shown that regular exercise reduces the incidence of certain life-threatening diseases and thereby increases longevity. Regular jogging in previously sedentary middle-aged males produces consistent decreases in resting heart rate and increases maximum oxygen consumption, which typically declines with age (Kasch 1976; Paolone et al. 1976). Other studies have shown that regular jogging can improve the functioning of the cardiovascular and respiratory systems, retard deterioration, and prevent disease (Frederick 1970; Roby and Davis 1970). These psychological and physiological advantages of exercise seem especially pertinent to problems that often accompany the aging process.

Last is psychosomatic or behavioral medicine. Running and other aerobic exercises play a vital role in the rapidly expanding area of preventive health care and health maintenance. Here exercise serves as a preventive measure to assist the "worried well" in avoiding more serious psychological or medical problems. The inclusion of exercise in programs for cessation of smoking, weight management, dietary regulation with diabetics, and rehabilitation after myocardial infarction signals its importance. Stress management also incorporates running to help patients reduce the harmful effects of stress in their daily living. Schaefer (1978) listed several specific benefits of regular running in reducing stress.

These are only a few areas in which exercise can increase physical and psychological health. Through persistent and continued application springing from quality research, we can more definitively determine appropriate exercise prescriptions for each population. Other populations, settings, and problems certainly deserve further attention. For example, how could exercise be incorporated into programs to treat the mentally retarded, the psychotic, and headache victims?

## Summary

Current research in counseling, psychology, and medicine points to physical exercise's positive effect on mental health. Running and other forms of exercise seem to build confidence, alleviate moderate state anxiety and reactive depression, increase body awareness and image, reduce weight, promote habit control, and improve sleep. Other areas of application have yet to be discovered. Aerobic activities maintained over a period of time do appear to produce positive psychological changes with a number of problems commonly presented to clinicians. For this reason an exercise approach, involving one or several forms of activity, deserves consideration as a possible adjunct to more traditional therapy.

Despite these initial claims, there is a desperate need for higher-quality research and theoretical development. There are also very specific limitations on this type of treatment, which remains in its infancy. Before running therapy can be considered fully viable as a treatment alternative, these concerns and issues will have to be addressed. Only then can we begin to rely on exercise as yet another tool in the quest to help people improve the quality of their lives.

## References

Bahrke, M. S., and Morgan, W. P. 1978. Anxiety reduction following exercise and meditation. *Cognitive Therapy and Research* 2:323–33.

Bellack, A. S., and Hersen, M. 1977. *Behavior modification: An introductory textbook.* Baltimore: Williams and Wilkins.

Bennett, J.; Carmack, M. A.; and Gardner, V. J. 1982. The effect of a program of physical exercise on depression in older adults. *Physical Educator* 39(1):21–24.

Campbell, D. T., and Stanley, J. C. 1963. *Experimental and quasi-experimental designs for research.* Chicago: Rand McNally.

Davidson, P. O., and Davidson, S. M., eds. 1980. *Behavioral medicine: Changing health lifestyles.* New York: Brunner/Mazel.

DeFries, Z. 1981. "Running madness": A prelude to real madness. In *Psychology of running,* ed. M. H. Sacks and M. L. Sachs. Champaign, Ill.: Human Kinetics Publishers.

Dodson, L. C., and Mullens, W. R. 1969. Some effects of jogging on psychiatric hospital patients. *American Corrective Therapy Journal* 23:130–34.

Dunbar, J. M., and Stunkard, J. A. 1979. Adherence to diet and drug regimen. In *Nutrition, lipids and coronary heart disease,* ed. R. Levy, B. Rifkind, B. Dennis and N. Ernst. New York: Raven Press.

Folkins, C. H., and Sime, W. E. 1981. Physical fitness training and mental health. *American Psychologist* 36:373–89.

Frederick, J. 1970. How jogging improves body functions. *Journal of Physical Education* 67:124.

Gary, V., and Guthrie, D., 1972. The effect of jogging on physical fitness and self concept in hospitalized alcoholics. *Quarterly Journal of Studies on Alcohol* 33:1073–78.

Harris, D. V. 1973. *Involvement in sport: A somatopsychic rationale for physical activity.* Philadelphia: Lea and Febiger.

Holden, R. H. 1962. Change in body image of physically handicapped children due to summer camp experience. *Merrill-Palmer Quarterly of Behavior and Development* 8:19–26.

Hollandsworth, J. G., Jr. 1979. Some thoughts on distance running as biofeedback. *Journal of Sport Behavior* 2:71–82.

Howard, G.; Heaps, R. A.; and Thorstenson, C. T. 1972. Self-concept change following outdoor survival training. Mimeographed. Provo, Utah: Brigham Young University.

Johnson, W. R. 1962. Some psychological aspects of physical rehabilitation: Toward an organismic theory. *Journal of the Association for Physiological and Mental Rehabilitation* 16:165–68.

Kasch, F. 1976. The effects of exercise on the aging process. *Physician and Sportsmedicine* 4:64–68.

Kostrubala, T. 1976. *The joy of running*. Philadelphia: J. B. Lippincott.

———. 1978. The training of a running therapist. *Medicine and Sport* 12:111–15.

Lazarus, R. S. 1975. A cognitively oriented psychologist looks at biofeedback. *American Psychologist* 30:553–61.

Leitenberg, H.; Agras, S.; Butz, R.; and Wincze, J. 1971. Relationship between heart rate and behavioral change during the treatment of phobias. *Journal of Abnormal Psychology* 78:59–68.

Maslach, C. 1976. Burned-out. *Human Behavior* 12:16–18.

Michael, E. D., Jr. 1957. Stress adaptation through exercise. *Research Quarterly* 28:50–54.

Miller, A. 1981. Therapeutic jogging for the developmentally disabled. Paper presented at the Midwest Symposium on Exercise and Mental Health, Lake Forest College, Lake Forest, Illinois, 25 April.

Morgan, W. P. 1974. Exercise and mental disorders. In *Sports medicine,* ed. A. J. Ryan and F. L. Allman, Jr. New York: Academic Press.

———. 1979. Anxiety reduction following acute physical activity. *Psychiatric Annals* 9(3):36–45.

Oglesby, C. 1981. The women who run: Arbitrary limitation or freedom. In *Psychology of running,* ed. M. H. Sacks and M. L. Sachs. Champaign, Ill.: Human Kinetics Publishers.

Paolone, A. M.; Lewis, R. R.; Lanigan, W. T.; and Goldstein, W. J. 1976. Results of two years of exercise training in middle-aged men. *Physician and Sportsmedicine* 4:72–77.

Roby, R., and Davis, P. 1970. *Jogging for fitness and weight control*. Philadelphia: Saunders.

Sacks, M. H., and Sachs, M. L., eds. 1981. *Psychology of running*. Champaign, Ill.: Human Kinetics Publishers.

Schaefer, W. 1978. *Stress, distress and growth*. Davis, Calif.: Responsible Action.

Schwartz, G. E.; Davidson, R. J.; and Goleman, D. J. 1978. Patterning of cognitive and somatic processes in the self-regulation of anxiety: Effects of meditation versus exercise. *Psychosomatic Medicine* 40:321–28.

Sime, W. E. 1977. A comparison of exercise and meditation in reducing psychological response to stress. *Medicine and Science in Sports* 8:55.

Solomon, E. G., and Bumpus, A. K. 1978. The running-meditation response: An adjunct to psychotherapy. *American Journal of Psychotherapy* 32:583–92.

Stein, L., and Belluzzi, J. D. 1978. Brain endorphins and the sense of well-being: A psychobiological hypothesis. *Advances in Biochemical Psychopharmacology* 18:299–311.

Wein, K. S.; Nelson, R. O.; and Odum, J. V. 1975. The relative contribution of verbal extinction to the effectiveness of cognitive restructuring. *Behavior Therapy* 6:459–74.

# Section 2

## Running and Psychology

# Introduction

The psychology of running has experienced rapid growth in the past decade. Concomitant with the "running boom," in which millions have taken up running, research has been conducted in numerous related areas. Five that have received particular attention are reviewed here: addiction to running, the effect of running on personality, the "runner's high," cognitive strategies used during running, and research in the psychology and therapeutics of running.

Michael L. Sachs and David Pargman (chap. 13) explore the relation of runners to their activity. For most, running is what Glasser has termed a positive addiction, supportive of the runner's psychology and physiology. For these people running is an important but considered part of life. Morgan has noted, however, that for some people it becomes a negative addiction; running becomes a controlling factor, eliminating other choices in life. In addition to running addiction, chapter 13 examines the related areas of commitment to running and motivation.

In chapter 14 Richard A. Dienstbier discusses the effect of exercise on personality, presenting a logical analysis of mediators of personality change including physiological effects, perception of physical changes, and changes in patterns of socializing and liking. He surveys research evidence on how running affects personality, pointing out problems with studies in this area (more fully explored by Silva and Shultz in chap. 17). Dienstbier concentrates on those personality dimensions most studied by researchers: anxiety (including "neuroticism"), depression, and the dimensions of Cattell's Sixteen Personality Factor

Questionnaire. In spite of flaws, research has shown personality changes after exercise programs of only four months or less. This chapter focuses on the commonality of the physiological systems involved in aerobic exercise and in emotional states and on the expectation that running will influence both short-term emotional functioning and temperament.

Perhaps the aspect of running that is most exciting but most difficult to study is the "runner's high." In this altered state of consciousness—a euphoric sensation during running, usually unexpected—the runner may feel heightened well-being, enhanced appreciation of nature, and transcendence of barriers of time and space. Reports on the percentage of runners who experience this differ considerably, with some studies indicating that 77 to 78 percent of the runners have experienced the runner's high while others estimate only 9 to 10 percent. In chapter 15 Michael L. Sachs discusses the characteristics of the runner's high and gives examples of the peak experience (what one might call a "super" runner's high). Additionally, Sachs discusses the theory that the endorphins are related to the runner's high and suggests possibilities for research.

Of particular importance are the cognitive strategies used during running. In chapter 16 Sachs discusses the concepts of association and dissociation first developed by Morgan. In the former, runners focus on bodily sensations, whereas in the latter they focus on anything else. Morgan noted that elite runners used associative strategies during a marathon competition while other competitors used primarily dissociative strategies. Further research has supported these findings and also suggested other ways to view the use of these strategies during training and competition. Related areas of the "wall" and the Tibetan art of lung-gom are discussed.

Research in the psychology and therapeutics of running is surveyed in a methodological and interpretive review by John M. Silva and Barry B. Shultz (chap. 17). They review certain studies on the value of running in treating anxiety and depression, then propose criteria for evaluating running research. They discuss problems of control in experimental designs and problems of analysis as well as methodological artifacts in behavioral research and make recommendations for improving research designs in this area.

MICHAEL L. SACHS AND DAVID PARGMAN

# 13

---

# Running Addiction

"I have run since infancy. . . . It's the passion of my life. Running as long as possible—I've made that into a sport. I have no other secrets. Without running I wouldn't be able to live." (Waldemar Cierpinski, in *Track and Field News,* 1980). Although most runners would not characterize their relationship with running this strongly, many would probably admit to similar sentiments. Cierpinski, an East German marathon runner and one of only two men to have won the Olympic marathon twice (in 1976 and 1980), illustrates the depth of involvement of some runners.

A number of terms have been used in the popular and research literature to describe this involvement with running. These terms include compulsion (Abell 1975), dependence (Sachs and Pargman 1979a), obsession (Waters 1981), healthy habit (Peele 1981b), and addiction (Glasser 1976; Kostrubala 1976). Eighteen years ago the World Health Organization suggested dropping the terms drug addiction and drug habituation in favor of the term drug dependence (Worick and Schaller 1977), in part owing to the frequently inappropriate use of the term addiction. The same criticisms may be offered today. Indeed, a term such as "healthy habit" (Peele 1981b) may be more appropriate for characterizing the relationship most runners have with their activity. But though the term "healthy habit" or "dependence" may be preferable, "addiction" remains in extensive use, so we will use that term.

Peele has written extensively in this area (1978, 1979, 1980, 1981a,b; Peele and Brodsky 1976) and raises a number of points to consider. Addiction is a process, rather than a condition. It is not an all-or-none state of being, unambiguously present or absent. Addiction is an extension of ordinary behavior—a pathological habit, dependence, or compulsion. It is characteristic not of drugs or activities per se (one is not necessarily addicted to heroin or to cigarettes), but of the involvement a person forms with these substances or events. Given this approach, addiction can certainly apply to participation in physical activity, including running, swimming, and playing tennis.

### Positive Addiction

The concept of addiction in relation to such salubrious experiences as exercise and meditation was first popularized by William Glasser in *Positive Addiction* (1976), an examination of addictions he considers supportive of the addict's psychology and physiology. Positive addictions, such as running and meditation, are thought to promote psychological strength and increase life satisfaction. This is in sharp contrast to negative addictions such as to alcohol or heroin, which often undermine psychological and physiological integrity. The thesis of Glasser's work is that "Many people, weak and strong, can help themselves to be stronger, and an important new path to strength may be positive addiction" (1976, 11).

While Glasser's work is not scientifically based in the sense of incorporating rigorous experimental design and statistical analysis, it includes useful clinical and psychiatric assessments. He reports the general feeling of "high" or euphoria experienced by regular runners (see Sachs, chap. 15). Classic descriptions of the state achieved in positive addiction include a loss of the sense of oneself, floating, euphoria, and total integration with running. Glasser recommends running for anyone, strong or weak psychologically, who seeks a positively addicting activity.

Glasser, as we noted, is generally credited with popularizing the concept of positive addiction to activities such as running and meditation. But Kostrubala, in *The Joy of Running* (1976), also used the term addiction: "Slow long-distance running is addictive" (p. 140). Although the question whether Glasser or Kostrubala first used the term is not really important here, the mid to late 1970s were the years when the concept of running addiction became a significant one in the psychology of running.

Research evidence on exercise addiction (and addiction to running in particular) is limited because of the relative newness of the concept and the difficulty of studying addicted exercisers, particularly in an experimental context. Baekeland (1970), for example, could not get regular exercisers to stop exercising for any amount of money. It is extremely difficult, if not impossible, to persuade addicted exercisers to stop so one can study the effects of exercise deprivation. The confounding effects of physical injury, often the only factor that will cause an addicted runner to stop, cloud interpretation of psychological reactions during this deprivation state.

## Addiction to Running

A number of studies have, however, examined psychological characteristics of exercise addicts. Sachs and Pargman (1979b) studied runners at several stages of addiction. Reasons for beginning to run varied and included the influence of others, concerns about general health, improvement of cardiovascular fitness, and weight reduction. These reasons, frequently cited in the literature, continued to be present as the participants maintained their running programs and addiction developed, but additional psychological considerations such as feeling better, relaxing, and getting away from things became manifest. Running became a significant part of their lives.

Running addiction may be defined as psychological and/or physiological addiction to a regular regimen of running, characterized by withdrawal symptoms after twenty-four to thirty-six hours without the activity. Withdrawal symptoms appear to be critical in determining the existence and degree of addiction. These include anxiety, restlessness, guilt, irritability, tension, bloatedness, muscle twitching, and discomfort. Some report suffering, apathy, sluggishness, weight loss owing to lack of appetite, sleeplessness, headaches, and stomachaches (Glasser 1976).

Addicted runners may suffer both psychological *and* physiological symptoms when they cannot run. The regular regimen is defined by the individual and may range from twice a day (or even more often) seven days a week, to only once a day a few times a week. However, such runners must have an expectation that they will run a certain number of times each week, and they generally plan these runs in advance (e.g., knowing one will run on Tuesdays, Thursdays, and Sundays, with the other days serving as rest days).

Finally, twenty-four to thirty-six hours is a general time frame, since most addicted runners run five, six, or seven days per week, so that missing a day brings on these withdrawal symptoms. However, these symptoms are expected only on those days when the individual had planned to run. In a "sensible" running program, a day or two of rest each week is built in. These rest days are preplanned, and the runner does not expect to run on these days. We should therefore not expect notable withdrawal symptoms on these "rest" days, and measurements taken then might well be misleading. However, if an individual has planned to run on a given day and found, for whatever reason (perhaps pressing familial or work responsibilities), that he or she could not run, then withdrawal symptoms would be expected.

The withdrawal symptoms are seen as a negative aspect of running. Harris (1981b), for example, tested 156 women and asked about their feelings during a period when they had stopped running. Only 10.3 percent of the woman had never stopped running. Of the rest, 71.4 percent felt less energetic, 67.9 percent felt guilty, 67.9 percent felt fatter, 40.0 percent felt depressed, and 38.6 percent felt tense when they stopped running. These negative changes were reported far more frequently than positive ones of feeling relieved (2.1 percent, thinner (1.4 percent), relaxed (1.4 percent), or more energetic (0.7 percent). In both this study and another (Harris 1981a) there was a preponderance of negative feelings correlated with not running. Summers et al. (1982) reported findings consistent with those of Harris.

The degree of these withdrawal symptoms remains to be fully investigated. Although Sachs (1981) has described these withdrawal symptoms, the degree of symptoms reported by the runners was only low to moderate. Robbins and Joseph (1982) note basically similar findings, though they report slightly higher levels of withdrawal symptoms. They state, as well, that women are more likely to associate themselves with withdrawal symptoms than are men, perhaps owing to greater sensitivity or greater willingness to report symptoms.

Although anecdotal reports indicate high levels of such withdrawal symptoms as guilt or anxiety in people deprived of exercise, it is possible that they will not be reported as so intense on paper and pencil tests. Furthermore, some symptoms might be more frequently cited because articles on exercise withdrawal in the popular literature lead runners to believe they should experience certain symptoms if they miss a run. Robbins and Joseph (1982) have termed this the *"Runner's World* effect'' (note also Thaxton 1982), and it may also be seen in other aspects of running such as the runner's high. It is clear from the social psychological literature that expecting to experience something may be all that is needed to cause that experience.

Withdrawal symptoms may be explained in a number of ways. Robbins and Joseph (1982) suggest two. The first is that withdrawal symptoms (or deprivation sensations, to use their term) indicate insufficient stress reduction or incomplete stress avoidance when a run is missed. For some people running masks sensations of stress; but as long as the sources of these sensations remain running will indeed only mask them (as opposed to "eliminating" them), and they will be experienced again when running ceases. For others running is a coping mechanism during periods of stress or times of anxiety and depression. A danger runners face is that exclusive reliance on running as a way of coping may cause other coping mechanisms to atrophy, leaving them without effective means of handling stress when running is not possible because of injury or for other reasons.

The second possibility Robbins and Joseph (1982) suggest is that withdrawal symptoms are explained by the "actual loss of the day to day reinforcement of positive self-feeling" (p. 6); "the psychological and psychophysiological distress experienced upon missing the daily run may simply reflect withdrawal of a self-esteem enhancing activity" (p. 7). Both these explanations are viable, and one or the other is probably applicable to individual runners.

In their study of the behavioral components of exercise addiction Robbins and Joseph (1982) found that the most consistent predictor of running deprivation sensations was general distress. They suggest that this finding supports a "misinterpretation" thesis of withdrawal symptoms (1982, 20–21); "Among runners for whom the activity serves to modify dysphoric mood states or psychophysiological distress, return of distress once the effects of the run have decreased may be misunderstood as symptoms of physiological withdrawal. In this instance, withdrawal may not be the pain associated with the body adjusting to the physiological changes of non-running, but a reexperience of the pain felt *before* the physiological changes of running." An example would be a runner with sleeping problems who is more likely to experience such problems after missing a workout. This might not be a deprivation effect but simply a recurrence of the previous problem.

Another finding of Robbins and Joseph (1982) was that fewer manifestations of distress were experienced by runners who used running primarily as an escape than by those for whom running was an important coping mechanism. They explain that escape is a means of avoiding life's stressors, but these stressors will not necessarily be present whenever the person cannot run. On the other hand, for those who use running to reduce the effect of stressors, an inability to run means that the effects are not reduced, so one would expect an increase in distress.

In examining runners who felt that mastery was their most important reason for running, Robbins and Joseph (1982) found withdrawal symptoms when running was not possible. They note that "frustration and irritability also appear to accompany withdrawal of a regular experience that acts to reinforce one's perception of competence and self-worth" (p. 23).

The time before exercisers report addiction varies. Glasser (1976) suggests that up to two years may be required, though some runners have reported addiction in as little as one to two months (Sachs 1981). Sachs (1981) has noted that some people report running for five, ten, and even twenty years before feeling addicted.

Carmack and Martens (1979) examined what they term "commitment to running," which we view as synonymous with running addiction. Runners scoring higher on a measure of commitment to running reported greater discomfort when they missed a run, had a higher level of perceived addiction, and ran for longer periods on their regular runs. In this study, as in those we have conducted (Sachs 1981; Sachs and Pargman 1979a,b), runners scoring high on commitment to running tend to give psychological reasons for continuing. Although a psychobiological framework (Morgan 1973) incorporating both psychological and physiological factors in addiction to exercise is most appropriate, predominantly psychological factors are reported in describing running addiction.

Combinations of running and meditation have been used in programs to develop positive addiction and promote psychological benefits. Solomon and Bumpus proposed a "running meditation response" as a viable adjunct to psychotherapy. They indicate that running regularly leads to addiction (1978, 585):

> We emphasize running three to five days a week simply because regularity leads to addiction, a key factor in the success of this method. The more frequently the patient runs, the more he will experience the pleasurable and desirable effects of running and, consequently, the more quickly he will become addicted. Addiction usually occurs in two to four months. Once the patient is "hooked," he will feel a compulsion to run. If he does not, he will experience withdrawal symptoms, such as anxiety, not feeling well, or insomnia.

### Measuring Addiction

The most popular instrument for measuring addiction to running is the "Feelings about Running" scale developed by Carmack and Martens (1979), which rates commitment to running (defined here as running addiction). The scale has acceptable validity and reliability and has been used extensively in subsequent research.

The "Feelings about Running" scale asks subjects to express how they feel most of the time (how they generally feel) toward twelve statements about running, employing a five-point scale from 1 (strongly disagree) through 5 (strongly agree). The scale includes such statements as "I look forward to running," "Running is vitally important to me," "Running is pleasant," "I would arrange or change my schedule to meet the need to run," and "Running is the high point of my day." Although the scale is valuable for researchers, we have found that runners tend to consistently score high (average in the middle to high 40s out of a possible 60—range of 12 to 60 on the scale). There appears to to be some desirability or demand factor inherent in the scale, since runners tend to agree with the statements about running, perhaps to avoid appearing to not really like an activity in which they participate extensively.

Furthermore, Thaxton (1982) found that the Commitment to Running (CR) score (on the "Feelings about Running" scale) was not significantly correlated with a measure of perceived addiction. Additionally, some measures of running involvement (race frequency and fast race times) correlated only with CR score and not with perceived addiction. Thaxton found that "several subjects with high scores (50 to 60) on the CR scale stated that they were not all physically and psychologically dependent on running and never experienced withdrawal" (p. 79). This suggests that Thaxton's method needs refinement, that the CR scale is not as strong a measure of commitment to running as it appears to be, or that both these possibilities are true. Researchers using the "Feelings about Running" scale of Carmack and Martens (1979) should consider further refining this instrument and possibly using it in conjunction with other appropriate psychological and physiological measures (e.g., Thaxton 1982).

Another instrument that may prove valuable was devised by Joseph and Robbins (1981), who incorporated the measurement of addiction to running into their "Running Survey." Unfortunately, no validity or reliability information has yet been published for this instrument.

J. M. Robbins (personal communication) has raised an important point concerning both his "Running Survey" and other measures in this area (such as the Sachs 1981 measure of withdrawal symptoms). In investigating withdrawal symptoms, it is important to examine both the frequency with which certain symptoms are reported *and* their severity. Current measures have not done so or differentiated adequately between the two measures. Sachs (1981), as was noted, has developed an instrument to measure runners' withdrawal symptoms, but its validity and reliability also remain to be determined.

## How and Why Does Addiction Develop?

Although numerous studies have investigated motivation for beginning to participate in physical activity, running in particular (Pargman 1980; Roth 1974; Sachs 1981), and have noted such factors as the influence of others, concern with general health, improvement of cardiovascular fitness and weight reduction, the process by which addiction develops in runners has not yet been identified. Sachs (1981), Sachs and Pargman (1979b), and Jacobs (1980), in three separate attempts to identify this process, all failed to uncover a personality typology of runners or to construct a general descriptive classification of the addiction process. Although it is evident that runners do become addicted to their activity, we cannot at present identify which factors predispose individuals to become addicted, nor can we pinpoint the environmental and situational factors critical to determining whether and when a person will become addicted to running.

Jacobs (1980), in particular, used depth interviews, survey questionnaires, and participant observation to investigate how people become addicted to running. He found that runners did indeed become addicted, and that the long-term effects were positive. Jacobs suggested that the basis for addiction might be the runners' perception that the effects of running were positive both physiologically and psychologically. However, no clear delineation of the process of addiction was provided—it remains for future research to uncover.

Addiction may be promoted by an environment that reinforces an "addicted lifestyle." Robbins (1982) has found evidence for this in the sociological literature. If, for example, a new runner joins a local track club, frequently participates in races, and gets "caught up" in the running lifestyle, the reinforcement derived from these interactions may promote addiction. Nash (1976, 1977, 1979, 1980) notes a number of intriguing aspects of running and weekend racing as eventful experiences in runners' lives. This "addicted lifestyle" must be considered in any comprehensive assessment of the addiction process.

A point made by Kostrubala (1976, 144) is relevant here:

> . . . the similarities of slow long-distance running to the addictive drugs named [alcohol, opiates, barbiturates] and to the hallucinogens. However, all these drugs, whether frowned upon by society or subtly supported (as in alcohol addiction), produce behavior which can best be described as conformity. The major difference in slow long-distance running as addictive is that its withdrawal symptoms are primarily insomnia and anxiety. But the most striking social aspect of this addiction is that, far from producing conformity, it seems to promote individuality.

The intrinsic nature of running as an individual sport may affect its addictive properties, but the point warrants investigation. Perhaps its promoting individuality makes it more difficult for the researcher to discover general characteristics of the process by which individuals become addicted to running.

An explanation of addiction may perhaps be found in the physiological components of exercise. The discovery of naturally occurring opiatelike peptides known as endorphins has raised speculation that these compounds may be related to altered states of consciousness during running (such as the runner's high) and to running addiction (see Sachs, chap. 15). Although initial research has not provided much support for such a relation, future investigation may still reveal a connection.

## Positive Addiction and Negative Addiction

Although at present we cannot specify what conditions are critical to running addiction, we can identify some factors important to the concept of negative addiction to running.

Addiction to running is generally positive. Glasser (1976) proposed that running builds psychological and physiological strength. Runners begin with some motivating factor, frequently internal and self-motivating (Dishman, Ickes, and Morgan 1980) but occasionally external (praise from others, the rewards of t-shirts at races, etc.). Before addiction can develop, however, they must be motivated to continue running for an extended period (at least one or two months).

A fair percentage of those who begin running soon find that it is not for them and revert to inactivity or try other sports. Runners who do continue are buoyed by positive and negative reinforcements. There are the inevitable positive comments on how well one looks or how much weight one has lost, interactions with newly met running friends and the social atmosphere at races and track club meetings, the feeling of being in better shape, sleeping better, and perhaps experiencing the "feel better" effect during and after running. Occasionally negative reinforcement contingencies arise, such as fear of what might happen if one misses a day or doesn't run enough on a given day. Robbins and Joseph (1982, 26) note, for example, that many runners may "tend to run more to avoid the negative sensations that come from not running." Other reasons for running may include mastery, novelty/stimulation, competition/recognition, and escape (Robbins and Joseph 1982).

Graham (1979) offered additional thoughts on the whys of running. He suggested grouping participants into competitors, "health nuts," and quiet-time seekers. He himself is a quiet-time seeker and says:

It seems that my crowd runs partly as an escape from the pressures of life. We're the ones for whom the change into ritual clothing, the pain of running, and the shower of cleansing constitute a daily rebaptism into newness of life.

For us, the time spent running is time no one else has a claim on, and the rewards are similar to those of prayer and contemplation. Indeed, such exercise may constitute a secular pietism. (p. 821)

Graham goes on to present an important concept in motivation for running: the anxiety of terminal helplessness. As one of the women in his study indicated: "I am going to run until I can't put one foot in front of another, and then I'll be dead. No geriatrics ward for me" (p. 821). A considerable number of runners may indeed be driven on their daily runs by a hope that running will save them from helplessness, by anxiety about incapacity at life's end, and by a hope that their runners' bodies will not decay in a convalescent home in old age.

Whatever the reason(s) for running, participation becomes a habit, a regular part of daily activity. At this stage the runner is hooked. For most runners this level of involvement represents a "healthy habit." Some may find that other aspects of life begin to be shaped around the daily run, including eating and sleeping schedules and time spent with family and old friends (the runner frequently makes new friends, almost all of whom are runners). These adjustments are in addition to changes in diet and in leisure activities, which frequently include races or long runs on Sunday mornings and voracious reading of books and magazines on running. Running becomes a compulsion, a habit, an addiction. When days are missed, powerful withdrawal symptoms may manifest themselves. Running occasionally becomes not merely a means to the end of getting in shape, but the end itself. The need to run may become constant (Sacks 1981).

There is a nebulous, idiosyncratic area here, in which addiction may be said to shift from positive to negative. Last this seem unimportant, note that running may move from an important but considered aspect of one's existence to become a controlling factor, eliminating other choices in life. The runner must learn where the fine line between positive and negative addiction lies.

Most runners will remain in the positive addiction zone where running remains important, adding to the quality of life, building physiological and psychological strength (Glasser 1976). Running complements and supplements the other aspects of existence that are important to most people: family, friends, and work. Responsibilities in all these areas are acknowledged, but running represents a positive addition to the lifestyle and an effective tool for managing stress, anxiety, and depression.

For a small percentage of others running begins to control their lives, eliminating other choices. Morgan (1979a,b) has presented evidence on this negative aspect of running, noting that the development of exercise addiction does not differ from addictive processes in general. Although running is generally positive, it can be abused (too much of a good thing). Morgan cites a number of case studies of runners who are virtually consumed by the need to run. These runners dramatically alter their daily schedules, continue to run even when seriously injured, and neglect the responsibilities of work, home, and family. Morgan suggests that the behavior of hard-core exercise addicts resembles that in other major addictions.

Runners may recognize symptoms of negative addiction in themselves or in other runners. The toll of such strenuous training shows itself in decreased ability to concentrate, listlessness, fatigue, lapses in judgment, impaired social activity and work productivity, constant thought about running, and other subtle signs. More obvious symptoms include skipping appointments because of the need to run. Hailey and Bailey (1982) have made an initial attempt at quantifying negative addiction that may prove helpful in this area in the future. Because runners tend to be well educated, many negatively addicted runners can acknowledge these symptoms and recognize the effects of running on their lives. But accepting help is another matter.

We must be aware, though, of the implicit moral judgment being made here. Given the characteristics described above, we can suggest certain criteria for determining whether a person is positively or negatively addicted to running. But if an individual is "diagnosed" as negatively addicted, is this necessarily negative? For some people, a lifestyle centered on running—running bums, as Merrill (1980) calls them—might be positive. Sheehan further clouds the issue:

> I have learned there is no need for haste, no need to worry, no need to agonize over the future. The world will wait. Job, family, friends will wait; in fact, they must wait on the outcome. And that outcome depends upon the lifetime that is in every day of running. . . . Can anything have a higher priority than running? It defines me, adds to me, makes me whole. I have a job and family and friends that can attest to that. (1979, 49)

Clearly, for Sheehan, though running may control his life it enhances his existence to the degree that from his perspective it may indeed be positive. Many runners, however, are not as introspective or as analytical as Sheehan and may not realize that, as Waters (1981) suggests, running can pass from dedication to obsession. Waters believes that for most runners this transition from positive to negative addiction is a transient overindulgence—that most runners find it uncomfortable and may be forced to reorder their priorities.

Although this may be true for a large percentage of negative addicts, there certainly are others who do not comprehend the level of their involvement or realize the extent to which running controls their lives.

The effect that running addiction has on family life remains unclear. Some studies report that running may improve family relations and increase harmony and cohesion (Jorgenson and Jorgenson 1978) and that runners score lower on a standardized scale of marital conflict than a normative sample (Jones and Jones 1977). But these same studies indicate that running can interfere with social life (Jones and Jones 1977) and markedly affect the scheduling of time (Jones and Jones 1977; Jorgenson and Jorgenson 1978). Robbins and Joseph (1980, 98) found that:

> Direct conflict between the runner and his or her spouse or partner over such issues as neglect, loss of shared interests and friends, fatigue, and neglect of work was found to be consistently related to commitment to running. Higher levels of time and intensity commitment, subcultural involvement, and cognitive identification are associated with more intense complaints of the runner by his or her partner. Significantly, 42 percent of Full-time runners reported to have reappraised a relationship because of their commitment to running.

They suggest that there is a complex interaction between relational happiness and commitment to running. On the one hand, committed runners may neglect family and partner because of their running. On the other hand, conflict within the family may lead a person to use running as an outlet. Perhaps disagreements lead to running, leading to more disagreements, leading to more running, and so forth. The cycle could just as easily begin with running, however, leading to disagreements, and so on. This complex process must be assessed for each individual.

Robbins and Joseph (1980) also report that, in contrast to findings from research on leisure in general, relationships in which both partners ran did not appear to differ in intensity of conflicts. However, they note that couples where both ran did "report happier overall relationships than single runner couples" (p. 98). The interaction of running with family life and interpersonal relation must certainly be considered in dealing with negatively addicted runners (as well as with positively addicted runners who are having difficulty in relationships owing to involvement in running).

We need to give thought to programs of therapy designed to return addiction to the positive end of the continuum. What form might such programs take? One program already in operation is the Toronto Runner's Clinic (*Runner's*

*World* 1981), which employs specialists in sports medicine, nutrition, fitness, and training. However, psychological aspects of addiction may not be directly addressed, and some suggestions for programs of therapy with a psychological emphasis are appropriate here.

Initially, general information about negative addiction must be provided in an effort to make negatively addicted runners aware of their dependence. Meetings can be held to discuss addiction to running in general, and they should focus specifically on behaviors that characterize the negatively addicted runner. Written material can highlight important points. At this juncture the runners, now educated as to the nature and degree of their addiction, must decide whether they wish to continue at the same level or try to decrease their involvement.

For those seeking help, the key at this point is getting them to decrease their running and learn to cope with their initial withdrawal symptoms. The assistance of a skilled running therapist is desirable (Kostrubala 1976, 1978; see also Kostrubala, chap. 7). As Robbins and Joseph (1982) have noted, if running has been used as the sole coping mechanism, other coping skills may have atrophied and the runner may need help in redeveloping them.

Eventually, running should be incorporated as an integral part of the lifestyle, but a part that blends well with the responsibilities of work, friends, and family. Some runners, as Waters (1981) and Morgan (1979a,b) report, can accomplish this restructuring on their own. But many need the help of psychologists, psychiatrists, or friends who understand this condition, are aware of the importance of running to these individuals, and can help them regroup and become "human" again.

What happens to the addicted runner who cannot run? Usually this is the result of an injury, which almost always must be serious to make an addicted runner stop. In some cases a period without running may be part of a program of therapy. A number of withdrawal symptoms were cited earlier, including feelings of guilt, irritability, anxiety, tension, and restlessness. Clearly, these runners need coping strategies to use when exercise deprivation occurs. If the injury (if this is the reason for not running) does not restrict participation in other sports, then activities such as swimming or bicycle riding may be recommended. Even this may not satisfy the "true" addict, however. As one women said when a pulled Achilles tendon forced her to stop running for a time and substitute bicycling, "It was like methadone maintenance for a heroin addict."

For others who cannot run, the effects of inactivity may be more serious. Little (1969, 1979, 1981) reports on what he terms "the athlete's neurosis":

"in the forty-four athletic subjects a direct threat to their own physical well being, in the form of illness or injury, had initiated the neurotic breakdown in 72.5 per cent of cases, while in the twenty-eight neurotics of non-athletic personality such physical threats had preceded the onset of symptoms in only 10.7 per cent—a highly significant difference'' (Little 1969, 189).

In the great majority of athletic subjects the neurotic symptoms developed almost immediately after injury. Little goes on to say that ''the athlete's neurosis, which is no rare, trivial or short-lived reaction, can, and usually does, provoke prolonged and crippling psychological, domestic and economic strains, as many of these men despite previous sound work records subsequently remained unemployable for years'' (1969, 194).

Without being unduly alarming, I must caution that the prevalence of athlete's neurosis in those devoted to physical activity (fitness fanatics, as it were) in Little's study is reflected in anecdotal reports of times when running is not possible among some hard-core (negatively addicted?) runners. Certainly these considerations are worthy of further examination in assessing addiction to running.

### Commitment to Running

However, regular, even daily, participation does not necessarily mean a person is addicted. Sachs and Pargman (1979b) proposed a model to clarify motivation for running. We conceptualize two axes, one indicating psycho-biologic dependence (addiction), and the other cognitive-intellectual commitment, speculating that motivation for running is best examined through a two-factor, rather than a unidimensional, model. This model has received some support from our research, but further work is needed to establish its utility in this area of study.

Psychobiologic dependence may be defined, as earler, in terms of addiction to running and the presence of withdrawal symptoms. Commitment to running may be viewed as multifaceted in that numerous social, psychological, and physiological factors appear to underlie it. Time spent thinking and reading about running, distance traveled to races, frequency of competition, money spent on books and magazines about running and on equipment and accessories, changes in eating, sleeping, and other lifestyle patterns to accommodate the daily run, and the intensity and duration of running itself are all aspects of participation in running. (Note that our use of the term commitment to running differs from that of Carmack and Martens 1979, who make it synonymous with our concept of addiction.)

The model of participation in running is presented in figure 1. Four quadrants are proposed to define the relation of commitment to addiction, each hypothe- sized to categorize a different "type" of runner. See Joseph and Robbins (1981), in particular, and Morgan (1979a), Pargman (1980), and Sime (1979) for other descriptions of types of runners.

The truly addicted exerciser as described in the literature, found in quadrant A, is characterized by high levels of both commitment and addiction. Such a person's lifestyle centers on regular (usually daily) running, and motivational factors have progressed beyond interest in keeping in shape or reducing stored body fat. Persons in quadrant A seek psychological well-being through running and also try to avoid the withdrawal symptoms manifest when they stop.

An individual who is addicted to running but not totally committed to a regular schedule would be in quadrant B. Whereas social-environmental agents such as family, work, or school may take priority and impede regular running, addiction is still characteristic of those in this quadrant.

Quadrant C contains the occasional runner, characterized by low levels of commitment and addiction. This person may feel occasional twinges of guilt if running is not possible but does not suffer the acute withdrawal symptoms of the highly addicted person. Quadrant C runners run occasionally, with conveni- ence and the absence of other physical activity options dictating frequency.

Individuals in quadrant D deserve special attention because, to date, little in the literature acknowledges them. These runners are highly committed but not addicted to participation. It is possible that, owing to the absence of a number of

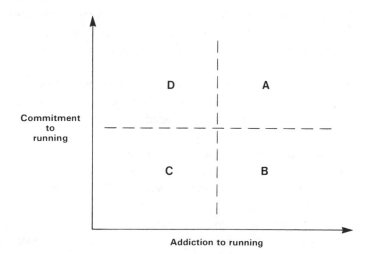

Figure 1. Model of participation in running.

Glasser's conditions for the development of a positive addiction, addiction has not yet developed. Glasser (1976, 93) has cited six criteria for a positive addiction:

(1) it is something noncompetitive that you choose to do and you can devote an hour (approximately) a day to it. (2) It is possible for you to do it easily and it doesn't take a great deal of mental effort to do it well. (3) You can do it alone or rarely with others but it does not depend upon others to do it. (4) You believe that it has some value (physical, mental, or spiritual) for you. (5) You believe that if you persist at it you will improve, but this is completely subjective—you need to be the only one who measures that improvement. (6) The activity *must* have the quality that you can do it *without criticizing yourself. If you can't accept yourself during this time the activity will not be addicting.*

Most runners begin running for health, weight reduction, or social reasons, but the addicted runner continues primarily because of the perceived psychological benefits of participation. These benefits include feeling better after a run, experiencing the runner's high, reducing stress, and avoiding withdrawal symptoms.

However, quadrant D runners do not progress to this stage, but remain committed for the health and social reasons that motivated them initially. One might run regularly to forestall a heart attack, owing to a history of heart attacks in his family. Another might run regularly because a boss or a friend runs, and reinforcement comes from these significant others rather than from running.

Quadrant D runners, therefore, do not run for mind-bending experiences, escape from depression, or euphoria. Their motives include health and social reasons, money (athletes on scholarship, professionals), prestige, power, and narcissism.

The proposed model of commitment and addiction is a dynamic one, with potential movement through its quadrants, but such movement does not occur freely. Indeed, there appear to be patterned directions for change of location within the model, as illustrated in figure 2.

All runners begin in quadrant C, at low levels of commitment and addiction. Before addiction can increase, commitment must increase, generally through an increase in how many days a week the person runs. Therefore movement from quadrant C can only be to quadrant D.

From quadrant D runners may move to quadrant A or C. As commitment remains high, addiction to running may develop, and the individual moves toward (into) quadrant A. If commitment decreases for any reason, movement

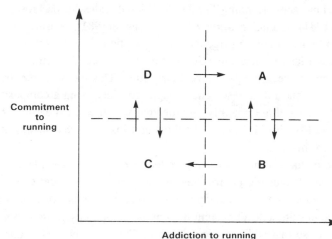

Figure 2. Potential movement patterns in the model of participation in running.

is toward quadrant C, with a low level of addiction remaining constant but commitment decreasing from high to low.

Movement from quadrant A can only be to quadrant B. Addiction will not decrease unless commitment first decreases, precipitating withdrawal symptoms. As commitment decreases, the person moves toward (into) quadrant B.

The runner in quadrant B will, within a matter of days or weeks, show a decrease in addiction and move toward quadrant C. At this point there are two possibilities for movement. If commitment remains constant (low), addiction will continue to decrease and movement into quadrant C will occur. If commitment increases, however, the runner will return to quadrant A.

That position in quadrant B is unstable is reinforced by the research of Conboy (1981). Conboy found that type B runners had the greatest mood change among runners in the four quadrants on a day when subjects could not run.

Despite the model's dynamic quality, position in quadrants A, C, and D tends to remain stable unless there are changes in motivation, with concomitant shifts in level of commitment or adherence to criteria for addiction (Glasser 1976). Position in quadrant B tends to be basically unstable, since low levels of commitment do not appear to be associated with high levels of addiction for longer than a few days or weeks. If movement does occur within the model, it takes the form(s) indicated earlier.

In evaluating the model, we must consider the measurement of the two factors. In the past, addiction has been measured using Carmack and Martens's

(1979) ''Feelings about Running'' scale. Additional scales, such as Joseph and Robbins's (1981) ''Running Survey'' and Sachs's (1981) measure of withdrawal symptoms, might be effective in conjunction with or instead of the Carmack and Martens measure. Commitment has been measured by the number of days a week the person regularly runs. This measure may be too basic, however, and future researchers might consider using a composite of factors representing those cognitive-intellectual variables cited earlier. Work by Joseph and Robbins (1981) and Robbins and Joseph (1980) makes useful initial steps in this area.

The value of the various distinctions cited in the model is evident as one considers what therapeutic approaches to use with addicted and committed individuals, and as one formulates programs to promote positive addiction to running. One must first develop commitment by maintaining participation at a sufficient level so that addiction can develop. The task, then, is to discover what factors move people from the state of committed but not addicted to committed *and* addicted and to promote this transfer.

This approach is preferable because a positive addiction to running presupposes that the activity is providing psychological and physiological strength and that the runner is therefore deriving positive benefits. Some of these benefits, particularly the psychological ones, may not be present if the runner is only committed (participating at a certain level) but not addicted. By promoting addiction, we endeavor to enhance the positive effects, primarily psychological, that positive addiction to running apparently offers.

### Healthy Habits versus Addiction

The relationship a person forms with a certain experience is critical in the development of addiction, with the emphasis on the process of the formation of this relationship. We have been using the term addiction herein because this term is used extensively in both the popular and the research literature. There is concern, however, that the term addiction is inappropriate here, since in its ''stricter'' application it has more limited usage than the broader definition Glasser (1976) has imparted to it with his concept of positive addiction. Indeed, the term addiction with respect to running may be appropriate only in discussing what Morgan (1979a,b) has termed negative addiction to running.

Peele (1981b) describes addiction as a pathological habit or dependency. He notes that an addiction impairs functioning, and that a habit cannot be simultaneously healthy and addictive. The ability to make decisions is a critical element here — when one can no longer make choices, then an addiction can be said to exist. The addiction controls the person's life, as opposed to the person controlling the addiction. Additionally, Peele states that "the keynote of an addiction is that it destroys a person's ability to cope with or gain gratification from anything else" (p. 28). Life is structured around the activity, and all emphasis is placed on and pleasure derived from it.

Although the concept of negative addiction (or just addiction) might therefore be appropriate in certain cases, it might be best to use another term for what we now think of as positive addiction to running. Peele suggests the term "healthy habits." These healthy habits enhance people's sense of themselves and their feeling of being in control of their health and well-being. Healthy habits also make people feel better about themselves, improve ability to cope with challenges, help in relation with other people and in activities, increase self-esteem, bring pleasure, and incease confidence in one's competence—all characteristics one would expect from a positive addiction.

Peele suggests a number of strategies for counseling addicted individuals and helping them develop healthy habits. He notes that one must begin by understanding the function the addiction serves and identify the rewards sought. Therapy then can provide intermediate rewards that substitute for the rewards derived from the addiction. Eventually the person learns to obtain real-world gratification from the activity. Ultimately, a habit is seen as healthful if it helps one find more satisfaction in life, rather than itself serving as the entire source of satisfaction. Peele suggests that a nonaddicted lifestyle is characterized by balance and proportion, including other interests, moderate expectations, appropriate alternatives, and friends with a variety of interests.

It appears that positive addiction to running is indeed a "healthy habit." Although the term addiction is likely to remain in regular use, particularly in the popular literature, we should realize that habitual running in its positive state is healthful. Given the negative connotations associated with the concept of addiction, it might be best to use the term "healthy habit" as more appropriate for describing our involvement with running.

## References

Abell, R. 1975. Confessions of a compulsive. *Runner's World* 10:30–31.

Baekeland, F. 1970. Exercise deprivation: Sleep and psychological reactions. *Archives of General Psychiatry* 22:365–69.

Carmack, M. A., and Martens, R. 1979. Measuring commitment to running: A survey of runners' attitudes and mental states. *Journal of Sport Psychology* 1:25–42.

Conboy, J. K. 1981. The effects of exercise withdrawal on mood states in runners. Unpublished manuscript, Massachusetts School of Professional Psychology.

Dishman, R. K.; Ickes, W.; and Morgan, W. P. 1980. Self-motivation and adherence to habitual physical activity. *Journal of Applied Social Psychology* 10:115–32.

Glasser, W. 1976. *Positive addiction*. New York: Harper and Row.

Graham, W. F. 1979. The anxiety of the runner: Terminal helplessness. *Christian Century* 29 August–5 September 821–23.

Hailey, B. J., and Bailey, L. A. 1982. Negative addiction in runners: A quantitative approach. *Journal of Sport Behavior* 5:150–54.

Harris, M. B. 1981a. Runners' perceptions of the benefits of running. *Perceptual and Motor Skills* 52:153–54.

———. 1981b. Women runners' views of running. *Perceptual and Motor Skills* 53:395–402.

Jacobs, L. W. 1980. Running as an addiction process. Ph.D. diss., University of Alberta.

Jones, S. B., and Jones, D. C. 1977. Serious jogging and family life: Marathon and sub-marathon running. Paper presented at the annual meeting of the American Sociological Association, Chicago, 5–9 September.

Jorgenson, D. E., and Jorgenson, C. B. 1978. Perceived changes in intrafamilial relations: A study of runners/joggers. Paper presented at the annual conference of the Western Social Science Association.

Joseph, P., and Robbins, J. M. 1981. Worker or runner? The impact of commitment to running and work on self identification. In *Psychology of running,* ed. M. H. Sacks and M. L. Sachs. Champaign, Ill.: Human Kinetics Publishers.

Kostrubala, T. 1976. *The joy of running*. Philadelphia: J. B. Lippincott.

———. 1978. The training of a running therapist. *Medicine and Sport* 12:111–15.

Little, J. C. 1969. The athlete's neurosis: A deprivation crisis. *Acta Psychiatrica Scandinavica* 45:187–97.

———. 1979. Neurotic illness in fitness fanatics. *Psychiatric Annals* 9(3):49–51, 55–56.

———. 1981. Addendum to "The athlete's neurosis: A deprivation crisis." In *Psychology of running,* ed. M. H. Sacks and M. L. Sachs. Champaign, Ill.: Human Kinetics Publishers.

Merrill, S. 1980. Running bums. *Runner* 2(7):68–72.

Morgan, W. P. 1973. Efficacy of psychobiologic inquiry in the exercise and sport sciences. *Quest* 20:39–47.

———. 1979a. Negative addiction in runners. *Physician and Sportsmedicine* 7(2):56–63, 67–70.

———. 1979b. Running into addiction. *Runner* 1(6):72–74, 76.

Nash, J. E. 1976. The short and the long of it: Legitimizing motives for running. In *Sociology: A descriptive approach,* ed. J. E. Nash and J. P. Spradley. Chicago: Rand McNally.

———. 1977. Decoding the runner's appearance. In *Conformity and conflict: Readings in cultural anthropology,* ed. J. P. Spradley and D. W. McCurdy. Boston: Little, Brown.

―――. 1979. Weekend racing as an eventful experience: Understanding the accomplishment of well-being. *Urban Life* 8(2):199–217.

―――. 1980. Lying about running: The functions of talk in a scene. *Qualitative Sociology* 3(2):83–99.

Pargman, D. 1980. The way of the runner: An examination of motives for running. In *Psychology in sports: Methods and applications,* ed. R. M. Suinn. Minneapolis: Burgess.

Peele, S. 1978. Addiction: The analgesic experience. *Human Nature* 1(9):61–67.

―――. 1979. Redefining addiction II: The meaning of addiction in our lives. *Journal of Psychedelic Drugs* 11(4):289–97.

―――. 1980. Addiction to an experience (Comment). *American Psychologist* 35:1047–48.

―――. 1981a. Reductionism in the psychology of the eighties: Can biochemistry eliminate addiction, mental illness, and pain? *American Psychologist* 36(8):807–18.

―――. 1981b. *How much is too much: Healthy habits or destructive addictions.* Englewood Cliffs, N.J.: Prentice-Hall.

Peele, S., and Brodsky, A. 1976. *Love and addiction.* New York: Signet.

Robbins, J. M., and Joseph, P. 1980. Commitment to running: Implications for the family and work. *Sociological Symposium,* no. 30:87–108.

―――. 1982. Behavioral components of exercise addiction. Unpublished manuscript, Jewish General Hospital, Montreal.

Roth, W. T. 1974. Some motivational aspects of exercise. *Journal of Sports Medicine and Physical Fitness* 14:40–47.

*Runner's World.* 1981. Treating the non-stop runner. *Runner's World* 16(8):CAN3.

Sachs, M. L. 1981. Running addiction. In *Psychology of running,* ed. M. H. Sacks and M. L. Sachs. Champaign, Ill.: Human Kinetics Publishers.

Sachs, M. L., and Pargman, D. 1979a. Commitment and addiction to regular running. Paper presented at the annual convention of the American Alliance for Health, Physical Education, Recreation, and Dance, New Orleans, Louisiana, 19 March.

―――. 1979b. Running addiction: A depth interview examination. *Journal of Sport Behavior,* 2:143–55.

Sacks, M. H. 1981. Running addiction: A clinical report. In *Psychology of running,* ed. M. H. Sacks and M. L. Sachs. Champaign, Ill.: Human Kinetics Publishers.

Sheehan, G. 1979. Negative addiction: A runner's perspective. *Physician and Sportsmedicine* 7(6):49.

Sime, W. E. 1979. Psychological concomitants of running. In *American Alliance for Health, Physical Education, and Recreation Research Consortium symposium papers,* vol. 2, book 2, ed. R. Cox. Washington, D.C.: American Alliance for Health, Physical Education, and Recreation.

Solomon, E. G., and Bumpus, A. K. 1978. The running meditation response: An adjunct to psychotherapy. *American Journal of Psychotherapy* 32:583–92.

Summers, J. J.; Sargent, G. I.; Levey, A. J.; and Murray, K. D. 1982. Middle-aged, non-elite marathon runners: A profile. *Perceptual and Motor Skills* 54:963–69.

Thaxton, L. 1982. Physiological and psychological effects of short-term exercise addiction on habitual runners. *Journal of Sport Psychology* 4:73–80.

*Track and Field News.* 1980. Marathon. *Track and Field News* 33(9):41.

Waters, B. 1981. Defining the runner's personality. *Runner's World* 16(6):48–51.

Worick, W. W., and Schaller, W. E. 1977. *Alcohol, tobacco and drugs: Their use and abuse.* Englewood Cliffs, N.J.: Prentice-Hall.

RICHARD A. DIENSTBIER

# 14

# The Effect of Exercise on Personality

In this chapter I shall consider the relation between aerobic exercise and the personality changes that may result from it. I will not deal with personality differences between individuals who choose different sports.

Causal relations between systematic aerobic exercise training (hereafter "running" or "exercise") and personality have not been definitively proved. This statement holds even when "definitively proved" is given the relaxed definition used in most social and biological sciences. It is not that running programs have not been associated with statistically significant changes over time on personality dimensions as measured by standard personality inventories. Rather, such findings have not been totally consistent, nor are the research designs usually well controlled. (See Silva and Shultz, chap. 17.) The area is an extraordinarily difficult one in which to do definitive research. As in therapy outcome and program evaluation, problems abound concerning subject selection, attrition, expectation, and control groups.

Despite the lack of definitive proof of links between running and personality, at a normal level of scientific acceptability, there is a growing list of reasonably strong studies that demonstrate an interesting relationship. I shall review the more outstanding of these studies and draw inferences about personality effects from a wide range of literature that indirectly suggests running/personality links.

First, however, a word about "traits" and "personality." (Those who have an aversion to any mention of the well-worn trait/situation controversy may skip ahead.) For most of the past decade there has been an (initially interesting) argument concerning whether human behavior is determined by personality consistencies, usually termed "traits," or whether such predispositions account for very little of behavior. By denying the importance or even the relevance of "traits," those who made the latter argument effectively abolished the term "personality." After the polarized dialectic that normally character- izes such disagreements, a rather old-fashioned but sensible view of interaction between situational and personality determinants of behavior emerged, acquir- ing a moderate consensus by the end of the 1970s.

Supporting the common observation that most theorists and researchers have far less influence upon each other than they believe or hope, most of the research literature on the running/personality link avoids any "revisionist" thinking about "traits," depending instead upon some of the more traditional trait-based personality inventories. At our present state of sophistication that emphasis may be proper, for to employ complicated definitions of personality while still attempting to develop even mildly convincing proofs of running/ personality links might prove overwhelming. My use of the term "personality" will be close to the definition usually acepted before the trait/situation debate. Though we must now acknowledge that knowing a score on some trait dimen- sion (independent of situational considerations) allows very little predictive accuracy concerning a single instance of behavior, I shall assume that running- induced changes on trait measures of standard personality inventories are important. Studies demonstrating such relations will be presented without further qualification or apology. (Recent innovative approaches to this question have found strong correlations between responses to psychological inventories and behavior when behavior is aggregated over many instances; see especially Epstein 1979.)

## Mediators of Personality Change: Logical Analyses

Before considering the literature on the running/personality question, I would like to explore what mediators might exist between a running program and apparent personality changes. Each mediator suggests the likelihood of different personality changes and affects our faith that any apparent changes are "real." I will therefore explore what personality changes we might logically expect from each mediator. I shall consider four general classes of mediators: actual physiological changes resulting from running; changes in patterns of socializing and living resulting from a running program; and runners' specific expectations for running-induced changes in temperament or traits.

## PHYSIOLOGICAL CHANGES

When exercise physiologists speak of a "training effect," they mean the increased capacity induced by consistent use, exercise, or stress of parts of the body. Although the limits of adaptability of an organ, organ system, or muscle system may be fixed by heredity and by a combination of previous and present environmental effects, most systems that are taxed in regular running will improve in output capability. To posit that such physiological changes may directly cause changes in traits or temperament is to leap directly into the ancient question of the relation of mind and body. While decades of study of brain chemistry and physiology have obscured the mind/body division as conceived in prescientific times, our understanding of the interactions of central nervous system function and peripheral changes is still not sophisticated, especially when the causal question involves peripheral effects on central functioning.

Thought about this has been largely restricted to the area of emotion and is related to a theoretical system proposed by William James and C. Lange near the turn of the century, which emphasized the importance of feedback of peripheral changes in the experience of emotion. Although their theoretical system was thought to be discredited when Cannon, Bard, and others discovered brain-stimulated emotional behavior, the James-Lange theory has undergone a remarkable recovery in the past two decades (e.g., see Fehr and Stern 1970). It has been noted that a variety of drugs whose effect is largely or exclusively peripheral affect mood and emotional states (for a review, see Dienstbier 1979). Additional evidence comes from victims of spinal-cord accidents who have lost the ability to obtain feedback from peripheral physiological changes and who experience a change in emotional responsiveness that is apparently linked to their limited feedback (Hohmann 1966).

Keeping those literatures in mind while focusing on running leads to the conclusion that, insofar as running affects the organ systems involved in emotional experience, both shortterm (through priming or depletion of capacity) and longterm (through a training effect and the change in capacity for intensity or duration of function), exercise should influence mood and emotional experience. In fact, it appears that many of the physiological systems necessary to sustain extended physical effort are the same ones that change during (and influence the experience of) emotional arousal. (This commonality of systems in exercise and emotion is not only observed, but is logically consistent as well, since the main adaptive purpose of emotional arousal seems to be to motivate the organism to activities that change its relation toward the emotional stimulus.) If we define temperament as a long-term tendency toward certain moods or emotional dispositions, it is apparent that we should expect to see some effect upon such measures after extensive training. Thus there seems a strong probability that changes in depression, anxiety, and positive moods and emotions should follow directly (with no additional mediators) from physiological changes induced through running.

Although I have been addressing peripheral effects on centrally processed experience, it is also quite likely that running has short- and long-term direct effects on brain chemistry. Recent speculation about the role of the endorphins in the "runner's high" fits in here (see Sachs, chap. 15). However, more mundane effects may prove important. I shall present a more formal discussion of research evidence below, but consider the following brief chain of findings and ideas. Appenzeller and Schade (1979) have noted that peripheral catecholamines (such as noradrenalin) increase sixfold over resting levels during a marathon run (measured via blood samples). Porges (1976) has suggested that levels of brain neural transmitters such as noradrenalin and acetylcholine are directly related to the peripheral concentrations of those substances. This strongly suggests that the short-term concentration of neural transmitters in the brain may change with running. If so, it is possible that a "training effect" in the brain may be gained from running. It may be that the changes in balance between introversion and extroversion, discussed below, are caused by such direct effects of running on brain physiology.

In summary, it is likely not only that running-induced peripheral physiological changes may cause long- and short-term temperament and mood changes, but that central nervous system physiological changes may be similarly influenced by exercise and may similarly influence personality. Insofar as research assessments of exercise programs demonstrate personality changes caused by such factors, we should expect to consistently obtain similar results from similar exercise programs.

PERCEPTION OF PHYSICAL CHANGES

Changes that often develop from a running program include reduction in body fat, redistribution of weight, increased energy levels, a more youthful appearance, and the ability to run farther and faster. The individual's valuing of those physical developments will be influenced by the values expressed by the larger society and significant others.

If a runner experiences physical changes consonant with his or her physical values, then running should lead to an improved body image. One need not look deeply into the literature of personality and developmental psychology to determine that one of the most durable "truths" of those disciplines is that a positive body image contributes significantly to a generally positive self-concept, and that positive self-concept or high self-esteem correlates with general psychological health by almost any reasonable definition of that concept (see Berger, chap. 10). The only limitation on our ability to translate this general finding to running-induced physical changes is the possibility that such changes will not be highly valued.

Runners who voluntarily engage in systematic training either come from a background of significant social support for such activities (and for the concomitant physical changes) or are sufficiently inner-directed that lack of social support for their changing physique is unimportant. Since most research on improved body image as a dependent measure uses subjects who are already disposed to exercise programs (e.g., middle-class college students), findings contrary to the expectation of improved body image and improved self-esteem after a running program are unlikely. Several studies that I will not review affirm improved physical self-image from running; see Greist et al. (1979) for a review.

However, while modern American middle-class values are consonant with the physical changes that usually follow a running program, the picture is not so simple when we consider working-class segments of American society: often a mesomorphic or even portly masculine appearance and voluptuous female appearance are favored. (This may partially account for the often noted over-representation of professionals and the upper middle class in running events.) Victor Altschul (1981) recently discussed the conflict a running therapy client encountered between his new body image shaped by running and the image provided by his father that he should not be a "skinny shit." The problems therapy clients encounter through valuing running-induced physical changes less or having less social support for them may not be insurmountable if they are recognized and addressed early in therapy.

Even in our American spectator-sport culture, most segments of society value being a participant rather than a mere observer of sports. The amazing distances a healthy individual may be able to run after only a few months of training therefore can lead to an increased sense of one's ability to master challenges and to attain goals that seemed remote only months earlier. (At the University of Nebraska at Lincoln, my good friend Jim Crabbe normally saw his one-semester aerobic students run more than fifteen miles at semester's end.) One's entire belief system about the degree to which one's life is self-determined, or internal (versus other- or fate-determined, or external), may be influenced by such significant successes. One recent study, which will probably be a prototype for future studies, found that children between six and fourteen years old became more internal after attending a fitness camp (Duke, Johnson, and Nowicki 1977). A vast social psychological literature on this personality dimension confirms that success in skill-oriented (as opposed to luck-oriented) tasks does result in a more internal orientation. Increasing internality (within a normal range), like increased self-esteem, correlates with other generally positive aspects of personality.

Therapists who encourage clients to run may maximize these positive relations if they encourage them to keep their goals reasonable. Also, referring clients to the running programs of local organizations (YMCA, etc.) that "coach" gently and wisely may further the sense of accomplishment and mastery that fosters internality. Since research assessments of exercise programs may show personality changes based upon such factors, other programs that promote such positive perceptions of exercise-induced changes should stimulate similar results. However, not all programs will be equal in this respect and therefore their participants may show unequal degrees of personality change.

### CHANGES IN PATTERNS OF SOCIALIZING AND LIVING

As William Morgan (1976) suggested, runners often "get religion." That is, they begin to realize that if exercise can bring such substantial improvement in physical well-being, then changes in patterns of drinking, eating, smoking, and sleeping may add to those benefits or at least make running easier and more successful. The therapist can increase clients' access to information and motivation relevant to such life changes by exposing them to running publications, most of which discuss diet almost as much as running. While such concomitant changes may enhance running therapies, they may devastate research efforts that attempt to isolate the effect of running itself on personality-relevant dependent variables. That is, a causal chain from exercise through changes in lifestyle to personality change is likely to vary greatly between exercise programs and experiences. Insofar as postprogram assessments reveal personality changes based on these factors, they may not be easy to replicate. The running researcher who wishes to minimize his subjects from embracing such concomitant changes must keep them in a small box during their nonrunning hours or find another line of research.

In discussing the importance of running in a therapy program in San Diego, California, Thaddeus Kostrubala (1976) said that when client and therapist run together their relationship progresses far more quickly to positive transference and willing self-disclosure than with nonrunning client-therapist pairs (see Kostrubala, chap. 7). This supports the development of therapy programs that include running and also provides a clue to the benefits of running with other people. Although the development of social relationships during running (versus some control activity) has not been systematically investigated in the research literature, it does appear from less systematic observations that those who run together share an experience that quickly leads to closeness. Emotionally troubled people—particularly depressives, who otherwise may experience a debilitating sense of loneliness—may particularly gain from this aspect of an exercise program.

## CHANGES IN EXPECTATION

Once again the therapist's gain is the researcher's obstacle. With the popularization of running has come the spread of knowledge about its supposed benefits. William Morgan describes this as the "granola effect"—suggesting that it is so universally accepted that running "is good for you" that it is almost impossible to get research funds to explore its effects. When the client is convinced of the benefits, not only is motivation to remain in the running program increased, but the potential for a "placebo effect" is significant. In such circumstances people may experience real gains owing to their expectations for improvement rather than the running program itself. Even with nonrunning control groups matched on all measurable demographic and psychological characteristics, such expectancies provide a severe confounding problem for the researcher. Unless control groups can somehow be given expectations similar to those of the running groups, true control is not possible. (Similarly, subjects' expectations in single-group longitudinal studies present problems.) Insofar as observed changes following exercise programs reflect subject expectancies rather than more dependable causal or intervening variables, we should expect little replicability; however, even where replication is achieved most of us would agree that we are seeing the effect of a confounding variable rather than of exercise per se.

## Research Evidence

### PROBLEMS

In the various sections above, I have unsystematically mentioned several causal relations that could account for the apparent effect of a running program

on personality. To recapitulate briefly, causal factors could include real physiological changes, the perception of physical changes, the influence of other
lifestyle changes undertaken concomitantly with a running program, social
gains that occur easily during running but could also have occurred under other
less strenuous conditions, the development of a sense of mastery and internality
that could also result from other achievements, and the individuals' expectations for improvement along various dimensions after a serious running program. Whether these factors are seen positively by the researcher, therapist, or
scholar depends on the person's orientation. Some factors that therapists strive
to include in their exercise programs may be viewed by the researcher as diaboli-
cally confounding. The researcher who wished to investigate only the most re-
strictive definition of direct causality between exercise programs and personality
would have to construct research with the following control features:

1. The research would deal with changes in personality over time during the
course of a running program. Most studies of exercise and personality simply
compare people engaged in various sports with each other or with nonsporting
control groups. The direction of causation of the specific sport causing personality differences is confounded with the possibility that people with specific
personality characteristics self-select into specific sports. As an example of
how misleading such research can be if overinterpreted, compare the findings
of Gontang, Clitsome, and Kostrubala (1977) that distance runners are highly
introverted with the findings of Jones and Weinhouse (1979) that, when
personality change is measured across time for individuals in a running program, runners become more extroverted.

2. To control for differences on personality inventories that may be caused
by background changes ranging from world and economic conditions to
weather, nonrunning control groups must be simultaneously involved in the
before/after design.

3. Similarly, to control for changes in self-esteem based on feelings of
mastery (assuming one is interested in running's physiological effect on
personality), the control group should also be engaged in some systematic
activity capable of satisfying achievement or mastery motives. Furthermore,
the degree to which those feelings exist and change over time should be
measured and compared between the experimental and control groups.

4. To control for differences in social contacts between the running and
control groups, the controls should be involved in activities that are as socially
engaging for them as running is for the runners.

5. The changes in lifestyle that often accompany running must be closely
observed in the experimental group and either matched in the control group or

statistically appraised and accounted for by techniques such as analysis of covariance.

6. Perhaps most difficult of all, the control group must be given the same expectation for personality change, therapeutic improvement, and so on as the running group, so that the presence of those expectations in the running group only is not a biasing factor.

Of the criteria listed above, longitudinal change measurement (point 1) is so important that I shall review only studies that use it. Unfortunately, although a handful of published studies use control groups as suggested in point 2, very few have incorporated matched activities for controls, as suggested in point 3, and no studies exist, to my knowledge, that take account of any of requirements 4 through 6.

## Personality Dimensions

The personality dimensions studied in research on running are primarily anxiety (including "neuroticism"), depression, and the sixteen dimensions of Cattell's Sixteen Personality Factor Inventory (16 PF) (1965). Those specific dimensions are selected for a number of reasons. Clinically concerned researchers are interested in anxiety and depression because of their high frequency among nonpsychotic people in our society and because the sense of well-being many runners informally report suggests an antidote to those negative emotional states. The literature dealing specifically with the effect of exercise on anxiety (as measured by standard anxiety inventories) and on depression is covered in chapters 9 and 10 of this volume. I will focus on research with the 16 PF.

Interest in the 16 PF is related to the affection many researchers of running have for inventories derived and validated by factor-analytic methods. Additionally, the 16 PF includes factors related to various emotional states that, like anxiety and depression, seem likely to be affected by running, with its apparent mood-altering qualities.

My analysis of individual studies and my general conclusions are likely to be somewhat controversial rather than obvious and universally accepted. At a minimum, where I suggest significant limits on the interpretation of certain studies, it is likely that their authors would demur. A recent review by Folkins and Sime (1981) reviewed some of these same studies and concluded that "it appears that there is no evidence to support a claim that global changes on personality tests follow from fitness training." Without access to the more recent studies in this series, Morgan (1976) came to a similar conclusion.

There are several possible reasons for the conservative conclusions of

Folkins and Sime: First, they did not review what is by far the strongest study in this series (Jasnoski and Holmes 1981). Second, Folkins and Sime listed only four separate research projects in their 16 PF review, apparently assuming mistakenly that three articles about one study (which has been republished, with minor modifications in analysis, *many* times) discussed different research projects—an understandable oversight given the way the articles were presented. Finally, those reviewers did not focus upon the second-order factors of the 16 PF. That is, although they criticized the choice of the 16 PF as unfortunate, since "few of the 16 personality factors are theoretically expected to change following short-term intervention," several of the 16 PF dimensions constitute a second-order factor of emotionality—a factor likely to be influenced by exercise-induced physiological changes in both the short term and the long term (as discussed above).

### Findings from Research with the 16 PF

Each of five studies reviewed below, using the 16 PF, provides some new information by virtue of having employed a unique subject population or training program. Although all the studies employed a before/after format, they differ in their strengths and weaknesses. This diversity of design allows more generalization than would be possible from a series of very similar studies, not only because of the diverse programs and populations used, but also because alternative explanations for positive results of one study (owing to the unique weaknesses of that study) are usually not equally applicable to the other studies.

The data from the studies are presented in table 1 (p. 264). The table lists the sixteen bipolar dimensions of the 16 PF, and a plus sign, or positive correlation, means that in the study being considered exercise is associated positively (and statistically significantly) with the first of the two terms. The three dimensions followed by daggers (†) are those that constitute the second-order factor of emotionality or anxiety (extracted as the first second-order factor when principal components factor analysis is applied to all 16 PF dimensions). Those three followed by double daggers (‡) are additional dimensions that, together with the first three, are sometimes found in a larger second-order emotionality or anxiety factor (hereafter "emotionality").

Consider first those studies that show correlations between fitness level and personality. Such correlational relationships are subject to many causal hypotheses, but they may appear either when pre- and post-test designs are used or when fitness change is correlated with personality change across a training program. Data from two studies that examined such correlations are presented in the first two columns of table 1. Young and Ismail (1976) demonstrated personality differences on seven of the sixteen dimensions between fourteen highly fit and fourteen unfit middle-aged men drawn from their total sample of fifty-six. Jasnoski and Holmes (1981) examined the relation between initial fitness level and personality for their sample of 103 college women, finding statistically significant relations on three of the sixteen dimensions. Note that seven of the ten relationships identified in the two studies indicate reduced emotionality associated with fitness.

The next two columns show correlations between changes in fitness level before and after exercise training and changes in personality measures across the same period. Designs that use this procedure can partially overcome the problem of no control group or an insufficient control group. That is, (substantial) change correlations indicate that expectancies and lifestyle changes are unlikely to cause the observed personality changes (since it is unlikely that there would be substantial correlations between fitness change and either expectancies or lifestyle changes).

Hammer and Wilmore (1973) studied fifty-three men participating in a ten-week jogging program. Although the study had no control groups and did not control for lifestyle changes or expectations, the use of change correlations gives the findings some credibility. Change in aerobic capacity correlated with becoming more *trusting* (vs. suspicious) and more *shrewd* or sophisticated (vs. forthright); being trusting is related to low emotionality.

Janoski and Holmes (1981) studied 103 women college students in a fifteen-week aerobic training program. Aerobic exercise consisted of jumping rope, running, or dancing and involved more than the usual class period by requiring thirty aerobic points each week. Although no control groups were used, analyses looked not only at before/after changes, but also at change of aerobic capacity compared with change in personality dimensions. Increases in aerobic capacity correlated with becoming more *placid or self-assured,* increased *liberalness* (or being more experimenting), and *decreased tension.*

Besides the Jasnoski and Holmes study described above, two other studies that looked at pre- and post-training changes on the 16 PF are noteworthy. Jasnoski and Holmes found that (comparing only before and after personality scores) subjects became more *imaginative, less shy,* and *less apprehensive.* Additionally, approaching statistical significance were changes in being more *experimenting or liberal* and more *tenderminded or sensitive.*

Buccola and Stone (1975) constructed a study with a control group consisting of men who undertook cycling rather than the jogging of the experimental group. Older men aged sixty to seventy-nine participated for

Table 1. Relations between Measures on Cattell's Sixteen Personality Factor Inventory (16 PF) and Fitness or Fitness Changes

| 16 PF Measure | Correlations between Fitness Level and 16 PF Measures | | Correlations between Changes in Fitness and in 16 PF Measures | | Differences between Pre- and Post-training on 16 PF Measures | | |
|---|---|---|---|---|---|---|---|
| | Young and Ismail 1976 | Jasnoski and Holmes 1981 | Hammer and Wilmore 1973 | Jasnoski and Holmes 1981 | Jasnoski and Holmes 1981 | Buccola and Stone 1975 | Jones and Weinhouse 1979 |
| Outgoing vs. reserved | | | | | | | |
| More intelligent vs. less intelligent | − | | | | | | |
| Emotionally stable vs. emotionally unstable† | + | +.28* | | | | | |
| Assertive vs. humble | | | | | | | |
| Happy-go-lucky vs. sober | | | | | | | |
| Conscientious vs. expedient | | | | | | | |
| Venturesome vs. shy‡ | + | | | | + | | |

| | | | | | | | |
|---|---|---|---|---|---|---|---|
| Tenderminded vs. toughminded | | | | | | | |
| Trusting vs. suspicious‡ | + | | + | | | | |
| Imaginative vs. practical | + | | | | + | | |
| Forthright vs. shrewd | | +.20* | − | | | | |
| Placid vs. apprehensive† | + | +.26* | | +.49*** | + | | |
| Experimenting vs. conservative | | | | +.37** | | | |
| Self-sufficient vs. group-dependent | | | | | | + | |
| Undisciplined vs. controlled‡ | | | | | | | |
| Relaxed vs. tense† | + | | | +.24* | | | + |

*p<.05.  **p<.01.  ***p<.001.  + = positive correlation  − = negative correlation.

†, ‡ Emotionality factor; see page 262 for explanation.

fourteen weeks in either activity. Although the men self-selected themselves into the two groups, the before/after format allowed comparison of change over time between the groups. While both groups showed increased aerobic capacity and reduced blood pressure, only the joggers changed significantly on any 16 PF dimensions, becoming more *self-sufficient* and *less surgent* or less "happy-go-lucky" (more sober). Since aerobic capacity improved for the cyclists too, there is no obvious reason why 16 PF changes occurred only for the joggers. It is therefore comforting that the significant changes for the joggers, described above, were mirrored in similar but nonsignificant changes for the cyclists.

Jones and Weinhouse (1979) provide the only really long-term study of this series, following twelve runners (seven males and five females) through a one-year training program. Although no control group was used, no controls for expectations or lifestyle changes were recorded, and no change correlations were offered, the long-term nature of the study makes it noteworthy. The subjects were in a counselor-training program. Since only twelve participated, fairly large changes were required to be statistically significant; therefore I will mention some of those nonsignificant changes that were substantial. The subjects became significantly more *relaxed,* scored nonsignificantly higher on the "*intelligence*" dimension (which really reflects an intellectual orientation rather than measured intelligence), became more *assertive* (vs. humble), and became more *surgent* or happy-go-lucky (vs. sober). Although these subjects started out very high on *emotional stability* (as might be expected for this population), they improved moderately but not significantly (from 7.5 to 7.8).

One study using the 16 PF with null findings should also be mentioned. Tillman (1965) compared high-school boys in a high-activity physical education class with another class of less active boys. While no statistically significant 16 PF differences appeared between the two groups, no means are presented in the article, leaving the "null" results difficult to interpret. Additionally, since only fifty boys participated in the two classes, and since some physical activity occurred in the "control" class this cannot be regarded as a strong study.

I will mention one particularly weak study because it is so frequently cited as demonstrating personality changes following aerobics training. In a number of articles, Ismail and Young have presented the results of a study of fifty-six middle-aged faculty members who responded to the 16 PF before and after an exercise program including jogging and various competitive and noncompetitive sports. The strength of the study lies in its nontraditional subject group, but the mix of competitive sports with aerobic training is problematic. The data have been as thoroughly examined and analyzed as possible (in at least six journal articles and sundry other publications reporting analyses ranging from correlations and analyses of variance through canonical correlations and multiple-order factor analyses on the entire sample and on various subgroups). The authors discuss at length analyses of pretraining *or* posttraining personality differences between individuals at different levels of fitness (e.g., Young and Ismail 1977). Such correlational analyses, subject to various causal interpretations, do not have the inferential power of those that correlate *changes* in pre/post fitness with *changes* in personality scores. While those researchers do not provide a clear analysis of pre/post personality changes in their total group in most of their articles, they do report (Young and Ismail 1976) statistically significant pre/post increases in conscientiousness and control for a *selected sample* of twenty-eight (seven subjects in each of four groups composed of old or young and "fit" or "unfit"). However, another of their several publications on this research effort (Ismail and Young 1977) presents a table of means without statistical analyses that indicates that, for the *total group* of fifty-six subjects, the pre/post change in conscientiousness is very small (and obviously far from significant); no comparable data for control are presented in their table of "selected" personality variables. Thus, although this research is frequently cited to answer the relatively simple question being addressed in this chapter, the Young and Ismail research must be considered merely suggestive.

Of the studies reviewed above, that by Jasnoski and Holmes is clearly superior to the others; it used a rigorous training program of sufficient length and a large number of subjects, and it documented both pre/post personality changes and changes in fitness correlated with changes in personality.

## Summary of 16 PF Results

Of the four major studies that show correlations between fitness change and personality change, personality differences from pretraining to post-training, or both, there is so little agreement on specific dimensions that one could make quite different conclusions for each study if they were reviewed singly. This explains why I have not reviewed studies whose before/after designs use relatively special personality measures. The design inelegancies forced upon researchers in this area are such that we should simply not trust findings established by single studies.

Despite the considerable inconsistencies in the findings of the studies summarized above, there are some strong overall trends. Before we look at individual dimensions, consider again that the 16 PF is not composed of sixteen independent factors. The factors are interrelated in complex ways (not being based upon orthogonal factor rotation) so that patterns of support may emerge from several different factors suggesting similar underlying changes.

Looking first at the three dimensions most associated with emotionality and anxiety, although correlations exist in two studies between being fit and demonstrating emotional stability, no support in change correlations or absolute change is found in the four stronger studies. Support is found for exercise programs' leading to being placid and relaxed, however, with both change correlations and pre/post changes appearing in the four studies on those dimensions. Similarly, two of the other three dimensions that are more weakly associated with the second-order factor of emotionality receive confirmation as associated with conditioning. Overall, of the eleven changes noted in the four studies, four are in predicted directions on two of the three strongest anxiety dimensions, and two more are in predicted directions on two of the three weaker anxiety dimensions.

## Conclusions

Personality psychologists tend to think of personality traits as largely established by a combination of hereditary dispositions and very long-term learning resulting from the interaction of people and their environments. While there has been considerable disagreement between theoretical systems about what "critical periods" might exist in the establishment of various personality traits (e.g., ranging from Freud's emphasis on experience in the first few years of life to the social learning theorists' view of lifelong input), a significant new research project by Loehlin and Nichols (1976), using twins, suggested that personality traits as measured by personality inventories are often heavily influenced by heredity. Based upon empirical research, the 16 PF dimensions related to emotional tension (upon which change has been noted, above) have a very strong hereditary component (Cattell 1965; Buss and Plomin 1975).

A common thread through all these systems of thought is the assumption that during the adult years most personality dimensions will change slowly, if at all. In short, insofar as we acknowledge any of those systems, our expectations for significant changes on personality dimensions from short-term running programs should be minimal. Resistance to change should be particularly strong for the emotion-relevant dimensions, with their strong heritability. Yet the research reviewed above, albeit flawed, has shown personality changes in a relatively coherent and mutually supporting pattern through exercise programs that typically are conducted for only four months or less. If we had similarly reviewed the anxiety and depression studies, the results would have been even more consistent.

Earlier I suggested that there is enough commonality of physiological systems involved in aerobic exercise and in the experience of emotional states that we should expect running to have an effect on short-term emotional functioning and on temperament. I shall accept the moderately strong confirmation of that expectation in the research reviewed above as providing license to speculate further on the nature of the physiological changes that are induced by running and that in turn affect temperament. (With several colleagues I have discussed this potential link more extensively elsewhere [Dienstbier et al. 1981], and so I will review that thinking only briefly.)

A number of exercise physiologists (e.g., Edington and Edgerton 1976; Moorehouse and Miller 1971) have speculated that exercise may increase the capacity of the adrenal glands to respond to physical stress. Similarly, psychological stress, calling for very similar physiological reactions, may be influenced by those changes. Evidence supporting this relation between glandular capacity and temperament includes Frankenhaeuser's (1979) recent finding that more emotionally stable schoolchildren show greater catecholamine responses to classroom challenges than less emotionally stable children. While common sense suggests that a larger or more prolonged physiological response to stress might be uncomfortable, Gal and Lazarus (1975) have noted that more intense stress reactions (measured physiologically) are more uncomfortable only when no activity is undertaken. Other supporting evidence from animal research indicates that animals who have had their sympathetic nervous systems and associated glandular responses "well exercised" through daily stress during infancy (which increases adrenal-cortical size and capacity) are less easily disturbed emotionally as adults. To turn to Selye's (1976) system, it may be that such increased glandular capacity allows the stage of resistance in the general adaptation syndrome to be prolonged, so that the individual does not as quickly enter the stage of exhaustion; this may reduce the experience of stress in response to stressors.

In summary, running may stimulate the development of the capacity of the sympathetic nervous system and associated glandular responses; in turn, this increased physiological capacity may be the major cause for the reduced emotional tension shown in both state and trait studies, as well as the major cause of reduced anxiety. Similarly, a major theoretical approach to depression, often called the catecholamine hypothesis (Schildkraut, Davis, and

Klerman 1968), suggests that a decline in central catecholamines, especially noradrenalin, is a major cause of depression. The effectiveness of noradrenalin-stimulating drugs (or monoamine-oxidase inhibitors) in combating depression is strong evidence for this hypothesis. The strong evidence reviewed by others in this volume linking running to reduced depression suggests either that the peripheral changes induced by running cause similar central changes (as suggested by Porges 1976) or that the central changes in catecholamine levels follow directly from running.

Many of the most interesting running-induced changes (those that may follow from direct physiological changes) may substitute for psychoactive drugs that aid in controlling negative emotional states. Unlike those chemical aids, the well-designed exercise program holds the promise of other positive changes: on the physical side, increased cardiovascular fitness and weight loss; on the psychological side, improved self-esteem and an enhanced sense of mastery and internality. In light of the well-established negative features associated with chemical dependence, running provides an extraordinarily appealing option for the psychotherapist. It should not be restricted to the client but should be used by client and psychotherapist alike.

### References

Altshul, V. A. 1981. Should therapists encourage their depressed clients to run? In *Psychology of running,* ed. M. H. Sacks and M. L. Sachs. Champaign, Ill.: Human Kinetics Publishers.

Appenzeller, O., and Schade, D. R. 1979. Neurology of endurance training. III. Sympathetic activity during a marathon run. *Neurology* 29(4):542.

Buccola, V. A., and Stone, W. J. 1975. Effects of jogging and cycling programs on physiological and personality variables in aged men. *Research Quarterly* 46:134–39.

Buss, A. H., and Plomin, R. 1975. *A temperament theory of personality development.* New York: Wiley.

Cattell, R. B. 1965. *The scientific analysis of personality.* Baltimore: Penguin.

Dienstbier, R. A. 1979. Emotion-attribution theory: Establishing roots and exploring future perspectives. In *Nebraska symposium on motivation, 1978,* ed. H. E. Howe and R. A. Dienstbier. Lincoln: University of Nebraska Press.

Dienstbier, R. A.; Crabbe, J.; Johnson, G. O.; Thorland, W.; Jorgensen, J. A.; Sadar, M. M.; and LaVelle, D. C. 1981. Exercise and stress tolerance. In *Psychology of running,* ed. M. H. Sacks and M. L. Sachs. Champaign, Ill.: Human Kinetics Publishers.

Duke, M.; Johnson, T. C.; and Nowicki, S., Jr. 1977. Effects of sports fitness camp experience on locus of control orientation in children, ages six to fourteen. *Research Quarterly* 48:280–83.

Edington, D. W., and Edgerton, V. R. 1976. *The biology of physical activity.* Boston: Houghton Mifflin.

Epstein, S. 1979. The stability of behavior. I. On predicting most of the people much of the time. *Journal of Personality and Social Psychology* 37:1097–1126.

Fehr, F. S., and Stern, J. A. 1970. Peripheral physiological variables and emotion: The James-Lange theory revisited. *Psychological Bulletin* 74:411–24.

Folkins, C. H., and Sime, W. E. 1981. Physical fitness training and mental health. *American Psychologist* 36:373–89.

Frankenhaeuser, M. 1979. Psychoneuroendocrine approaches to the study of emotion as related to stress and coping. In *Nebraska symposium on motivation, 1978,* ed. H. E. Howe and R. A. Dienstbier. Lincoln: University of Nebraska Press.

Gal, R., and Lazarus, R. S. 1975. The role of activity in anticipating and confronting stressful situations. *Journal of Human Stress* 1:4–20.

Gontang, A.; Clitsome, T.; and Kostrubala, T. 1977. A psychological study of fifty sub-three-hour marathoners. *Annals of the New York Academy of Sciences* 301: 1020–28.

Greist, J. H.; Klein, M. H.; Eischens, R. R.; Faris, J.; Gurman, A. S.; and Morgan, W. P. 1979. Running as treatment for depression. *Comprehensive Psychiatry* 20:41–54.

Hammer, W. M., and Wilmore, J. H. 1973. An exploratory investigation in personality measures and physiological alterations during a ten-week jogging program. *Journal of Sports Medicine and Physical Fitness* 13:231–37.

Hohmann, G. W. 1966. Some effects of spinal cord lesions on experienced emotional feelings. *Psychophysiology* 3:143–56.

Ismail, A. H., and Young, R. J. 1977. Effect of chronic exercise on the personality of adults. *Annals of the New York Academy of Sciences* 301:958–69.

Jasnoski, M. L., and Holmes, D. S. 1981. Influence of initial aerobic fitness, aerobic training and changes in aerobic fitness on personality functioning. *Journal of Psychosomatic Research* 25:553–56.

Jones, R. D., and Weinhouse, S. 1979. Running as self therapy? A research study. *Journal of Sports Medicine* 19:397.

Kostrubala, T. 1976. *The joy of running.* Philadelphia: J. B. Lippincott.

Loehlin, J. C., and Nichols, R. C. 1976. *Heredity, environment, and personality.* Austin: University of Texas Press.

Moorehouse, L., and Miller, A. T., Jr. 1971. *Physiology of exercise.* Saint Louis: C. V. Mosby.

Morgan, W. P. 1976. Psychological consequences of vigorous physical activity and sport. In *The Academy papers: Beyond research—solutions to human problems,* ed. M. G. Scott. Forty-seventh Annual Meeting of the American Academy of Physical Education, 31 March–1 April 1976. Iowa City: American Academy of Physical Education.

Porges, S. W. 1976. Peripheral and neurochemical parallels of psychopathology: A psychophysiological model relating autonomic imbalance to hyperactivity, psychopathy, and autism. In *Advances in child development and behavior,* vol. 2. New York: Academic Press.

Schildkraut, J. J.; Davis, J. M.; and Klerman, G. 1968. Biochemistry of depression. In *Psychopharmacology: A review of progress, 1957–1967,* ed. D. H. Efron, J. O. Cole, J. Levine, and J. R. Wittenborn. Washington, D.C.: U.S. Public Health Service.

Selye, H. 1976. *The stress of life.* New York: McGraw-Hill.

Tillman, K. 1965. Relationship between physical fitness and selected personality traits. *Research Quarterly* 36:483–89.

Young, R. J., and Ismail, A. H. 1976. Personality differences of adult men before and after a physical fitness program. *Research Quarterly* 47:513–19.

———. 1977. Comparison of selected physiological and personality variables in regular and nonregular adult male exercisers. *Research Quarterly* 48:617–22.

# 15

# The Runner's High

Unlike a lot of runners, this one chooses to run at noon, when the sun over the shimmering blue Pacific burns hottest. The first half hour, as he trots through the seaside parks of La Jolla, is pure agony, "exaggerated body pain and philosophical crisis." But he knows there's relief: "Thirty minutes out and something lifts. The fatigue goes away and feelings of power begin. I think I'll run 25 miles today. I'll double the size of the research grant request. I'll have that talk with the dean and tolerate no equivocating." Then, another switch, from fourth gear into overdrive. "Sometime into the second hour comes the spooky time. Colors are bright and beautiful, water sparkles, clouds breathe, and my body, swimming, detaches from the earth. A loving contentment invades the basement of my mind, and thoughts bubble up without trails. I find the place I need to live if I'm going to live." (Black 1979, 79)

This effusive description of the runner's high comes not from a mystical "running bum," but from noted psychopharmacologist Arnold Mandell. Many runners can tell of times when their experience of the runner's high has been similarly exhilarating.

In reading the popular literature, one may get the impression that every runner who puts on running shoes and runs gets high, but this is not so. The findings of a number of studies that noted what percentage of runners experienced the runner's high differ dramatically. Lilliefors (1978), in *The Running*

*Mind,* dealt with a select group of runners and indicated that 78 percent reported experiencing a sense of euphoria during their runs. Furthermore, 49 percent said the euphoria was occasionally spiritual in nature. I found that 77 percent of the sixty runners interviewed in a study (Sachs 1980) had experienced the runner's high.

On the other hand, some studies report very low percentages of runners as having this experience. After giving a talk to a group of forty runners on psychological aspects of running, I asked how many had experienced the runner's high (Sachs 1978). Only 10 percent said they had done so. Similarly, Weinberg (1980) found that only 9 percent of the runners he studied reported experiencing the runner's high.

I will propose reasons for these drastically different percentages later, but it is clear that the runner's high is not experienced by all runners. Indeed, basic problems still exist in constructing a suitable definition of it.

The literature on the runner's high uses at least twenty-seven adjectives or phrases in describing the runner's high. This long list includes euphoria, strength, speed, power, gracefulness, spirituality, sudden realization of one's potential, glimpsing perfection, moving without effort, and spinning out. I attempted a major study on the runner's high (Sachs 1980), incorporating interviews and questionnaires to determine its nature and predict in whom it would occur and when and where it was most likely. I constructed a preliminary definition of the runner's high as "a euphoric sensation experienced during running, usually unexpected, in which the runner feels a heightened sense of well-being, enhanced appreciation of nature, and transcendence of barriers of time and space."

Research evidence on the runner's high is virtually nonexistent, primarily owing to the difficulty of studying a phenomenon that supposedly occurs unexpectedly. But one study has provided interesting findings. Wagemaker and Goldstein (1980) used electroencephalograph readings before and after runs. The EEG readings of the runners before exercise were similar to those of subjects with emotional fatigue, but running reversed the fatigue. After running, the EEG patterns indicated the normal waxing and waning between the right and left hemispheres. Subjects said that they could think more clearly and that their fatigue had disappeared. They felt better, were more rested, and could concentrate and study more effectively. Wagemaker and Goldstein suggested that the runner's high develops after twenty-five to thirty-five minutes of running.

With research evidence lacking, I formulated a number of hypotheses and conducted the study noted earlier (Sachs 1980). I considered several variables in examining the runner's high.

## On the Trail of the Runner's High

An initial set of variables of particular interest included addiction and commitment to running, which had been the focus of earlier work by myself and others (Carmack and Martens 1979; Jacobs 1980; Morgan 1979a, b; Sachs 1979; Sachs and Pargman 1979a, b; see also the review in chap. 13). These researchers have noted the increased significance of psychological factors in research on running, particularly on increases in addiction to running. The runner's high has consistently been cited in the literature as a positive aspect of running. It seemed likely that experience of the runner's high, representing this positive factor, would be related to increases in addiction and commitment to running. One of the key factors in Glasser's (1976) initial development of the positive addiction concept was the "positive addiction state," closely related to the concept of the runner's high.

A particularly interesting explanation of the runner's high concerns differences in laterality of brain dominance (right/left) among runners. Glasser has suggested (Johnson 1978) that the state of mind during a run might be termed "right-brain consciousness." Running may provide a classic meditation state in which the left side of the brain is left alone and may "turn off," permitting the right brain to "take over." Ornstein and Galin (1976) note that when tasks require use of one hemisphere there is an increase in the level of alpha waves (essentially a decrease in information processing) in the other hemisphere.

Mandell (Black 1979, 87) has also suggested that running increases right-brain dominance. Clearly, the runner's high as described earlier is characteristic of right-brain function. Numerous researchers have indicated functional differences between the cerebral hemispheres (e.g., Bever 1975; Bogen 1969; Gazzaniga 1970; Ornstein 1972). The left hemisphere is characterized by activities such as verbal, analytic, abstract, rational, and objective. The right hemisphere's activities are depicted as preverbal, holistic, symbolic, spatial, and subjective.

Although both Glasser and Mandell are careful to note that their speculations are tentative, the descriptions of the runner's high suggest that right-brain dominant individuals are more likely to experience it. Since it is clear that many runners do not experience the runner's high, perhaps those with left-brain dominance have difficulty shifting to the right brain.

To test this hypothesis, one would have to assess right/left brain dominance within a sample of runners, then tap their perceptions about the running high. Ideally, runners' brain-wave patterns would be monitored during their perception of the high. Unfortunately this was not feasible in my study (Sachs 1980) for several reasons, including the difficulty of monitoring EEG function and obtaining reliable data during strenuous gross motor activity.

Another potentially important factor is training style. "Gentle" running, as Henderson (1974) termed it, may be sacrificed in favor of speed-oriented high mileage, in preparation for competitive races. For most runners participation means running a certain number of miles. Too often the emphasis is on speed. Running as fast as possible for a certain distance appears to be the training goal for most runners, and running "gently" is apparently not popular. It has been suggested, however, that the key to experiencing the runner's high may lie in the quality of the run—in the training style the runner adopts. This training style may include type of run (such as long, slow distance) and "perceptual set" (such as gentle or hard).

In discussing a phenomenological aesthetic of body awareness, Ravizza (1979) notes components of the consciousness of experience: a quiet mind, total involvement in the movement, letting play be aesthetic, and entering into the experience. He suggests that the attitude toward participation is critical to heightened experience of an activity. It might be said that the runner's attitude toward the run may underlie perceptions about the activity as well as feelings during it. The runner's high, being unexpected, must be "allowed to happen." This can be achieved only if the runner "lets go," as Ravizza notes. Kleinman (1979) points out that the emphasis must be on *process* (rather than product) in dealing with qualitative aspects of movement and sport.

The runner straining against the clock does not "let go." The judgmental self, highlighting preconceived ideas of time and distance to be covered, restricts the possibility of a heightened experience (Glasser 1976). As Lilliefors (1978) observes, relaxation is necessary for the runner's high to occur.

### The Study: Following the Hypothesized Trail

The goals of my research were twofold. First, to get a broader description of the runner's high; second, to specify characteristics that would differentiate experiencers and nonexperiencers of the runner's high.

The variables noted earlier were measured with a number of questionnaires and tests. Cerebral dominance was assessed by both the Conjugate Lateral Eye Movement Test (CLEM) (Bakan 1978) and the Your Style of Learning and

Thinking Test (SOLAT) (Torrance et al. 1977). Addiction, commitment, training style, the runner's high, and other aspects of the running experience were assessed by questionnaires developed by Carmack and Martens (1979) and Sachs (1980).

The subjects were sixty regular runners from Tallahassee, Florida. A regular runner was defined as someone who had run an average of at least thirty minutes a day four days a week for the past two months.

The runners averaged thirty-two years old and had been running for an average of 5.7 years. Over the past twelve months they had averaged 49.9 minutes and 6.4 miles per run, with these figures increasing to 53.5 minutes and 6.8 miles for the past two months. They averaged 5.8 days a week running. Thirty-nine of the runners were married, and the other twenty-one were single (including divorced). Only six were not college graduates, and four of these were still in school. Almost half had gone beyond the bachelor's degree, and most had received the master's degree or the Ph.D. (thirteen). Occupations included twenty-six job categories, with professors (nine) and graduate students (nine) the most numerous.

As I noted earlier, 77 percent (forty-six of the sixty runners) said they had experienced the runner's high. Thirty-seven said they experienced it during a certain percentage of their runs, averaging 29.4 percent. The nine who noted experiencing the runner's high a number of times averaged 3.5 times. Half of the runners who experienced it said there were meaningful degrees or levels of the runner's high for them.

The next step was to test the ability to predict the runner's high from the variables tested, specifically cerebral dominance, addiction and commitment to running, training style, and several descriptive characteristics of the running experience (such as mileage and number of races). Stepwise multiple regression and discriminant function analyses were used. Although the runner's high did not appear to be as elusive as once thought, since thirty-six of the sixty runners were reporting it on 30 percent of their runs, I found that, given the variables tested, I could not predict who would experience it. Addiction to running and number of years a person had been running did correlate positively with experience of the runner's high, however, and this suggests possibilities for future research. But there were conflicting findings, such as that the more minutes or miles run, the less likely one was to experience the runner's high. Clearly, predicting experiencers and nonexperiencers is much more difficult than it first appears.

When these attempts at prediction did not prove fruitful, I turned to further descriptive material. Clearly the runner's high was not experienced until the runner had achieved a high degree of physiological preparedness and could run a fairly long distance without pain. Evidently a runner must be able to run easily and comfortably for five to ten miles, depending on the individual, before the runner's high becomes a part of the running experience.

The runners appeared to agree on a number of factors about the runner's high, though there were some notable differences. Many indicated that they had no conscious control over the experience—that it was not possible to predict when it would occur. For example, one said that "You can't decide to feel like this," and another noted that "You can't bring it on, control it, predict it."

Many of the runners also noted that absence of problems, little anxiety about day-to-day affairs, and no pressure about time during the run were prerequisites. For example, one reported that the runner's high occurred when he was "not concerned about time and [there were] no major personal or job concerns on hand." Another runner echoed the idea that "you need only be relaxed and unconcerned about pace, time, or other factors requiring concentration."

Environmental and climatic conditions suggested as prerequisites included cool, calm weather, absence of hills, and running in familiar areas with few distractions (traffic, bumps). Although long runs were said to be necessary for experience of the runner's high, consideration of the quality of the run was mixed, with some runners needing to run slowly and comfortably, while others spoke of "only during and after hard runs." But some runners reported they could experience the runner's high in any conditions—in the rain, or in areas where they had never run before.

The picture presented is of a phenomenon that cannot be predicted, that is promoted by cool, calm weather with low humidity and few distractions, and that requires a relatively long distance (six miles or more, at least twenty to thirty minutes of running) at a comfortable pace (though there must be no concern with speed or time). But there are notable individual differences between runners, and for each a slightly different set of conditions may be necessary. (See the appendix to this chapter for some of the runners' descriptions of the runner's high.)

Although half (twenty-three) of the runners reported experiencing different levels or degrees of the runner's high, descriptions of these levels were not clear. A dichotomous approach to understanding experience of the runner's high suggests that there are lesser feelings of general well-being that are frequently encountered and also much different euphoric states that are experienced rarely. In a continuous approach the general feeling of well-being would be at one end of the continuum and what one runner called a "super high" would be at the other.

The general feelings of well-being were described as "floating, effortless running," and as relaxation, pleasant sensations, and drifting. Others spoke not only of these reactions but also of the "super high," the highest degree being calm jubilation. The "super high" was further described as when "you're really into a flow, all systems are go, you're running fast but feeling effortless, there's no strain, you're almost part of the environment." A number of the runners indicated that they rarely reached the highest levels of this euphoric state.

### The Peak Experience

W. E. Sime (personal communication) provided a report by a national-caliber runner, describing the runner's high as a rare and exotic experience:

A highly unique transcended state wherein the other senses (sight, sound, and smell) took on peculiar degrees of sensual acuity. He described his visual experience as being somewhat similar to that which a blind man might go through shortly after having an operation which provided him with the miracle of sight, that is, a very sudden and astounding experience.

Another fascinating example of the peak experience was given to me by a woman runner (personal communication):

Antecedents were: 18 mos. of running, had not yet run a marathon, weekly mileage at 25–30 mi. This occurred in the midst of the APA 1977 S.F. convention—got up early one morning and caught a bus to Golden Gate Park and began what I'd expected to be a fairly typical, 6 mi. run. I ran from the main gate of the park a couple of miles to the "end" of the park and turned around to return. As I was running back, I suddenly became aware of the environment in an unusual way—the sun and shade and trees and grass and sky were becoming part of me, or better yet—me part of them. My awareness and sensitivity took a quantum leap into a place I'd never been before.

The next sensation was one that I hope to have again because it was incredible. There was an incredibly strong sense that my whole life was leading up to that very moment—all the anguish, all the joy, all the work—everything—had been pointing me toward being there, at that time, running. About the time that I grasped the past and present, the future began unfolding—no specifics but a sense of flow, a sense of me in time and space that went beyond that moment into a future. It was both awesome and comfortable, reassuring.

I kept running the whole time and found myself deviating from a straight path to run to a tree that seemed to reach out to me. There were squirrels and rabbits and birds everywhere, and they also seemed tuned in to me in a way I'd never experienced before. There must be a word for that but I don't know what it is.

The final piece of this that I remember acutely is that my mother was there. She was just there. A strong sense of her presence. I knew she knew what I was doing and experienced it with me. I don't often think about my mother any more—she died in 1956.

As I reached the top of the park, I jogged into a Japanese garden, sat on a rock and wept uncontrollably. As I wept, all the strong sensations began fading and I returned to "normal." I started to run back to the bus stop and filled with unbelievable energy, I couldn't stop running and ran all the way back to the hotel at Union Square.

Nothing else in my five years of running even approaches that. The invincible feeling after my first marathon was good but it wasn't metaphysical. The feelings of well-being that overcome me in running are also good (if infrequent: about 1 in 20 runs) but seem related to the rest of my life—how things are going on the job, how much sleep, diet, weight, and the like.

It appears that the runner's high, as described by most of the subjects, is a relatively mundane experience compared with those described above. The notion of the second and third wind, of feeling better during the run, may explain what most runners characterize as the runner's high. Indeed, a number of the runners spoke of the high in physiological terms, though most described it as having a psychological basis. It is important to realize that each person's interpretation of his or her own experience is a valid one. It is inappropriate for an observer/judge to decide that a runner is or is not "getting high." But we need to clarify the nature of this phenomenon and emphasize the different "types" of high that have emerged. At one end of an apparent continuum there occurs a general feeling of well-being, a vague sense of effortlessness, floating, and elation; at the other end are peak experiences such as those described by Sime, Mandell, and the woman runner.

Most of the runners supported the definition offered earlier, with occasional disagreement about selected aspects such as transcendence of barriers of time and space and enhanced appreciation of nature. Future research may help refine the definition to include experiences at different points along the proposed continuum.

What can one say about the runner's high after examining these findings and those in the literature, talking with runners, and thinking about personal experiences? It appears that we are dealing with something real. The runner's high does exist, though not everyone experiences it, and though individuals are affected in different ways. It is likely that the different percentages cited earlier are due to differing characteristics of the groups of subjects, perhaps beginners contrasted with experienced runners, or significant differences in level of addiction or number of years of running, the two variables that were shown to be related to experience of the runner's high.

As I noted, we are not in a position to pass judgment that one individual is experiencing the runner's high and another is not in spite of reporting euphoria. Many runners probably interpret the "feel-better" phenomenon as a runner's high, but if they see this as positive and it enhances their involvement, this interpretation should be encouraged.

Maslow (1962, 1964, 1968) has described peak experiences, such as those cited earlier, as involving the following characteristics of the individual: greater integration than at other times; more ability to fuse with the world; feeling oneself at the peak of one's powers; using capabilities to their fullest; effortlessness and ease of functioning; being a center of activities and perceptions; being more creative; and being more spontaneous, expressive, and natural. Occasionally, as with Mandell, Sime's runner, and the woman runner, runners report an altered state of consciousness that one might term a peak experience. These experiences may more truly reflect the state we think of as the runner's high. Given the comparative frequency of the "feel-better" phenomenon, it might be well to examine the peak experience in greater detail in the future.

### The Endorphins

Although the investigations discussed here have for the most part been psychological studies, there is psychophysiological research in progress that may eventually provide the key to understanding the runner's high. A number of articles have summarized research into "the brain's own opiates" (Durden-Smith 1978; Snyder 1977a, 1980; Villet 1978). In the past few years, naturally occurring opiatelike peptides known as endorphins have been discovered. Snyder notes (1977a, 26):

> The chemical identification of the endorphins has major relevance both for practical medical practice and a fundamental understanding of brain function. Since opiates such as morphine both cause euphoria and relieve pain, clarification of how these opiate-like peptides function will greatly advance our understanding of how the brain regulates emotions and the perception of pain. Already, it is clear that neurons containing these compounds are highly localized in "emotional" and "pain sensing" parts of the brain.

Glasser (1978, 2) suggested that the endorphins might be the "missing link in my research for the addictive factor in Positive Addiction." He conducted research (Glasser 1979) on how blocking the action of the endorphins (through chemical means, with the drug naltrexone) affected subjective evaluations of running. No positive relation was obtained between taking naltrexone and reduced pleasure from the run. Glasser suggested, however, that it was likely that not enough naltrexone was given to adequately block the effects of the endorphins.

Mandell (1979) also considered possible relations of neurotransmitters to the runner's high in his discussion of the "second second wind," and Riggs (1981) provided an excellent review of endorphins, neurotransmitters, and neuromodulators and their relation to exercise. Furthermore, enkephalin (one of the endorphins) has been "indicted" by Pargman and Baker (1980) as perhaps playing a significant role in the runner's high.

Recent work directly relevant to this area has been conducted by Appenzeller and his colleagues (Appenzeller 1980, 1981; Appenzeller and Schade 1979; Appenzeller et al. 1980). Appenzeller and Schade (1979) found that, contrary to previous findings, the autonomic nervous system showed no sign of exhaustion throughout a marathon in well-trained endurance athletes. Furthermore, total plasma catecholamines and norepinephrine had increased by 300 percent at seven miles, remained unchanged to twenty miles, and increased to 600 percent of baseline levels by the end of the race.

Additional work by Appenzeller et al. (1980; also note Appenzeller 1980, 1981) showed tremendous increases in serum beta-endorphin levels after a 45.9 kilometer (28.5 mile) race, reaching approximately 200 percent of prerace figures. Although beta-endorphin levels for runners forty and older were lower than levels for those thirty-nine and younger, increases for both groups from pre- to postrace were statistically significant and proportionally similar.

Appenzeller et al. (1980, 419) note the following: "Endurance running produces a marked increase in β-endorphin. Whether this increase persists after physical activity and is responsible for the 'runner's high,' the behavioral alterations of endurance-trained individuals, improved libido, heightened pain threshold, absence of depression, and other anecdotal effects of endurance training remains conjectural."

It should be noted, however, that Appenzeller's work has been criticized for methodological shortcomings and (like that of others in this area) should be carefully scrutinized. For example, though Colt, Wardlaw, and Frantz (1981) found that running stimulated the secretion of beta-endorphin, they "do not believe the decrease in anxiety which has been reported after running . . . , or other mood changes such as the 'runner's high,' can be attributed to the small changes which occurred in peripheral plasma β-endorphin concentrations'' (p. 1640).

Colt, Wardlaw, and Frantz (1981) found a rise in beta-endorphin levels for 45 percent of their runners after an easy run, and for 80 percent of their runners after a strenuous run. Additionally, the percentage increase in beta-endorphin over baseline was negatively correlated with the number of years the runners had been training. This may be related to the findings of Appenzeller et al. (1980) if one assumes that the older (forty and over) runners had more years of training than the younger ones (thirty-nine or less). This information was not available from their original study.

These significant increases in endorphin levels after exercise have been shown in other studies (Bortz et al. 1981; Carr et al. 1981b; Moretti et al. 1981). Related work with naloxone (an opiate blocker) has both supported (Haier, Quaid, and Mills 1981) and failed to support (Markoff, Ryan, and Young 1982) these research findings. Of particular interest here, however, is that research on the endorphins has for the most part been concerned with endorphins at the peripheral level. These measurements of endorphins taken from the blood-stream raise the question of what effects the endorphins in the brain, at the central level, have on the runner's high, on addiction to running, or on other aspects of running and exercise. The explanations suggested for the effects of the endorphins have concentrated on the central level. Are the effects of increased endorphins at the peripheral level the same? In a letter responding to the article of Carr et al. (1981b), Hawley and Butterfield (1981, 1591) note, in particular, that "It is doubtful that plasma levels influence or reflect levels in the central nervous system, where the primary action of the opioids is known to occur. Only if central-nervous-system levels of β-endorphin are shown to be elevated in response to exercise can the endogenous opioid be implicated in such subjective phenomena as the euphoria or anti-nociception frequently reported during exercise." They further point out that "In human beings, ACTH does not cross the blood-cerebrospinal fluid barrier, and β-endor-phin . . . seems to be likewise impermeable: intravenous injection of the opioid does not affect perception of pain or mood and does not alter β-endorphin levels in the cerebrospinal fluid, whereas injection into the cerebral ventricle and intrathecally causes profound analgesia."

In reply, however, Carr et al. (1981a, 1592) note that "Until the passage of peptides across the blood-brain barrier during exercise is evaluated, assertions about the impermeability of this barrier that are based on observations in unstressed subjects are premature."

It appears clear, though, that the point made by Appenzeller et al. (1980) cited earlier is well taken, and that the answers to the question of the relation of the endorphins to the runner's high (and to other facets of the running experience) have yet to be determined. We need to find causal, as opposed to correlational, explanations. A question immediately arises about those who do not experience the runner's high. Does the mechanism of the endorphins somehow work differently for these runners, if the endorphins are indeed important to the runner's high? Further research in this area promises to be exciting, for it is here that the answers may lie.

For the moment the runner's high remains a particularly personal experience, not readily accessible to scrutiny by researchers. Some studies report that most runners experience it. It is described as very positive, enhancing the quality of the run. Whether what most runners term the runner's high is just a generalized feeling of well-being or whether it approaches the exalted regions of the peak experience remains to be determined. The euphoric runner's high can and should be used to increase the benefits of running. Though it remains as elusive as ever, its trail is enticing and will surely be followed by increasing numbers of researchers in coming years.

## Appendix: Descriptions of the Runner's High

M. R.: Lift in the legs, mental awareness, physical excellence, ability to suppress pain or discomfort.

H. G.: Euphoria – free of worry, guilt, tension. Feel as if I can run forever, and fast too; hear crowds cheering as if at the end of a race.

K. H.: Feeling of self-assurance and power; rhythmic breathing without strain; gliding through air and only lightly touching down; feeling of accomplishment, that one could run forever without breathing hard or aching.

J. F.: Field of awareness narrows, appreciate common sensations more. See colors more distinctly on long runs. Mind wanders to pleasant things, daydream only about positive experiences.

J. S.: Feel like could nearly leave feet and fly. Gone as fast as could during a race, but very little discomfort.

R. H.: Mind very alert, and feel acutely aware of environment. Body moving in perfect rhythm with no jerks. Ease, sense of exhilaration, joy, and liberation.

B. R.: Feel free and natural in your surroundings. At peace with being a human animal in the world.

B. W.: Complete joy in the run; no fatigue.

C. P.: Euphoria, laughing and crying at the same time.

R. E.: Calm, feeling good, no cares at all.

# References

Appenzeller, O. 1980. Report from Otto Appenzeller, M.D. *AMJA Newsletter*, July, 31.
————. 1981. Does running affect mood? (Reader's Forum) *Runner's World* 16(4):13.
Appenzeller, O., and Schade, D. R. 1979. Neurology of endurance training. III. Sympathetic activity during a marathon run. *Neurology* 29(4):542.
Appenzeller, O.; Standefer, J.; Appenzeller, J.; and Atkinson, R. 1980. Neurology of endurance training. V. Endorphins. *Neurology* 30:418–19.
Bakan, P. 1978. Two streams of consciousness: A typological approach. In *The stream of consciousness: Scientific investigations into the flow of human experience*, ed. K. S. Pope and J. L. Singer. New York: Plenum Press.
Bever, T. G. 1975. Cerebral asymmetries in humans are due to the differentiation of two incompatible processes: Holistic and analytic. In Developmental psycholinguistics and communication disorders, ed. D. Aaronson and R. Reiber. *Annals of the New York Academy of Sciences* 263:251–62.
Black, J. 1979. The brain according to Mandell. *Runner* 1(7):78–80, 82, 84, 87.
Bogen, J. E. 1969. The other side of the brain: Parts I, II, and III. *Bulletin of the Los Angeles Neurological Society* 34:73–105, 135–62, 191–203.
Bortz, W. M., II; Angwin, P.; Mefford, I. N.; Boarder, M. R.; Noyce, N.; and Barchas, J. D. 1981. Catecholamines, dopamine, and endorphin levels during extreme exercise. *New England Journal of Medicine* 305(8):466–67.
Carmack, M. A., and Martens, R. 1979. Measuring commitment to running: A survey of runners' attitudes and mental states. *Journal of Sport Psychology* 1:25–42.
Carr, D. B.; Bullen, B. A.; Skrinar, G. S.; Arnold, M. A.; Rosenblatt, M.; Beitins, I. Z.; Martin, J. B.; and McArthur, J. W. 1981a. Exercise and the endogenous opioids. *New England Journal of Medicine* 305(26):1592.
————. 1981b. Physical conditioning facilitates the exercise-induced secretion of beta-endorphin and beta-lipotropin in women. *New England Journal of Medicine* 305(10):560–63.
Colt, E. W. D.; Wardlaw, S. L.; and Frantz, A. G. 1981. The effect of running on plasma β-endorphin. *Life Sciences* 28:1637–40.
Durden-Smith, J. 1978. A chemical cure for madness? *Quest/78* 2(3):31–36, 38.
Gazzaniga, M. S. 1970. *The bisected brain.* New York: Appleton-Century-Crofts.
Glasser, W. 1976. *Positive addiction.* New York: Harper and Row.
————. 1978. The positive addiction experiment. *Starting Line* 2:2.
————. 1979. Glasser experiment: Results. *ARC,* no. 4:7.
Haier, R. J.; Quaid, K.; and Mills, J. S. C. 1981. Naloxone alters pain perception after jogging. *Psychiatry Research* 5:231–32.
Hawley, L. M., and Butterfield, G. E. 1981. Exercise and the endogenous opioids. *New England Journal of Medicine* 305(26):1591.
Henderson, J. 1974. *Run gently, run long.* Mountain View, Calif.: World Publications.
Jacobs, L. W. 1980. Running as an addiction process. Ph.D. diss., University of Alberta.

Johnson, G. 1978. Researching the running mind. *On the Run,* no. 10:11–17.

Kleinman, S. 1979. Qualitative aspects of the sport experience: An experiential guide for performers and teachers. Paper presented at a symposium on Aesthetics and Sport Art, annual convention of the American Alliance for Health, Physical Education, and Recreation, New Orleans, 15 March.

Lilliefors, J. 1978. *The running mind.* Mountain View, Calif.: World Publications.

Mandell, A. J. 1979. The second second wind. *Psychiatric Annals* 9:57–69.

Markoff, R. A.; Ryan, P.; and Young, T. 1982. Endorphins and mood changes in long-distance running. *Medicine and Science in Sports and Exercise* 14:11–15.

Maslow, A. H. 1962. Lessons from the peak experience. *Journal of Humanistic Psychology* 2:9–18.

———. 1964. *Religions, values, and peak-experiences.* New York: Viking Press.

———. 1968. *Toward a psychology of being.* Princeton, N.J.: D. Van Nostrand.

Moretti, C.; Cappa, M.; Paolucci, D.; Fabbri, A.; Santoro, C.; Fraioli, F.; and Isidori, A. 1981. Pituitary response to physical exercise: Sex differences. *Medicine Sport* 14:180–86.

Morgan, W. P. 1979a. Negative addiction in runners. *Physician and Sportsmedicine* 7(2):56–63, 67–70.

———. 1979b. Running into addiction. *Runner* 1:(6): 72–74, 76.

Ornstein, R. E. 1972. *The psychology of consciousness.* San Francisco: W. H. Freeman.

Ornstein, R. E., and Galin, D. 1976. Physiological studies of consciousness. In *Symposium on consciousness,* ed. P. R. Lee, R. E. Ornstein, D. Galin, A. Deikman and C. T. Tart. New York: Viking Press.

Pargman, D., and Baker, M. C. 1980. Running high: Enkephalin indicted. *Journal of Drug Issues* 10(3):341–49.

Ravizza, K. 1979. The body aware: A phenomenological aesthetic. Paper presented at a symposium on Aesthetics and Sport Art, annual convention of the American Alliance for Health, Physical Education, and Recreation, New Orleans, 15 March.

Riggs, C. E. 1981. Endorphins, neurotransmitters, and/or neuromodulators and exercise. In *Psychology of running,* ed. M. H. Sacks and M. L. Sachs. Champaign, Ill.: Human Kinetics Publishers.

Sachs, M. L. 1978. Selected psychological considerations in running. Invited presentation, Running Clinic (Temple Israel Brotherhood, Gulf Winds Track Club, and Athletic Attic—sponsors), Tallahassee, Florida, 8 August.

———. 1979. An examination of the relationship of commitment to and dependence upon running to a model for participation in running and personality typology of regular runners. Unpublished manuscript, Florida State University.

———. 1980. On the trail of the runner's high: A descriptive and experimental investigation of characteristics of an elusive phenomenon. Ph.D. diss., Florida State University.

Sachs, M. L., and Pargman, D. 1979a. Commitment and addiction to regular running. Paper presented at the annual meeting of the American Alliance for Health, Physical Education, and Recreation, New Orleans, 19 March. In *Abstracts: Research papers*

*1979 AAHPER Convention.* Washington, D.C.: American Alliance for Health, Physical Education, and Recreation.

———. 1979b. Running addiction: A depth interview examination. *Journal of Sport Behavior* 2:143–55.

Snyder, S. H. 1977a. The brain's own opiates. *Chemical and Engineering News* 55(48):26–35.

———. 1977b. Opiate receptors and internal opiates. *Scientific American* 236:44–56.

———. 1980. *Biological aspects of mental disorder.* New York: Oxford University Press.

Torrance, E. P.; Reynolds, C.; Riegel, T.; and Ball, O. E. 1977. Your style of learning and thinking, forms A and B: Preliminary norms, abbreviated technical notes, scoring keys, and selected references. *Gifted Child Quarterly* 21:563–73.

Villet, B. 1978. Opiates of the mind. *Atlantic* 241(6):82–89.

Wagemaker, H., Jr., and Goldstein, L. 1980. The runner's high. *Journal of Sports Medicine and Physical Fitness* 20:227–29.

Weinberg, W. T. 1980. Relationship of commitment to running scale to runners' performances and attitudes. Paper presented at the annual convention of the American Alliance for Health, Physical Education, Recreation, and Dance, poster presentation session, Detroit, 12 April. In *Abstracts: Research papers 1980 AAHPERD Convention.* Washington, D.C.: American Alliance for Health, Physical Education, Recreation, and Dance.

MICHAEL L. SACHS

# 16

---

# The Mind of the Runner: Cognitive Strategies Used during Running

The cognitive aspects of running are critical to understanding the psychology of running. The earlier chapters in this section—on running addiction, the effect of exercise on personality, and the runner's high—addressed some of these cognitive aspects. The "mind of the runner" encompasses not only these areas, but also particular cognitive strategies used during running. By a particular psychological or perceptual set the runner may enhance or impair performance and the perceived quality of the run.

Other authors have discussed cognitive skills and athletic performance (see in particular an excellent review by Mahoney 1979). Here I am concerned with the psychological preparation of runners (particularly for competition) and the coping strategies of association and dissociation they use in training and competition. After a detailed examination of these strategies and the presentation of a study of them conducted at Florida State University (Sachs 1980), I will address a number of related areas. These include attention and the experience of physical symptoms (in which the strategy of dissociation assumes particular significance), the "mind game" (mental preparation for running a marathon and strategies used during marathon competition), the famous (or infamous) "wall" associated with the marathon, and the Tibetian art of lung-gom (perhaps the ultimate use of dissociation). Most of the work on cognitive strategies has dealt with the marathon, so this chapter will also focus on the marathon, but the information here is also applicable to shorter and longer distances.

## Psychological Preparation

Although innumerable sources in the literature deal with physical preparation for running (training schedules, diet, footwear; see, for example, Fixx 1977, 1980), psychological factors have rarely been addressed. The few articles that do exist relate to psychological preparation for running the marathon.

Orlick (1980), in one of the few "practical" guides available, discusses psyching for marathons. He cites a number of strategies that are effective in both long- and short-term preparation for the event. These include self-assessment, listening to one's body, talking to one's body, relaxing, using imagery, dealing with pain (by associative and dissociative strategies), and employing multiple goals and self-reinforcement. Additionally, Orlick suggests that preplanning strategy and simulating performance conditions in training are important aids in psychological preparation.

The importance of mental preparation in achieving success in the marathon, for both the elite and the nonelite runner, has also been noted by Friedman (1980), who cites the strategies of goal setting and visualization (described by Orlick) and also includes studying the upcoming race and memorizing the desired mile splits.

Pelletier and Sachs (1981) examined motivation and psychological preparation for marathon running, testing twenty runners with in-depth interviews. Their subjects reported that preparation for the marathon was at least 50 percent psychological, emphasizing the importance of mental factors, in addition to physical preparation, for completion of the marathon distance (and achieving desired goals). The runners identified the challenge of the marathon as important and reported using strategies of concentration and visualization in preparing for it.

Psychological preparation for running, particularly for distances other than the marathon, has not received the attention it deserves. Further study of the strategies identified by Friedman (1980), Orlick (1980), and Pelletier and Sachs (1981) will deepen our understanding of how they can enhance preparation for and performance in both competitive races and noncompetitive runs.

## Coping Strategies: Association and Dissociation

Coping strategies represent a particularly intriguing, but relatively unexplored, area of research. Morgan (1978; Morgan and Pollock 1977) used the terms "association" and "dissociation" to categorize cognitive strategies during running. In association, runners focus on their bodily sensations and stay aware of physical factors critical to performance. In dissociation runners think of anything but bodily feelings. In Morgan's examples, marathon runners intentionally used dissociation to "think away" pain during the latter stages of the race (Morgan 1978).

These strategies have been clarified further. In association runners focus continuously on bodily sensations such as "respiration, temperature, heaviness in the calves and thighs, abdominal sensations" (Morgan 1978, 39) in an effort to maximize performance while minimizing pain or discomfort. This strategy enables them to approach that fine line between maximum performance and overextension, giving the edge to maximum performance. Popular descriptions of this strategy tend to include attention paid to others in a race as part of general association to racing conditions. However, in the "truest" sense, association appears to be restricted to focusing on one's own bodily sensations.

Dissociation occurs when the runner "purposely cuts himself off from the sensory feedback he normally receives from the body" (Morgan 1978, 39). In other words, runners think about anything except how they feel at that point. Morgan cites a number of dissociative strategies that runners use, including mentally writing letters, listening to a stack of Beethoven records, building a house, and doing complex mathematical problems. One problem with dissociation, however, is that it can be carried to the extent that signals of pain from injuries are disregarded (Colt and Spyropoulos 1979) or signs of oncoming hypo- or hyperthermia are not perceived. Runners may also misjudge their capabilities and have too much or too little left at the end of a race.

Attentional diversion ("focusing attention on a natural or pleasant stimulus rather than on a stressful stimulus"; Bloom et al. 1977, 83) is directly related to dissociation. Bloom et al. (1977) demonstrated that attentional diversion was effective in reducing stress (threat of painful shocks). Similarly, Popkin, Stillner, and Pierce (U.S. Department of Health and Human Services 1981), who have been studying racers in the annual Iditarod Trail Sled Dog Race (a 1,049 mile race across Alaska) since 1975, found that racers "used a strategy of "inattention,' focusing attention externally, away from themselves and their condition" (p. 9) to best cope with the effects of stress. Runners certainly may also have learned that dissociation, or attentional diversion, is effective in reducing stress during training and competitive runs.

In chapter 15 I discussed research on the runner's high, focusing in particular on work conducted with a group of sixty runners at Florida State University (Sachs 1980). In further work on the runner's high I attempted to manipulate the cognitive strategies of these runners. In chapter 15 I discussed the potential importance of differences in right/left brain function in the runner's high. It is of particular interest that the strategies of association and dissociation may entail differential functioning of the right and left hemispheres. Association, being a continuously analytical task, appears to involve left-brain activity. Dissociation, however, may involve either right- or left-brain activity. To use Morgan's examples, the letter writer and mathematics enthusiast would be engaging in left-brain functions, while the music lover would probably be emphasizing right-brain activity. It therefore seemed that any attempt to manipulate right/left brain functioning while running would encompass one of three strategy groupings: association; dissociation emphasizing right-brain activity; and dissociation emphasizing left-brain activity.

The effects of these strategies on perception of the run had yet to be determined. It seemed likely that enhancing right-brain activity would promote experience of the runner's high (see chap. 15) and, concomitantly, enhance the perceived quality of the run. To test these potential effects, therefore, I used an intervention involving the three strategy groupings. I hypothesized that the dissociators using right-brain activities would increase the quality of the run significantly more than the other groups, and that their experience of the runner's high would be significantly greater.

A primary finding in this study was that the concepts of association and dissociation do serve as functional general categories for discussing the thought processes of runners. But, simple categorization of runners as associators or dissociators may not be meaningful. Although the sixty runners employed primarily associative or dissociative strategies, all runners reported frequent shifts during the run from association to dissociation and back again. This frequent "slipping in and out" of the strategies made it difficult for the runners to classify themselves as associators or dissociators, though they could say which strategy they used most of the time. In this group of runners, 68 percent (forty-one) categorized themselves as using dissociative strategies most of the time, 25 percent (fifteen) used mostly associative strategies, and 7 percent (four) used associative and dissociative strategies equally often.

Previous research with marathon runners has proposed three categories of the dissociative state: diversions (meditating, fantasizing), problem solving, and spontaneity ("it just happens") (Lorentzen and Sime 1979). Spontaneity and problem solving were most frequently used among the sixty runners in the Florida State study (Sachs 1980). Spontaneity was characterized by descriptions such as free flow of thoughts, drifting, aimless thinking, random thoughts, letting the mind wander, letting the mind freewheel, free floating, and absence of set thought patterns. In general the mind was permitted to move freely from thought to thought (or focus on "nothing at all"), with no particular pattern.

This aspect of spontaneity may also be characteristic of ultramarathoners, those runners who participate in races longer than the marathon distance. Sacks et al. (1981) examined mental status and psychological coping during a one-hundred-mile race and found that the participants tended to engage in "meditative thinking," in which the "runners are focusing neither on themselves nor on some distracting thought, but rather they are not particularly focusing at all" (p. 173). Meditative thinking would be classified as spontaneous thinking in the Lorentzen and Sime (1979) categorization of dissociative states.

Problem solving for the runners in the Florida State study (Sachs 1980) was characterized by expressions such as becoming reflective, working out problems, sorting out things, day's activities, and whatever's troubling me mentally. Diversions were reported less often, but they generally featured expressions of daydreaming. Two sets of fantasies in particular were noteworthy, with one runner reporting a daydream of becoming the first to run the marathon in less than two hours (the current world record is 2:08:13), and another dreaming of victory in the Olympics.

Within these categories, many "themes" were present, depending to some extent on the reasons for running, but also on factors in everyday existence. Some runners used the run to "get away" and were therefore less likely to focus on problems and difficulties. Others considered the run a time where thinking was particularly clear, presenting a good opportunity to sort through the day's activities, plan future events, and work out problems. Problems noted involved work, home, school, and interpersonal relationships. Berger and Mackenzie (1980) noted that running, among other sports, is conducive to introspection and to thinking in general (see also Berger, chap. 10). This was clearly true for many of the runners in the Florida State study (Sachs 1980).

Lorentzen and Sime (1979) state that the 217 runners they studied identified association as including "monitoring body signs, and reducing anxiety, pain and effort sense" (p. i). These benefits were reported by the runners in the Florida State study as well, but reports of anxiety reduction were infrequent. There was a continuous monitoring of the self, reviewing the body's state from head to toe, and a desire to stay in tune with "what's going on." Other runners reported being aware of the self, rarely getting out of touch, and concentrating on form and maintaining pace. In particular, runners reported concentrating on sensations from various parts of the body, level of fatigue, form being maintained, and striking of the pavement with each step. The legs and feet were primary, though assessment of breathing rate and level of exertion was also characteristic. This agrees with Lorentzen and Sime's statement that "runners utilized association in order to monitor general condition of the legs, general body functioning, and muscle tightness" (1979, i).

Let me emphasize again that these characterizations of association and dissociation represent cognitive strategies runners employed at given points during their runs. There was, as noted, frequent shifting back and forth between association and dissociation as conditions warranted. For example, a shift to an uneven surface, or running in particularly hot and humid weather, prompted a shift to associative strategies to maintain a safe pace, careful footing, and appropriate form. In particular, the excessive summer heat and humidity in Florida placed a premium on maintaining awareness of body functions stressed by adverse climatic conditions.

Many runners indicated a tendency to associate more during the early and late parts of the run and to dissociate during the rest of the time. During the first mile(s), the runner would monitor feet, legs, breathing, form, and so on, to be aware of the progress of the body and to facilitate the desired relatively effortless state. Toward the end of the run association was used to maintain form and assess fatigue. The onset of pain was interpreted as a sign to associate. At the first awareness of pain, association was used to identify the source and nature of the discomfort and assess possible courses of action (i.e., stop, slow down, speed up).

In contrast to Morgan's (1978) runners who reported using dissociation to think about anything but the pain during the marathon run (at least the nonelite competitors), for the runners in the Florida State study pain served as a stimulus to associate. However, a critical difference between the context in which Morgan's runners and the runners in this study reported their reactions to the stimulus of pain may explain these opposing findings. Morgan's runners reported the feelings they had during a race; the Florida State runners reported strategies they used during training. Training runs are generally less stressful and intended for different purposes then racing (e.g., relaxation, social interaction, sharpening, conditioning, pleasure), though racing may include some of these components. Indeed, the runners reported that during races and harder runs they tended to associate more than during "regular" training, to maintain performance at the upper limits of their capabilities. It is possible that examining strategies toward the end of the marathon run with these runners would provide findings like Morgan's.

In summary, the runners in the Florida State study tended to dissociate most of the time during their training runs but shifted frequently between association and dissociation. It is clear that we cannot provide a simple characterization of the cognitive strategies of runners and that the pattern of strategies they use and the nature of their thought processes are complex.

## Strategy Experiment

Runners were instructed to implement the strategy assigned to their group—association, dissociation/right-brain activities, or dissociation/left-brain activities—during the next-to-last mile of the middle four of eight runs (the first two runs and last two runs served as baseline measures). This was done so that each runner employed the strategy at approximately the same point during a run. Emphasis was placed on interfering as little as possible with the runner's schedule, to avoid confounding the results of the manipulation. The strategies assigned to each group are described in detail in the appendix to this chapter.

Ratings were obtained of perceived quality of the run and experience of the runner's high (see chap. 15). There was only one significant finding, concerning evaluation of the quality of the run, but this not clearly explained by follow-up tests of the effect.

The failure of the strategy manipulation may have been due to a number of factors. For example, most of the runners who had to use a strategy different from the one(s) they normally used reported having difficulty. Some runners reacted negatively to interference with their thought processes even during a relatively small segment of the run. One runner said, "I was glad I didn't have to count anymore. The forced strategies had become a real intrusion into my 'private hour.'" A few of the runners said they might not have participated had the experiment required a greater number of trials.

If manipulating the quality of the run and experience of the runner's high through changes in cognitive strategies is to be effective, it is likely that more specific training in these strategies will be needed. Runners not familiar with the strategies assigned to them discussed their precise use with the experimenter and in some cases practiced them at or near the testing site. Most runners appeared fairly "set in their ways," voicing preferences for their habitual thought processes. For example, one runner said, "I don't use any other strategy really because I have been running for a few years and my thought processes are locked in." A training program would instruct the runners in the benefits and techniques of particular strategies. The strategies runners habitually use may not be the best for particular training or racing conditions. They should evaluate the available strategies in different situations (i.e., training, racing) and use those most appropriate at particular times. Let me emphasize that attempts to change "standard" thought processes may be met with resistance, and such efforts must be carefully planned and carried out.

Further evidence is needed on the effectiveness of particular strategies and on whether intraindividual differences significantly influence the magnitude of strategy effects. The benefits of use of dissociative/right-brain strategies in enhancing the quality of the run and experience of the runner's high must be demonstrated before training programs emphasizing these strategies can be honestly supported. Note also that association is commonly used during racing to enhance performance. Perhaps dissociative strategies should be recommended only for improving the quality of training runs, while harder runs and race performance are enhanced by associative strategies.

An alternative approach might be the system suggested by Sime (1980). Sime discusses the strategies of association/dissociation in offering the Pace-Assisted Dissociation/Association (PADA) approach. This approach aims to synchronize respiration rate and depth with frequency of leg movements by adjusting length of stride. Synchrony is maintained by counting. Sime suggests that PADA may help keep the respiratory system slightly ahead of metabolic fatigue. The use of dissociation as a self-hypnotic diversion, within the context of the PADA approach, may result in relaxed running, improved performance, and higher-quality runs.

There may also be a physiological component inherent in runners' successful use of cognitive strategies and in their pain tolerance. Freischlag (1981), drawing upon work by Landers, Obermeier, and Wolf (1977), Melzack (1973), and Worthy and Markle (1970), suggested the fascinating hypothesis that perhaps eye color (iris pigmentation), a measure of neuromelanin (which inhibits reactivity of the nervous system), is related to pain tolerance and marathon performance. Freischlag found that the fastest 20 percent of the runners in his study had lighter eye color than the slowest 20 percent (subjects ranked according to marathon time performance). Worthy (1974) suggested that "light-eyed animals tend to excel in behaviors requiring delay, self-pacing, or nonreaction (low reactivity)" (Landers, Obermeier, and Wolf 1977, 95). Perhaps the effectiveness of the various cognitive strategies runners employ is affected by eye color. This hypothesis warrants further investigation.

Future research on manipulating cognitive strategies in runners will require work in several areas. First, the strategies used in both association and dissociation (right and left brain) must be developed so the runner can clearly grasp the principles behind given strategies. Second, the differential effectiveness of strategies across levels of running (elite, nonelite; training, racing) must be determined. Third, differences in the use and effectiveness of strategies across individuals must be investigated, to identify the level of training and difficulty involved for those accustomed to using different cognitive strategies during their runs.

## Attention and the Experience of Physical Symptoms

Pennebaker and his colleagues at the University of Virginia have conducted a number of studies dealing with the relation of attention to the perception of internal states. Pennebaker et al. (1978), for example, examined the effects of attention on the experience of physical symptoms. They suggested that, since most symptoms are negatively valenced, "the more an individual focuses attention on a given symptom, the more painful or disliked the symptom should become" (p. 1).

They conducted two experiments. In the first, a distraction (dissociation) strategy was significantly more effective in increasing time of pain onset from immersing the hand in cold water (1° C), compared with strategies designed to focus attention on the painful stimulation (either on the hand or on the water). In a second experiment, examining muscle fatigue on a hand dynamometer task, subjects instructed to associate with pain or soreness symptoms after the task reported significantly greater stiffness/soreness than subjects instructed to think of a waterfall, the distraction (dissociation) strategy. Pennebaker et al. (1978, 5) concluded that the results "confirm the general prediction that attention to physical symptoms tends to exaggerate, or heighten, their occurrence."

Of even more direct significance to the general focus of this chapter is work by Pennebaker and Lightner (1980) examining competition between internal and external information during exercise. In the first of two experiments, subjects exercised on a treadmill, with exercise intensity held constant. While exercising, subjects listened either to a tape of a series of street sounds, to their own breathing, or to nothing. Results indicated that attention to distracting sounds produced a significant decrease in perceptions of fatigue and related symptoms. On the other hand, perception of these symptoms was magnified when attention was focused internally (listening to breathing). Pennebaker and Lightner attribute the results to differences in the degree to which subjects encoded internal sensations, specifically increasing when attention was focused on the subjects' own breathing.

The second experiment extended the investigation to a field setting, testing joggers on cross-country and circular lap courses (Pennebaker and Lightner 1980). Subjects jogged alternately on the two types of courses for ten days, and time for course completion and symptom and fatigue measures were recorded each day. Times were significantly lower on the cross-country course than on the lap course (both were eighteen hundred meters), though there were no differences in reports of fatigue or symptoms between runs. Pennebaker and Lightner suggest that: "Subjects set and maintained their jogging pace in accord with their perceptions of fatigue-related symptoms. Given that subjects were focusing on external factors to a higher degree on the cross-country course, their processing of internal sensations was restricted. Consequently, they could increase their pace before feeling maximally fatigued" (1980, 171).

The research by Pennebaker and his colleagues (Pennebaker and Lightner 1980; Pennebaker et al. 1978) suggests that dissociative strategies may improve performance as well as decrease perception of fatigue and related symptoms. Perhaps the associative strategies used by elite runners are not the most effective in maximizing performance and reducing reported symptoms. However, further work clearly is needed to determine whether these findings from nonelite runners can be generalized to runners—especially elite runners—in competition. Pennebaker's research supports the efficaciousness of the strategies used by the nonelite marathoners as reported by Morgan (1978).

The concept of arousal-induced attention to self is important here. Wegner and Giuliano (1980), for example, reported that subjects who ran in place were more self-focused than subjects who waited in a chair or reclined in a lounge chair. Running or other physical activities may focus attention inward, and therefore predispose the individual toward associative strategies. Hollandsworth (1979) has suggested that long-distance running and other forms of aerobic exercise may provide biofeedback training. Individuals may learn to control their physiological responses to some degree to improve performance.

A final point is the interpretive set used with respect to painful/nonpainful symptoms. Painful symptoms are inherently interpreted as negative, but the interpretation of nonpainful symptoms is not so clear. "For nonpainful symptoms, . . . the interpretive context determines whether the experienced sensations are defined as symptomatic at all" (Pennebaker and Skelton 1978, 528). These findings bear on the use of running to cure psychological problems. Orwin's (1973) work, for example, focused on patients' *reinterpreting* physiological reactions as due to the physical exertion of running rather than to the presenting agoraphobia. This "misattribution" approach (see Zillmann 1978), seen in other related psychological research (see Pennebaker 1980 for a good analysis of this area), may prove of great significance in running therapy and the psychology of running. Clearly, interpretive sets must be considered in future work with perception of bodily sensations and cognitive strategies for enhancing performance.

## The Mind Game

Further insight into mental preparation for running the marathon and strategies used during marathon competition is provided in a number of studies by Orlick, Power, and Partington (1979, 1980a,b), who examined sixty-four experienced marathon runners attending a marathon clinic in Ottawa, Canada. The fastest 5 percent of the runners (marathon time range 2:30 to 2:55, mean 2:46) were compared with the slowest 5 percent (marathon time range 4:16 to 4:43, mean 4:37). The faster runners' primary objectives were to run well, improve previous times, and beat opponents. During the race these runners concentrated on pace, strategy, awareness of effort, and improving position. The slower runners had as their main objective "just finishing" and concentrated on keeping the pace slow, holding back, and finishing.

Orlick, Power, and Partington found that the runners "talk themselves through their own difficulties" (1979, 37), in that they used key phrases or thoughts to bring themselves through any difficult times they might experience during the race. Some examples of self-talk are:

"I have come this far, I can go a few more miles."

"Must not walk! Must not fail! Pain is not too bad, it could be worse."

"If others can do it, so can I."

"One mile at a time."

"Everyone hurts as much as I do." (1979, 37)

It is interesting to compare the runners' internal dialogue, their self-talk, with the manipulations used in cognitive therapy (Buffone 1980; see Buffone, Sachs, and Dowd, chap. 11).

Orlick, Power, and Partington (1980b) also studied runners' thoughts during training runs. Thinking about the running experience (association) was noted in 17.5 percent of the responses, while thinking of other things (dissociation) was cited in 13.2 percent. Most of the responses included "thinking about how to manage their lives" (p. 34), including solving general problems (29.5 percent), work problems (15.9 percent), or personal problems (9.9 percent), time planning (7.9 percent), and interpersonal relations (7.2 percent)—responses similar to reports from some of the runners in my earlier study (Sachs 1980). However, these latter responses (dealing with "life management") might be classified as dissociative strategies according to the earlier definitions. If this scheme is adopted, the difference in degree between associative (17.5 percent) and dissociative (83.6 percent) thinking during training runs is noteworthy. In contrast with my study however, no precise indication is given of the degree of shifting between the two strategies during the run or the prevalence of the different strategies during different parts of the run. Nevertheless, the findings of Orlick, Power, and Partington (1979, 1980a,b) do point out the importance of dissociative strategies during running.

### The Wall

The use of associative and dissociative strategies has been highlighted in discussing the infamous "wall." The wall is a barrier, with both psychological and physiological components, that runners supposedly encounter at the twenty-mile mark of the marathon. The word "supposedly" is important here, because a number of elite marathoners have averred that the wall is a myth, that no such barrier exists (Merrill 1981). But there are many marathoners, mostly the nonelite, who swear to its existence and claim they have "hit the wall" in their races.

The most plausible explanation for the wall appears to be the changeover from primarily glucose to primarily fat metabolism after approximately twenty miles for most runners. Why don't the elite experience the wall (assuming it exists)? This likely is due to training, inherent physiological advantages, and psychological preparation. Merrill (1981, 46) talks about the use of association in running the marathon: "Faster times and less trouble with the Wall seem to be the dual benefits of associative marathoning. The lesson: Keep your mind on the race—a constant monitoring of body and environment will probably get you through the Wall with greater speed, safety, and comfort."

Merrill suggests that the associative strategies used by elite runners will improve competitive performance. While this may be sound advice, the findings of Pennebaker and his colleagues (Pennebaker and Lightner 1980; Pennebaker et al. 1978), and the reports of Orlick, Power, and Partington (1979, 1980a,b) and of Morgan (1978; Morgan and Pollock 1977) suggest a place for dissociative strategies as well. It is likely that a clear understanding of the nature of the wall will be required before we can give effective advice on the use of associative and dissociative strategies. An initial hypothesis might be that associative strategies are best used to avoid the wall in the first place, but that if the wall is encountered dissociative strategies may enhance the runner's chances of completing the marathon.

## The Art of Lung-gom

Perhaps the ultimate in the effective use of dissociative strategies is the art of lung-gom practiced in Tibet. David-Neel (1965) provides a fascinating discussion of this art, which includes "a large number of practices which combine mental concentration with various breathing gymnastics and aim at different results either spiritual or physical" (p. 199). The practice of lung-gom permits the lamas (monks) to travel at relatively high speeds for long distances, day and night, across difficult terrain in the mountains of Tibet.

David-Neel describes seeing one lama engaged in lung-gom (1965, 202–3): "I could clearly see his perfectly calm impassive face and wide-open eyes with their gaze fixed on some invisible far-distant object situated somewhere high up in space. The man did not run. He seemed to lift himself from the ground, proceeding by leaps. It looked as if he had been endowed with the elasticity of a ball and rebounded each time his feet touched the ground."

The lamas usually fix their gaze on a particular star in the sky (lung-gom is most effectively practiced at night), and after long experience the lama reaches the stage where he "does not feel the weight of . . . [his] body" (p. 215). Although the training is over a long period (at least thirty-nine months), the results for those who become adept at lung-gom are clearly exceptional.

The relevance of this experience for the runner may be difficult to ascertain, but it appears to lie in training for successful use of meditation and a dissociative strategy. The runner who practices particular strategies during training may find them successful during races.

## Conclusion

It is clear that we cannot yet provide definitive recommendations on the use of associative and dissociative strategies. Most runners use both during their training and frequently shift between the two as environmental and physical conditions warrant.

The efficacy of dissociative strategies seems clear, but better runners appear to profit from careful use of associative strategies. The term "better" may be important, as opposed to "elite," because though Morgan's (1978) work was with elite competitors, that of Orlick, Power, and Partington (1979, 1980a,b) was with very good, rather than elite, runners. These runners, though, still reported using associative strategies during the marathon.

Each runner may need to experiment to choose the particular strategies within each grouping that prove most effective in different training and racing situations. The specific blend of strategies for a training run may differ from that mix most effective in a ten-mile race, and also from the best for the marathon.

## Note

I would like to express my appreciation to Dr. David Pargman, Florida State University, for his guidance and assistance in the work that forms the basis for this chapter. I also thank Dr. Bonnie G. Berger, Brooklyn College, for her comments on an earlier draft of this chapter.

## Appendix: Cognitive Strategies for Runners in the Florida State Study

Association: Concentrate on how your body feels during this part of your run. Analyze your stride, posture, respiration, feeling of your feet, calves, thighs. Be as aware as possible of the sensations of your body at this time.

Dissociation/right-brain activities:
1. Thinking of music (without the words): for example, the music of a song you particularly like, or a classical piece you're familiar with.
2. Painting a picture: paint a picture, perhaps of a landscape, a face, or an action scene.
3. Thinking of faces: think of faces, perhaps of family or friends, focusing on their features, colors, textures.
4. Focusing on colors of the environment: focus on the colors of various features of the environment in which you run, such as the green of the grass and trees, the gray or black of the streets and sidewalks, or the yellow of the line in the middle of the road.
5. Concentrating on a spot in front of you: look at a forty-five-degree angle toward the ground and maintain your attention on an imaginary point. The point will, of course, move as you progress, but your focus will be on the point rather than on specific characteristics of the surface or terrain upon which you're running.

Dissociation/left-brain activities:
1. Problem solving: think of a problem you are currently faced with (for example: a project to be completed at work or school; an argument with a spouse, co-worker, girl friend, or boyfriend; what to do this weekend), and logically attempt to solve the problem. Think of alternative courses of action, and pros and cons of each.
2. Counting: count the number of objects of a particular type that you see, such as trees, cars, mailboxes, people, birds, or your breaths or foot strikes.
3. Issues: pick a controversial issue, such as nuclear power or drinking-age laws, and play the role of a judge, listening to presentations from both sides of the issue. Make a decision based on a rational, logical approach rather than an emotional one.

4. Arithmetic: solve some arithmetic problems, such as division and multiplication.
5. Letter writing: imagine yourself writing a letter to a friend you haven't written in a while. What would you include in the letter, and how would you structure it?

## References

Berger, B. G., and Mackenzie, M. M. 1980. A case study of a woman jogger: A psychodynamic analysis. *Journal of Sport Behavior* 3:3–16.

Bloom, L. J.; Houston, B. K.; Holmes, D. S.; and Burish, T. G. 1977. The effectiveness of attentional diversion and situation redefinition for reducing stress due to a nonambiguous threat. *Journal of Research in Personality* 11:83–94.

Buffone, G. W. 1980. Psychological changes associated with cognitive-behavioral therapy and an aerobic running program in the treatment of depression. Ph.D. diss., Florida State University.

Colt, E. W. D., and Spyropoulos, E. 1979. Running and stress fractures. *British Medical Journal*, no. 6192:706.

David-Neel, A. 1965. *Magic and mystery in Tibet*. New Hyde Park, N.Y.: University Books.

Fixx, J. F. 1977. *The complete book of running*. New York: Random House.

———. 1980. *Jim Fixx's second book of running*. New York: Random House.

Freischlag, J. 1981. Selected psycho-social characteristics of marathoners. *International Journal of Sport Psychology* 12:282–88.

Friedman, P. 1980. Mental preparation and achievement. *New York Running News* (special marathon issue) 24(5):40–41.

Hollandsworth, J. G., Jr. 1979. Some thoughts on distance running as training in biofeedback. *Journal of Sport Behavior* 2:71–82.

Landers, D. M.; Obermeier, G. E.; and Wolf, M. D. 1977. The influence of external stimuli and eye color on reactive motor behavior. In *Psychology of motor behavior and sport—1976*, vol. 2, ed. D. M. Landers and R. W. Christina. Champaign, Ill.: Human Kinetics Publishers.

Lorentzen, D., and Sime, W. E. 1979. Association/dissociation and motivation in marathon runners. Unpublished manuscript, University of Nebraska.

Mahoney, M. J. 1979. Cognitive skills and athletic performance. In *Cognitive-behavioral interventions: Theory, research, and procedures,* ed. P. C. Kendall and S. D. Hollon. New York: Academic Press.

Melzack, R. 1973. *The puzzle of pain*. New York: Basic Books.

Merrill, S. 1981. How to beat the wall. *Runner* 3(4):42–46.

Morgan, W. P. 1978. The mind of the marathoner. *Psychology Today* 11(11):38–40, 43, 45–46, 49.

Morgan, W. P., and Pollock, M. L. 1977. Psychologic characterization of the elite distance runner. *Annals of the New York Academy of Sciences* 301:382–403.

Orlick, T. 1980. *In pursuit of excellence*. Ottawa: Coaching Association of Canada.

Orlick, T.; Power, C.; and Partington, J. 1979. The mind game. Part I. *Canadian Runner,* December, 36–37.

———. 1980a. The mind game. Part II. *Canadian Runner,* January, 20–22.

———. 1980b. The mind game. Part III. *Canadian Runner,* February, 32–35.

Orwin, A. 1973. "The running treatment": A preliminary communication on a new use for an old treatment (physical activity) in the agoraphobic syndrome. *British Journal of Psychiatry* 122:175–79.

Pelletier, D., and Sachs, M. L. 1981. La motivation et la préparation psychologique des marathoniens. Unpublished manuscript, University of Quebec at Trois-Rivières.

Pennebaker, J. W. 1980. Self-perception of emotion and internal sensation. In *The self in social psychology,* ed. D. M. Wegner and R. R. Vallacher. New York: Oxford University Press.

Pennebaker, J. W., and Lightner, J. M. 1980. Competition of internal and external information in an exercise setting. *Journal of Personality and Social Psychology* 39:165–74.

Pennebaker, J. W., and Skelton, J. A. 1978. Psychological parameters of physical symptoms. *Personality and Social Psychology Bulletin* 4:524–30.

Pennebaker, J. W.; Skelton, J. A.; Wogalter, M.; and Rodgers, R. J. 1978. Effects of attention on the experience of physical symptoms. Paper presented at the annual meeting of the American Psychological Association, Toronto.

Sachs, M. L. 1980. On the trail of the runner's high: A descriptive and experimental investigation of characteristics of an elusive phenomenon. Ph.D. diss., Florida State University.

Sacks, M. H.; Milvy, P.; Perry, S. W., III; and Sherman, L. 1981. Mental status and psychological coping during a one hundred-mile race. In *Psychology of running,* ed. M. H. Sacks and M. L. Sachs. Champaign, Ill.: Human Kinetics Publishers.

Sime, W. E. 1980. Cognitive strategies in running. Paper presented at the Third Annual Psychology of Running Seminar, Cornell University Medical College, New York City, 24 October.

U.S. Department of Health and Human Services. 1981. Mushing from Anchorage to Nome: A race against the effects of stress. *Research Resources Reporter* 5(11):8–9.

Wegner, D. M., and Giuliano, T. 1980. Arousal-induced attention to self. *Journal of Personality and Social Psychology* 38:719–26.

Worthy, M. 1974. *Eye color, sex, and race.* Anderson, S. C.: Droke House/Hallux.

Worthy, M., and Markle, A. 1970. Racial differences in reactive versus self-paced sports activities. *Journal of Personality and Social Psychology* 16:439–43.

Zillmann, D. 1978. Attribution and misattribution of excitatory reactions. In *New directions in attribution research,* vol. 2, ed. J. H. Harvey, W. Ickes, and R. F. Kidd. Hillsdale, N.J.: Lawrence Erlbaum Associates.

JOHN M. SILVA AND BARRY B. SHULTZ

# 17

# Research in the Psychology and Therapeutics of Running: A Methodological and Interpretive Review

Historical records show that physical activity has been viewed as a fundamental aspect of total well-being since before 776 B.C. (Robinson 1955). Plato, a student of Socrates, argued strongly in the *Republic* for proper care of the body and the mind. Plato contended that the essence of a person, the soul or spirit, benefits from regular vigorous activity. Robinson (1955) reports that Plato's original name of Aristocles was changed by his teacher Aristo in honor of his physical condition. Plato means "broad-shouldered."

The cathartic effects of vigorous exercise were mentioned as a great benefit by philosophers and scientists from Aristotle to Freud. The belief that direct or vicarious physical activity can, in and of itself, purge one's psychological or emotional problems has generally been discarded by social scientists as unproved, but contemporary research supports physical activity, running in particular, as a psychiatric adjunct and in some instances as a primary intervention strategy. The therapeutic value of running or other exercise is a serious issue in clinical psychology. Any therapy or adjunct prescribed on a large scale to those seeking professional help should withstand the most rigorous and systematic tests. Without such scrutiny the therapist may do a disservice both to the client and to the profession. This chapter will examine representative literature on running as therapy. The effects of running on anxiety and depression will be briefly reviewed and summarized. The final sections will point out various methodological shortcomings of research in the psychotherapeutics of running and offer suggestions for stronger experimental designs. The systematic assessment of running as therapy should be the criterion by which this now popular intervention strategy is determined to be meaningful or a fad.

## Research on the Therapeutic Value of Running

### RUNNING AND ANXIETY

Vigorous physical activity like running has been both indicated and contraindicated as a treatment for anxiety. Research by Pitts and McClure (1967), Fink, Taylor, and Volanka (1969), and Kelly, Mitchell-Heggs, and Sherman (1971) has suggested that vigorous physical activity that creates a lactate accumulation may actually bring on anxiety and irritability. Such an effect is accentuated in anxiety neurosis and was cited by Pitts and McClure as promoting an anxiety attack reaction in neurotic patients. Research countering the Pitts-McClure position was advanced by Grosz and Farmer (1969), who argued that infusing sodium lactate as Pitts and McClure did creates a metabolic alkalosis. Exercise-induced lactic acid buildup, however, induces acidosis. Several studies have used various levels of exercise as the independent variable and measures of anxiety as the dependent variables. In most of this research, walking or running has been the exercise prescription. Research by Morgan, Roberts, and Feinerman (1971) and more recent work by Sime (1977) indicated that state anxiety, as measured by objective paper-and-pencil techniques, was not reduced after mild walking.

State anxiety has also been assessed after more vigorous exercise. Morgan (1973) and Morgan and Horstman (1976) reported significant drops in state anxiety in subjects with both high and low anxiety levels when measurement was taken twenty to thirty minutes after exercise. There were some design problems in these studies that will be addressed later in this chapter. In any case, the question whether running is effective as a therapy or adjunct for anxiety-related problems cannot be answered by research that evaluates only state anxiety at one point after exercise. The enduring effect of the exercise on ongoing anxiety and the source of the anxiety are not addressed in research limited to an observational base of one. There is also the problem of discriminating fatigue from anxiety. Such contamination could certainly be manifested when anxiety is measured by a test such as the Spielberger State-Trait Anxiety Inventory (Spielberger 1966). The state of the literature in the area of anxiety reduction through running or walking is such that as yet no strong position can realistically be taken. Further examination should be directed toward the long-term effects of the exercise, toward ensuring adequate control designs, and toward appropriate measures of both state and trait anxiety.

## RUNNING AND DEPRESSION

Depression is often a complex pathology characterized by feelings of stress, helplessness, and low self-esteem and by the persistence of self-defeating behavior (Anderson 1973). Since depression is often accompanied by some psychomotor incapacitation, it is not surprising that physical activities such as running have been used to try to inspire a sense of accomplishment and self-regulation in mildly and moderately depressed patients. Several studies have been conducted on the relation between running and depression. Blue (1979) provided case-study evidence of the positive effect of running in reducing moderate depression in patients who had previously received ineffective treatments of empathy, cognitive behavior therapy, and antidepressant medication. The antidepressant quality of running has also been demonstrated by Brown, Ramirez, and Taub (1978), who found that running three or five days a week for ten weeks significantly lowered depression scores for both depressed and nondepressed subjects as measured by a checklist. Folkins (1976) also found increases in positive moods and decreases in depression after exercise therapy that included some running.

The relation between running and depression has been evaluated in various studies by John Greist and his colleagues. Greist et al. (1978) randomly assigned moderately depressed subjects to either running treatment ($n = 8$), time-limited psychotherapy ($n = 9$), or time-unlimited psychotherapy ($n = 7$). After twelve weeks of treatment the running group had dramatically reduced depression scores, which compared favorably with those of the time-limited therapy group. The depression scores of the running group and the time-limited therapy group were considerably lower than those of the time-unlimited therapy group after twelve weeks of therapy. Follow-up measurement of depression one, three, six, nine, and twelve months after treatment showed that the running group continued to have low depression scores. The authors conclude that running may be as effective as other therapies because it creates feelings of mastery and improved self-image in individuals who may be experiencing lowered feelings of self-worth and competency. Greist et al. (1979), drawing upon previously published studies, expanded upon the reasons why running may alleviate mild depression. Factors such as self-determination, positive bodily changes and sensations, symptom relief, consciousness alteration, and biochemical changes, including the appearance of norepinephrine and morphinelike endorphins, may be significant in countering depressive states. The authors strongly recommended continued study of running as a therapeutic aid and recognized the need for controlled experimental research in this area.

Most of the literature on depression and running tends to find running very effective in reducing depression. The justifications for this appear reasonable from a clinical standpoint. The literature in this area, however, is not unlike that on anxiety in that few studies have employed sound design strategies or statistical tests of the differences found among treatment groups. It is remarkable and worth noting, however, that virtually all studies have found that regular running coincides with reduced levels of depression. Few published studies have not found this effect. In the rest of this chapter we will address various methodological concerns that have profound implications for the appropriate interpretation of research in the psychotherapeutics of running and will offer examples of how these concerns relate specifically to that research. We hope that future research will incorporate sound design principles and thus provide the clinician with a more definitive and defensible statement on the role of running as an adjunct or primary therapy for anxiety and depression.

## The Efficacy of Running as a Psychiatric Adjunct: Methodological and Interpretive Problems

Certain methodological and interpretive problems may seriously call into question the conclusions of investigations of the efficacy of running as a mode of psychotherapy. In evaluating the literature we will adopt Kerlinger's (1973) general guidelines for sound research, placing special emphasis on threats to internal and external validity, since this is a common failing of the literature. We will note selected problems of experimental design and analysis and suggest improvements. Additionally, we will briefly present the potential for methodological artifacts, which can contaminate experimental findings, and suggest various changes in method. The final section presents future directions that may advance research in the study of running as a psychotherapeutic aid.

### CRITERIA FOR EVALUATING RUNNING RESEARCH

Kerlinger (1973) has developed three criteria for evaluating research, most easily put in the form of questions. First, can the research design unambiguously answer the researcher's question? Second, is the independent variable responsible for the covariation in the dependent variable? And third, to whom and what can the findings of the study be generalized? A good design should eliminate as many competing or plausible rival hypotheses as possible (Campbell 1969a). A single-group before/after design may indicate that a group undergoing running therapy experienced a significant reduction in anxiety, but is running the only plausible explanation? Other factors during the pre/post interval may have lowered anxiety levels, or the attention of the investigators could have accounted for the results. Much of the running literature deals with self-selected subjects and with subjects in need of therapy (e.g., Dodson and Mullens 1969). In such a sample some changes may be expected regardless of the treatment. Campbell (1969b) indicated that psychotherapy can be a cosymptom treatment; that is, the treatment may be a cause, but it is also an effect. Thus these and other plausible hypotheses often render the findings equivocal. The source of many of these problems can be traced to the design. Kerlinger's (1973) second and third criteria deal essentially with concerns for internal and external validity. Because of the importance of these factors we will discuss these criteria at some length.

*Internal Validity*

Several authors have compiled inventories on threats to experimental validity. The most prevalent threats to the internal and external validity of research on running as a mode of therapy will be highlighted. Internal validity is concerned with whether the experimental treatment made a difference in this specific instance. Threats to internal validity that are particularly relevant to the running literature include history, instability, testing, regression artifacts, selection, and selection-maturation interaction (Campbell 1969b; Stanley 1973). As we noted previously much of the running literature utilizes simple before/after designs and thus history—events other than the treatment occurring during the pre/post interval—becomes a possible rival explanation. Some studies have allowed participants to elect to run either three or five times a week. A lack of control is built into such a study and can invalidate findings. Because of the prevalence of pre/post designs, initial testing may alert subjects to the purpose of the study, and this sensitizing may interact with the treatment and produce larger effects than shown by a group that was not pretested.

Regression artifacts are pseudoshifts toward the mean. Since patients who need help are often selected for running therapy, they are usually outside the limits that define normal scores on anxiety or depression scales. Some movement toward the mean (norm) would be expected on retesting, being more likely the greater the extremity of the scores. Selection and selection/maturation interaction can also create interpretive problems that obscure treatment effects. Selecting comparison groups that differ on pretest measures (e.g., Folkins, Lynch, and Gardner 1972) can bias results and create problems for the investigators. A selection bias also implies differential rates of maturation or change. It is possible that running may reduce depression but that the rate of change may be greater on self-selected depressed participants than on randomly selected participants. The rate of change may actually be totally unrelated to the treatment. When the research design is a simple two-group comparison, the study might generate an inappropriate conclusion.

## External Validity

Campbell and Stanley (1966) state that external validity is concerned with the populations, settings, and variables to which these specific findings can be generalized. Bracht and Glass (1968) subdivided external validity into population validity and ecological validity. Population validity is concerned with the two inferential leaps, first from the sample to the accessible population, and second from the accessible population to a target population. Advocates of running as an important therapy for reducing anxiety and depression would probably have a very large target population—most anxious or depressed people. However, much experimentation has involved volunteer subjects and patients identified as having problems.

Ecological validity, on the other hand, deals with the setting of the research and the nature of the variables under investigation. Bracht and Glass (1968) and Campbell (1969b) developed inventories for threats to external validity, which can include variable representativeness, testing effects, interaction of selection and treatment, reactive effects of experimental arrangement, experimenter effect, and multiple-treatment interference. Kerlinger (1973) referred to variable representativeness in terms of the consistency or constancy of the effect. Would a running therapy program found effective in one study work the same way in another study? This is a question of replication of treatments across studies (Campbell 1969b; Sidman 1960).

Variable representativeness also refers to the nature of the independent and dependent variables. Is running the independent variable (the therapy being manipulated), and is it explicitly defined? Or would any vigorous activity, competitive or noncompetitive, produce a similar reduction in anxiety and depression? Similar concerns exist for the dependent variable. Is a researcher investigating the same kind of anxiety with the State Trait Anxiety Inventory (STAI) as with several other measures that have anxiety components, such as the Profile of Mood States (POMS), the Eight State Questionnaire (8 SQ), and the Institute of Personality and Ability Testing (IPAT) Anxiety Scale? Similar questions may be asked about the use of behavioral assessment and clinical observations of patient behavior. These are all questions of ecological validity, and unfortunately they are seldom attended to. As Lana (1969) noted, pretesting can sensitize participants to treatment effects. Would the treatment effects of running therapy be as effective in reducing depression if subjects were not made aware that they were depressed and that running might be useful in lowering their depression levels? How generalizable are the findings in the running therapy literature to people who are not tested before treatment? The concerns created by the interaction of selection and the experimental treatment have been highlighted previously. Essentially, this is a question of whether people within "normal" limits on anxiety and depression scales would show similar reductions after running or whether positive findings are generalizable only to the maladjusted.

Another threat to external validity is the experimenter effect. Experimenter effects can also bias internal validity, and they will be dealt with in more detail later. Finally, multiple-treatment interference can confound research findings when each subject receives several treatments. This is a problem when running is used as an adjunct. Having already experienced one treatment, will participants respond to a second treatment as if the first had never occurred? Results in such research would be generalizable only to similar settings—that is, to other multiple-treatment programs.

The importance of ensuring internal and external validity cannot be overemphasized. Such rigorousness is essential in assessing any technique that purports to influence psychological states or ameliorate mental health problems.

EXPERIMENTAL DESIGNS: PROBLEMS OF CONTROL

Anecdotal reports, case studies, and correlational studies permeate the running literature. This section, however, will be primarily concerned with the conclusions drawn from experiments. Stanley (1973) has listed four basic kinds of experiments: controlled, quasi-experimental, natural, and pseudoexperimental. Most of the running literature can be classified as either controlled experimental or quasi-experimental in design. There are relatively few threats to internal and external validity in controlled experiments; hence such designs are the goal of most researchers. Most research in the behavioral sciences, however, is based on quasi-experimental designs. Not all situations lend themselves to controlled experiments, and quasi-experimental designs are often advocated (Campbell 1963, 1969b; Campbell and Stanley 1966).

Controlled experimental designs emphasize experimenter control of sources of bias and experimental contamination. Boring (1969) traced the history of the concept of control in research and pointed out that the term "control" has at least four separate meanings. It can refer to constancy of conditions, a means of calibration, a comparison group, or a way to shape behavior. The running research in general has evidenced a lack of control, especially with respect to establishing constancy of conditions and employing proper and sufficient control groups. The experimenter gains control by preventing extraneous variables from unduly influencing the dependent variable. Systematic protocols and randomization generally ensure that variation in the dependent variable was caused by variation in the independent variable. Much of the current literature fails in both these categories.

The most fundamental controlled experimental design would be the experimental group/control group (randomized subjects) design (Kerlinger 1973). An accessible population would be identified, preferably one in which systematic exercising was not prevalent, and subjects would be randomly selected. The subjects would then be randomly assigned to either an experimental or a control group. Ideally, the number of subjects would have been determined by a power analysis (Cohen 1969). A running program protocol would be followed for a predetermined period, and then both groups would be measured to determine if there were differential levels of anxiety or depression between them.

This basic design is most often violated in the way subjects are selected. Most studies use samples of convenience and volunteers. The resultant quasi-experimental design is permissible but requires caution. Campbell (1969a) has pointed out the need for new control groups in behavioral research. He especially advocates using expanded-content control groups, of which the sham-operation and placebo control groups are special cases. Studies that use running as an adjunct to medication especially need placebo control groups. Studies in which knowledge of the hypothesis might bias results need demand-character control groups. Additionally, many research reports can barely conceal the investigator's position about the benefits of running. To guard against experimenter bias, expectancy control groups seem most appropriate. Other control procedures and control group designs have been suggested by several authors, including Morgan (1972), whose work is relevant to sport psychology.

A design common in the literature is the nonequivalent control group design (Campbell and Stanley 1966). Unlike a true experimental design where subjects are randomly assigned from a common population, subjects from naturally assembled collectives (e.g., classrooms, therapy groups) become the experimental and control groups. Randomly assigning the groups to either treatment or control can mitigate threats to internal and external validity. Both groups are pretested, one receives the treatment, such as a running program, and both are measured by a post-test.

As noted earlier, threats to internal validity come from intrasession history, interaction of selection and maturation, and possibly regression. Since most of these studies involve self-selected subjects from nonequivalent groups, there may be differences on the pretest that would confound the treatment effects. Even when no differences exist on the pretest, one group may change faster (maturation), thus producing pseudodifferences. It is also possible that regression may occur if one group was selected for its extremity on the variable of interest and the other was a "normal" group. Spontaneous remission in the experimental group could be expected on retesting regardless of treatment (Campbell and Stanley 1966).

Pretesting is generally used to ensure the equality of groups. However, additional experimental control procedures may be used, and artifacts may be caused by the pretesting. The pretest may differentially sensitize the groups, causing a more reactive situation between the pretest and the treatment. Some studies have used talks about the positive benefits of running as part of the pretreatment protocol. Pretesting for anxiety or depression may be more easily linked to the "hoped for" positive benefits of running. Researchers can guard against this presensitization by using the Solomon four-group design to test for treatment effects as well as a pretest/treatment interaction. The Solomon design can be represented as follows:

$$
\begin{array}{cccc}
 & Y_b & X & Y_a & \text{(Experimental)} \\
R & Y_b & \bar{X} & Y_a & \text{(Control 1)} \\
 & & X & Y_a & \text{(Control 2)} \\
 & & \bar{X} & Y_a & \text{(Control 3)}
\end{array}
$$

$R$ indicates that the subjects have been randomly assigned to groups. $Y_a$ is a measure of the dependent variable *after* treatment. $Y_b$ is the pretest on the dependent variable *before* treatment. The independent or experimental variable is $X$, with the symbol $\bar{X}$, indicating that this variable has not been manipulated.

Many investigators inappropriately try matching to control for potential pretreatment differences. Matching may be a useful adjunct if randomization was used and the matching variables correlated at least .50 with the dependent variable (Kerlinger 1973). However, in the absence of randomization, matching controls only for the variables that are matched and those that correlate highly with them. This still leaves many other variables to confound the results. Additionally, matching results in correlated groups and hence in nonorthogonal partitioning of variance estimates. The Solomon four-group design is perhaps one of the best designs available to test the true effect of running upon psychological well-being.

One major problem in data analysis is selecting the wrong test of statistical significance. The experimental design should suggest the appropriate procedure for treating the data. The most common mistake is to use univariate statistics where multivariate procedures are required. Brown, Ramirez, and Taub (1978) for example, measured six scales from an adjective checklist, on two groups (normal and depressed), before and after jogging for ten weeks. Apparently, the twenty-four possible comparisons were made with individual t-tests. Some of the sixteen significant findings are obviously spurious results due to an inflated type I error. A type I error refers to the probability of falsely rejecting a true null hypothesis.

The diversity of sample sizes in the various cells is another common problem in statistical analysis. Disproportionate cell sizes cause nonorthogonal partitioning of variance sources and thus inappropriate variance estimates. To prevent such a situation, regression analysis should be used. Such a procedure orthogonalizes the data and allows for the appropriate partitioning of variance estimates. Unequal cell sizes occur frequently in the running literature, since treatment groups in clinical settings are often not equal or proportional in number.

Another analysis problem beginning to appear because of an increase in factorial designs is referred to as a type IV error. A type IV error is made "whenever a researcher offers an incorrect interpretation to a correctly rejected statistical hypothesis" (Levin and Marascuilo 1972, 368). Marascuilo and Levin (1970) have likened a type IV error to a physician's correctly diagnosing an ailment but prescribing the wrong medicine. The misinterpretation resulting from a type IV error is only a symptom, and it is important to understand the etiology of this statistical disease.

Type IV errors most commonly occur from a lack of consistency between the interaction contrasts and the omnibus interaction test. This inconsistency may be due to a failure to maintain the familywise type I error rate relative to the interaction test or to a failure to select an appropriate mathematical model to answer the researchers' questions (Marascuilo and Levin 1976). A type IV error is evidenced in a study conducted by Heaps (1978), who explored the effect of type of feedback (physical or social) on fitness levels and the effect of level of feedback (high or low) on selected self-attitudes, including one anxiety measure. The author did not report information concerning the interaction test but did state that the physical standards had a greater impact, thus implying a differential effect. The author reports a hypothesis error rate of .01. Thus any interaction post hoc tests must have an error rate equal to .01 to be logically consistent. Marascuilo and Levin (1970) recommend the Scheffé, but a Bonferroni $t$ on the six pairs of means with an error rate of .0016 would be logically consistent. The second problem for Heaps (1978) concerns whether he was interested in the interaction model, the simple effects model, or the cell means model. Since this appears to be an exploratory study, the most versatile ANOVA model, or the cell means analysis, is recommended (Marascuilo and Levin 1976).

The researcher must attend to common pitfalls that can lead to misinterpretation of research findings. The complexity of some of these analysis problems justifies adding a data analyst to the research team.

## METHODOLOGICAL ARTIFACTS IN BEHAVIORAL RESEARCH

Psychological research is merely a special case of social interaction in which people can be a source of error or bias that may contaminate the findings and invalidate the investigator's conclusions (Argyris 1968; Orne 1962). A number of authors have delineated potential sources of bias in behavioral research (Barber 1976; Rosenthal 1976; Rosenthal and Rosnow 1969a), but only those particularly relevant to the literature concerning running as therapy will be covered here. Social psychological sources of bias will be subdivided into experimenter effects, subject effects, and experimenter/subject interaction effects.

### Experimenter Effects

Rosenthal (1969) clarified a variety of personal and situational variables that are potential artifacts in behavioral research and thus require control. Three sources of experimenter contamination include experimenter bias, experimenter expectancy, and personal characteristics of the experimenter.

Experimenter bias can occur from differential treatment of the experimental and control groups that might favor one group. Double-blind techniques, tape-recorded instructions, and other standardized procedures can eliminate these problems (Singer 1973). Experimenter expectancy, or the Rosenthal effect (Barber 1973), is another form of experimenter bias in which the investigator's desires or expectations influence the dependent variable. Since many investigators are strong advocates of the benefits (or detriments) of running therapy, experimenter expectancy effects are strong possibilities. Expectancy control groups can guard against invalid inferences in cases where expectancy effects are suspected.

Personal characteristics of the experimenter can also influence the outcome of experiments. Factors such as sex (Rumenik, Capasso, and Hendrick 1977), attitude, warmth, personality, and status (Rosenthal 1976) can bias results. Differential interpersonal relations between therapists and patients, the status of medical personnel, and the cross-sex effect are likely candidates for bias in the running literature. Including these factors in the design (both male and female therapists), or using double-blind procedures, can control for these confounding influences.

### Subject Effects

Psychosocial characteristics of the subjects, subjects' attitudes toward research, and the Hawthorne effect are all possible subject artifacts. Most studies concerned with running as therapy use self-selected or nonrandom volunteer populations. This selection process may bring into question the external validity of some research findings. The important question is whether there may be any psychosocial characteristics that distinguish the subject population from a representative population and, if so, what influence they may have upon the dependent variable (Rosenthal and Rosnow 1969b; Williams 1973).

The attitudes or roles that subjects adopt can be a problem. Weber and Cook (1972) have identified four subject roles: good subject role, negativistic role, faithful subject role, and evaluation apprehension role. The apprehensive role has been shown by Rosenberg (1969) to be a threat capable of confounding research findings. The good role and negativistic role also exist, but they are confounded with subject anxiety (evaluation apprehension), according to Weber and Cook (1972). Subject roles are less likely to be a problem with field settings and naive populations (noncollege), but even children and noncollege adults may quickly learn roles. Thus it is important in running research either to not promote the development of a subject attitude toward the treatment conditions or to encourage a similar attitude toward all experimental conditions.

The Hawthorne effect occurs because subjects know they are in an experiment or because the experimental setting changes their environment. Both may affect their condition. Often it is the artificiality of the setting that produces changes in the subjects' behavior. This can threaten external validity unless proper designs are utilized. Field research can alleviate some of the problems of artificiality, and the Solomon four-group design can control for various threats including the Hawthorne effect. Since running may have considerable novelty for many psychotherapy patients, the Hawthorne effect should not be dismissed.

### Subject/Experimenter Interaction

The final behavioral artifact consists of the demand characteristics of the research setting. Orne (1962, 779) defined this as the "totality of cues which convey an experimental hypothesis to the subject." Demand characteristics can come from the experimental procedure or from experimenter expectancy. They can activate subject roles, and thus they threaten external validity. Orne (1969) suggested that quasi-controls be used to guard against the influence of demand characteristics. Some of these controls include postexperimental inquiry, the nonexperiment, and simulators. In the running literature many therapists have commented on their own commitment to running and expressed their strong belief in running as an effective treatment modality. When the therapist takes a positive position toward one therapy and not toward another, a demand characteristic is apt to develop in the patient, a subjective belief that if running is supposed to work it will work. The true effect of the exercise becomes confounded in such a situation. With proper planning and control this artifact, and most of the artifacts outlined in this section, can be effectively controlled or eliminated.

FUTURE DIRECTIONS FOR RUNNING THERAPY RESEARCH

In this section I shall suggest directions for research in running as a psychiatric adjunct or therapy. In part these suggestions are based on the perceived shortcomings of current approaches and represent an attempt to suggest potential research trends.

The literature on running therapy is becoming voluminous, but it must be characterized as an accumulation of isolated facts. Many behavioral scientists (Bock 1975; Dotson 1980) have recognized similar situations in related disciplines and have called for models to represent the phenomena in question. Bock (1975) has called for scientific inferences from the hypothetico-deductive paradigm. Essentially, this paradigm posits that a model is developed, observable consequences are deduced, and data are collected to determine "goodness-of-fit." Models are created not to explain data already collected, but rather to explain the adequacy of a priori predictions. Knowledge is most rapidly gained with the hypothetico-deductive paradigm when strong inferences are used to exclude competing hypotheses (Platt 1964). Dotson (1980) supports this position but also calls for greater complexity in research problems, reflecting on competing models and improving the soundness of statistical inference. Research of this type can be characterized as having "high logical density."

Running therapy is a complex phenomenon, and the interactive aspects of its influence, the exceptions, and the paradoxes require complex models and research designs. Many investigators are currently looking at physiological, biochemical, and psychological influences of running. Models built around these systems will require more complex analyses. Specifically, multivariate analyses are needed where there are two or more dependent variables. According to Harris (1975), any experimental manipulation that affects many different but partially related aspects of behavior is potentially suitable for multivariate procedures. Multivariate procedures can descriptively analyze patterns, determine optimal combinations of variables, or inferentially determine which of a set of multiple comparisons are significantly different. This inferential task is performed simultaneously on all variables, as opposed to cases where multiple $t$'s are used. Such an approach controls the type I error rate that I noted is frequently overlooked in running research. The suggestion is that investigators become more aware of multivariate techniques, so that both past statistical errors and new complex models can be appropriately analyzed.

Another trend that seems evident in the literature is an increased interest in running therapy by clinical psychologists and psychiatrists. Rather than relying on descriptive case studies (e.g., Blue 1979), single-case experimental designs are favored for investigating intervention programs on individual clients (Kazdin 1978). Within-subject designs are fairly flexible for investigating diverse outcomes or clinical problems that are not prevalent, as pilot studies for group research, and as an evaluative tool for psychotherapy (Gottman 1973; Kazdin 1978). One problem of single-case studies is often the method of analysis. Generally, visual analysis of graphs has been used. This is a rather subjective method except for extreme effect cases. One procedure recommended for both single-case and group research is time-series analysis (Gottman 1973). These designs are especially useful for data taken over a long period. Time-series designs can also serve as controls for threats to internal validity of quasi-experimental designs, such as the nonequivalent control group design discussed earlier. Specific designs and issues may be found in Glass (1977), Jones, Vaught, and Weinrott (1977), and Simonton (1977). Specific designs and the advantages and disadvantages of single-case experiments are beyond the scope of this section. Those who are interested can find valuable information in the writings of Craig and Metze (1979), Kazdin (1973), and Leitenberg (1973).

## References

Anderson, C. M. 1973. Assumption centered psychotherapy. In *Direct psychotherapy*, vol. 1, ed. R. M. Jurjevich. Coral Gables, Fla.: University of Miami Press.

Argyris, C. 1968. Some unintended consequences of rigorous research. *Psychological Bulletin* 70:185–97.

Barber, T. X. 1973. Pitfalls in research: Nine investigator and experimenter effects. In *Second handbook of research on teaching*, ed. R. M. W. Travers. Chicago: Rand McNally.

————. 1976. Pitfalls in human research: Ten pivotal points. New York: Pergamon Press.

Blue, F. R. 1979. Aerobic running as a treatment for moderate depression. *Perceptual and Motor Skills* 48:228.

Bock, R. D. 1975. Multivariate statistical methods in behavioral research. New York: McGraw-Hill.

Boring, E. G. 1969. Perspective: Artifact and control. In *Artifact in behavioral research*, ed. R. Rosenthal and R. L. Rosnow. New York: Academic Press.

Bracht, G. H., and Glass, G. V. 1968. The external validity of experiments. *American Educational Research Journal* 5:437–74.

Brown, R. S.; Ramirez, D. E.; and Taub, J. M. 1978. The prescription of exercise for depression. *Physician and Sportsmedicine* 6 (12):35–45.

Campbell, D. T. 1963. From description to experimentation: Interpreting trends as quasi-experiments. In *Problems in measuring change*, ed. C. W. Harris. Madison: University of Wisconsin Press.

————. 1969a. Prospective: Artifact and control. In *Artifact in behavioral research*, ed. R. Rosenthal and R. L. Rosnow. New York: Academic Press.

————. 1969b. Reforms as experiments. *American Psychologist* 24:409–29.

Campbell, D. T., and Stanley, J. C. 1966. *Experimental and quasi-experimental designs for research*. Chicago: Rand McNally.

Cohen, J. 1969. *Statistical power analysis for the behavioral sciences*. New York: Academic Press.

Craig, J. R., and Metze, L. P. 1979. *Methods of psychological research*. Philadelphia: W. B. Saunders.

Dodson, L. C., and Mullens, W. R. 1969. Some effects of jogging on psychiatric hospital patients. *American Corrective Therapy Journal* 23:130–34.

Dotson, C. O. 1980. Logic of questionable density. *Research Quarterly for Exercise and Sport* 51:23–36.

Fink, M.; Taylor, M. A.; and Volanka, J. 1969. Anxiety precipitated by lactate. *New England Journal of Medicine* 281:1429.

Folkins, C. H. 1976. Effects of physical training on mood. *Journal of Clinical Psychology* 32:385–88.

Folkins, C. H.; Lynch, S.; and Gardner, M. M. 1972. Psychological fitness as a function of physical fitness. *Archives of Physical Medicine and Rehabilitation* 53:503–8.

Glass, G. 1977. Topics in time-series experimentation. In *Proceedings of the Colorado Measurement Symposium,* ed. D. Mood. Boulder: University of Colorado.

Gottman, J. M. 1973. N-of-one and n-of-two research in psychotherapy. *Psychological Bulletin* 80:93–105.

Greist, J. H.; Klein, M. H.; Eischens, R. R.; and Faris, J. W. 1978. Running out of depression. *Physician and Sportsmedicine* 6 (12):49–56.

Greist, J. H.; Klein, M. H.; Eischens, R. R.; Faris, J.; Gurman, A. S.; and Morgan, W. P. 1979. Running as treatment for depression. *Comprehensive Psychiatry* 20:41–54.

Grosz, H. J., and Farmer, B. B. 1969. Blood lactate in the development of anxiety symptoms. *Archives of General Psychiatry* 21:611–19.

Harris, R. J. 1975. *A primer of multivariate statistics.* New York: Academic Press.

Heaps, R. A. 1978. Relating physical and psychological fitness: A psychological point of view. *Journal of Sports Medicine* 18:399–408.

Jones, R. R.; Vaught, R. S.; and Weinrott, M. 1977. Time-series analysis in operant research. *Journal of Applied Behavior Analysis* 10:151–66.

Kazdin, A. E. 1973. Methodological and assessment considerations in evaluating reinforcement programs in applied settings. *Journal of Applied Behavior Analysis* 6:517–31.

———. 1978. Methodological and interpretive problems of single-case experimental designs. *Journal of Consulting and Clinical Psychology* 46:629–42.

Kelly, D.; Mitchell-Heggs, N.; and Sherman, D. 1971. Anxiety and the effects of sodium lactate assessed clinically and psychologically. *British Journal of Psychiatry* 111:129–41.

Kerlinger, F. N. 1973. *Foundations of behavioral research.* 2d ed. New York: Holt, Rinehart and Winston.

Lana, R. E. 1969. Pretest sensitization. In *Artifact in behavioral research,* ed. R. Rosenthal and R. L. Rosnow. New York: Academic Press.

Leitenberg, H. 1973. The use of single-case methodology in psychotherapy research. *Journal of Abnormal Psychology* 82:87–101.

Levin, J. R., and Marascuilo, L. A. 1972. Type IV errors and interactions. *Psychological Bulletin* 78:368–74.

Marascuilo, L. A., and Levin, J. R. 1970. Appropriate post hoc comparisons for interaction and nested hypotheses in analysis of variance designs: The elimination of type IV errors. *American Educational Research Journal* 7:397–421.

———. 1976. The simultaneous investigation of interaction and nested hypotheses in two factor analysis of variance designs. *American Educational Research Journal* 13:61–65.

Morgan, W. P. 1972. Basic considerations. In *Ergogenic aids and muscular performance,* ed. W. P. Morgan. New York: Academic Press.

———. 1973. Influence of acute physical activity on state anxiety. *Proceedings of the National College of Physical Education Meeting,* 113–21.

Morgan, W. P., and Horstman, D. H. 1976. Anxiety reduction following acute physical activity. *Medicine and Science in Sports* 8:62.

Morgan, W. P.; Roberts, J. A.; and Feinerman, A. D. 1971. Psychologic effect of acute physical activity. *Archives of Physical Medicine and Rehabilitation* 52:422–25.

Orne, M. T. 1962. On the social psychology of the psychological experiment: With particular reference to demand characteristics and their implications. *American Psychologist* 17:776–83.

————. 1969. Demand characteristics and the concept of quasi-controls. In *Artifacts in behavioral research,* ed. R. Rosenthal and R. L. Rosnow. New York: Academic Press.

Pitts, F. N., and McClure, J. N. 1967. Lactate metabolism in anxiety neurosis. *New England Journal of Medicine* 277:1329–36.

Platt, J. R. 1964. Strong inference. *Science* 146:347–53.

Robinson, R. S. 1955. *Sources for the history of Greek athletics.* Cincinnati, Ohio: Privately published.

Rosenberg, M. J. 1969. The conditions and consequences of evaluation apprehension. In *Artifacts in behavioral research,* ed. R. Rosenthal and R. L. Rosnow. New York: Academic Press.

Rosenthal, R. 1969. Interpersonal expectations: Effects of the experimenter's hypothesis. In *Artifacts in behavioral research,* ed. R. Rosenthal and R. L. Rosnow. New York: Academic Press.

————. 1976. *Experimenter effects in behavioral research.* Enlarged ed. New York: Irvington.

Rosenthal, R., and Rosnow, R. L., eds. 1969a. *Artifacts in behavioral research.* New York: Academic Press.

————. 1969b. The volunteer subject. In *Artifacts in behavioral research,* ed. R. Rosenthal and R. L. Rosnow. New York: Academic Press.

Rumenik, D. K.; Capasso, D. R.; and Hendrick, C. 1977. Experimenter sex effects in behavioral research. *Psychological Bulletin* 84:852–77.

Sidman, M. 1960. *Tactics of scientific research.* New York: Basic Books.

Sime, W. E. 1977. A comparison of exercise and meditation in reducing physiological response to stress. *Medicine and Science in Sports* 9:55.

Simonton, D. K. 1977. Cross-sectional time-series experiments: Some suggested statistical analyses. *Psychological Bulletin* 84:489–502.

Singer, R. N. 1973. Methodological controls for social psychological problems in experimentation. *Quest* 20:32–38.

Spielberger, C. D. 1966. *Anxiety and behavior.* New York: Academic Press.

Stanley, J. C. 1973. Designing psychological experiments. In *Handbook of general psychology,* ed. B. B. Wolman. Englewood Cliffs, N.J.: Prentice-Hall.

Weber, S. J., and Cook, T. D. 1972. Subject effects in laboratory research: An examination of subject roles, demand characteristics, and valid inference. *Psychological Bulletin* 77:273–95.

Williams, H. G. 1973. Volunteerism, the beneficent subject and ecological validity. *Quest* 20:26–31.

# Part 3

---

# Running Therapy & Psychology
# A Selected Bibliography

A bibliography on psychological considerations in exercise, including exercise as psychotherapy, exercise dependence (addiction), and the psychology of running, has been in existence for seven years. A number of students were working on the psychology of running under the guidance of Dr. David Pargman at Florida State University, and the bibliography began with fewer than one hundred references derived from the reference list of the 1976 master's thesis of Sharon Burgess entitled "Stimulus-Seeking, Extraversion, and Neuroticism in Regular, Occasional, and Non-exercisers." The listing slowly grew under the "editorship" of Michael Sachs, and continued to increase as Gary Buffone also began working on it. Growth of the list has been exponential in the past few years, and the bibliography attained more than eleven hundred references by summer 1983.

The Sachs and Buffone bibliography is too long for publication here, but this volume includes a selected listing of more than one hundred references that appear to be of the highest quality or greatest interest and that are representative of different areas in running therapy and psychology. The works listed are published, including a number of valuable review articles and books, and should be readily available in a local or university library or through interlibrary loan.

We have not included unpublished papers (which are sometimes difficult to obtain), doctoral dissertations or master's theses (which are valuable for beginning research but frequently difficult and expensive to get), or articles from the popular running magazines such as *Runner's World* and *The Runner*.

These popular articles can be readily found by examining back issues of the magazines and are frequently useful to those interested in an introduction to an area, for anecdotal material on a given topic, or in identifying researchers on a particular subject (the author has usually tracked down a few "experts" in the area, talked with them, and quoted them in the article).

However, a number of these unpublished papers, doctoral dissertations and master's theses, and popular articles *will* be found in the reference lists for the chapters in this volume. The selected bibliography provides a good listing of reading in running therapy and psychology, in addition to the chapters in this book. The articles listed here and the reference lists to particular chapters will lead to other articles, so that a comprehensive literature review for a number of areas in the psychology and therapy of running can easily be achieved. Those interested in keeping abreast of literature in the areas presented in this book should regularly avail themselves of a number of valuable resources in their libraries, particularly *Current Contents* and *Dissertation Abstracts International*. Check with your local or university library for various indexes in psychology and the sport sciences as well.

Regular listings of recently published material may also be found through the organization called Running Psychologists (RP). Michael Sachs and Gary Buffone are currently official bibliographers for RP, which was founded at the 1978 American Psychological Association (APA) convention in New York and has grown steadily since that time. Running Psychologists serves the interests of its members through a regular newsletter (*The Running Psychologist*), activities at the annual APA national convention (get-togethers, fun runs, a race), and similar functions at some regional APA conventions, and constitutes a rallying point for individuals with similar interests. For more information write to:

Eugene E. Levitt, Ph.D
Director, Section of Psychology
Department of Psychiatry
Indiana University School of Medicine
Indianapolis, Indiana 46202

Information concerning the complete Sachs and Buffone bibliography on psychological considerations in exercise may be obtained from Michael Sachs at the following address:

Dr. Michael L. Sachs
Post Office Box 213
Reisterstown, Maryland 21136-0213

Altshul, V. A. 1978. The ego-integrative (and disintegrative) effects of long-distance running. *Current Concepts in Psychiatry* 4(4):6–11.

————. 1981. Should we advise our depressed patients to run? In *Psychology of running,* ed. M. H. Sacks and M. L. Sachs. In *Psychology of running,* Champaign, Ill.: Human Kinetics Publishers.

Aristides. 1979. Running and other vices. *American Scholar* 48(2):155–63.

Bahrke, M. S., and Morgan, W. P. 1978. Anxiety reduction following exercise and meditation. *Cognitive Therapy and Research* 2:323–33.

Barnes, L. 1980. Running therapy: Organized and moving. *Physician and Sportsmedicine* 8(6):97–100.

Bennett, J.; Carmack, M. A.; and Gardner, V. J. 1982. The effect of a program of physical exercise on depression in older adults. *Physical Educator* 39(1):21–24.

Berger, B. G., and Mackenzie, M. M. 1980. A case study of a woman jogger: A psychodynamic analysis. *Journal of Sport Behavior* 3:3–16.

Blue, F. R. 1979. Aerobic running as a treatment for moderate depression. *Perceptual and Motor Skills* 48:228.

Blumenthal, J. A.; Williams, R. S.; Williams, R. B., Jr.; and Wallace, A. G. 1980. Effects of exercise on the type A (coronary prone) behavior pattern. *Psychosomatic Medicine* 42:289–96.

Bolton, B., and Renfrow, N. E. 1979. Personality characteristics associated with aerobic exercise in adult females. *Journal of Personality Assessment* 43:504–8.

Borreson, P. M. 1980. The elimination of a self-injurious avoidance response through a forced running consequence. *Mental Retardation* 18(2):73–77.

Briggs, C. A.; Sandstrom, E. R.; and Nettleton, B. 1979. An approach to prediction of performance using behavioral and physiological variables. *Perceptual and Motor Skills* 49:843–48.

Browman, C. P. 1981. Physical activity as a therapy for psychopathology: A reappraisal. *Journal of Sports Medicine and Physical Fitness* 21:192–97.

Brown, J. C. 1979. *The therapeutic mile.* Irmo, S.C.: Human Growth and Development Books.

Brown, R. S.; Ramirez, D. E.; and Taub, J. M. 1978. The prescription of exercise for depression. *Physician and Sportsmedicine* 6(12):34–37, 40–41, 44–45.

Brownell, K. D.; Stunkard, A. J.; and Albaum, J. M. 1980. Evaluation and modification of exercise patterns in the natural environment. *American Journal of Psychiatry* 137:1540–45.

Buffone, G. W. 1980. Exercise as therapy: A closer look. *Journal of Counseling and Psychotherapy* 3(2):101–15.

Carmack, M. A., and Martens, R. 1979. Measuring commitment to running: A survey of runners' attitudes and mental states. *Journal of Sport Psychology* 1:25–42.

Colt, E. W. D.; Dunner, D. L.; Hall, K.; and Fieve, R. R. 1981. A high prevalence of affective disorder in runners. In *Psychology of running,* ed. M. H. Sacks and M. L. Sachs. Champaign, Ill.: Human Kinetics Publishers.

Cooper, A. M. 1981. Masochism and long distance running. In *Psychology of running*, ed. M. H. Sacks and M. L. Sachs. Champaign, Ill.: Human Kinetics Publishers.

Crocitto, J. A. 1982. Jogging: A holistic integrative experience. *Journal of Humanistic Education and Development* 21(2):58–64.

Curtis, J., and McTeer, W. 1981. Toward a sociology of marathoning. *Journal of Sport Behavior* 4(2):67–81.

DeFries, Z. 1981. "Running madness": A prelude to real madness. In *Psychology of running*, ed. M. H. Sacks and M. L. Sachs. Champaign, Ill.: Human Kinetics Publishers.

DeVries, H. A. 1981. Tranquilizer effect of exercise: A critical review. *Physician and Sportsmedicine* 9(11):48–49, 52–53, 55.

Dienstbier, R. A.; Crabbe, J.; Johnson, G. O.; Thorland, W.; Jorgensen, J. A.; Sadar, M. M.; and LaVelle, D. C. 1981. Exercise and stress tolerance. In *Psychology of running*, ed. M. H. Sacks and M. L. Sachs. Champaign, Ill.: Human Kinetics Publishers.

Dishman, R. K., and Gettman, L. R. 1980. Psychobiologic influences on exercise adherence. *Journal of Sport Psychology* 2:295–310.

Dishman, R. K.; Ickes, W.; and Morgan, W. P. 1980. Self-motivation and adherence to habitual physical activity. *Journal of Applied Social Psychology* 10:115–32.

Driscoll, R. 1976. Anxiety reduction using physical exertion and positive images. *Psychological Record* 26:87–94.

Egger, G. 1979. *Running high*. Melbourne: Sun Books.

Ewing, J. H.; Gillis, C. A.; Scott, D. G.; and Patzig, W. J. 1982. Fantasy processes and mild physical activity. *Perceptual and Motor Skills* 54:363–68.

Folkins, C. H., and Sime, W. E. 1981. Physical fitness training and mental health. *American Psychologist* 36(4):373–89.

Folkins, C. H., and Wieselberg-Bell, N. 1981. A personality profile of ultramarathon runners: A little deviance may go a long way. *Journal of Sport Behavior* 4(3):119–27.

Freischlag, J. 1981. Selected psycho-social characteristics of marathoners. *International Journal of Sport Psychology* 12:282–88.

Gary, V., and Guthrie, D. 1972. The effect of jogging on physical fitness and self-concept in hospitalized alcoholics. *Quarterly Journal of Studies on Alcohol* 33:1073–78.

Glasser, W. 1976. *Positive addiction*. New York: Harper and Row.

Graham, W. F. 1979. The anxiety of the runner: Terminal helplessness. *Christian Century*, 29 August–5 September, 821–23.

Greist, J. H.; Eischens, R. R.; and McInvaille, T. 1978. *Run to reality*. Madison, Wisc.: Madison Running Press.

Greist, J. H.; Klein, M. H.; Eischens, R. R.; Faris, J.; Gurman, A. S.; and Morgan, W. P. 1978. Running through your mind. *Journal of Psychosomatic Research* 22:259–94.

Hailey, B. J., and Bailey, L. A. 1982. Negative addiction in runners: A quantitative approach. *Journal of Sport Behavior* 5:150–54.

Harper, F. D. 1979. *Jogotherapy: Jogging as a therapeutic strategy*. Alexandria, Va.: Douglass Publishers.

Harris, D. V., and Jennings, S. E. 1977. Self-perceptions of female distance runners. *Annals of the New York Academy of Sciences* 301:808–15.

Harris, M. B. 1981. Women runners' views of running. *Perceptual and Motor Skills* 53:395–402.

Hendricks, G., and Carlson, J. 1982. *The centered athlete: A conditioning program for your mind.* Englewood Cliffs, N.J.: Prentice-Hall.

Henschen, K. P.; Edwards, S. W.; and Mathinos, L. 1982. Achievement motivation and sex-role orientation of high school female track and field athletes versus nonathletes. *Perceptual and Motor Skills* 55:183–87.

Hilyer, J. C., Jr., and Mitchell, W. 1979. Effect of systematic physical fitness training combined with counseling on the self-concept of college students. *Journal of Counseling Psychology* 26:427–36.

Hilyer, J. C.; Wilson, D. G.; Dillon, C.; Caro, L.; Jenkins, C.; Spencer, W. A.; Meadows, M. E.; and Booker, W. 1982. Physical fitness training and counseling as treatment for youthful offenders. *Journal of Counseling Psychology* 29:292–303.

Hollandsworth, J. G., Jr. 1979. Some thoughts on distance running as training in biofeedback. *Journal of Sport Behavior* 2:71–82.

Hollandsworth, J. G., Jr., and Jones, G. E. 1979. Perceptions of arousal and awareness of physiological responding prior to and after running 20 kilometers. *Journal of Sport Psychology* 1:291–300.

Holmes, D. S.; Solomon, S.; and Rump, B. S. 1982. Cardiac and subjective response to cognitive challenge and to controlled physical exercise by male and female coronary prone (Type A) and non-coronary prone persons. *Journal of Psychosomatic Research* 26:309–16.

Jasnoski, M. L., and Holmes, D. S. 1981. Influence of initial aerobic fitness, aerobic training and changes in aerobic fitness on personality functioning. *Journal of Psychosomatic Research* 25:553–56.

Jasnoski, M. L.; Holmes, D. S.; Solomon, S.; and Aguiar, C. 1981. Exercise, changes in aerobic capacity, and changes in self-perceptions: An experimental investigation. *Journal of Research in Personality* 15:460–66.

Joseph, P., and Robbins, J. M. 1981. Worker or runner? The impact of commitment to running and work on self identification. In *Psychology of running,* ed. M. H. Sacks and M. L. Sachs. Champaign, Ill.: Human Kinetics Publishers.

Keefe, F. J., and Blumenthal, J. A. 1980. The life fitness program: A behavioral approach to making exercise a habit. *Journal of Behavioral Therapy and Experimental Psychiatry* 11:31–34.

Kostrubala, T. 1976. *The joy of running.* Philadelphia: J. B. Lippincott.

Lance, L. M., and Antshel, D. 1981. Social factors associated with adoption of running as a sport innovation. *International Review of Sport Sociology* 16:79–86.

Ledwidge, B. 1980. Run for your mind: Aerobic exercise as a means of alleviating anxiety and depression. *Canadian Journal of Behavioral Science* 12:126–40.

Levin, S. J. 1982. Running: An adjunctive group therapy technique. *Group* 6:27–34.

Lichtman, S., and Poser, E. G. 1983. The effects of exercise on mood and cognitive functioning. *Journal of Psychosomatic Research* 27:43–52.

Lilliefors, J. 1978. *The running mind.* Mountain View, Calif.: World Publications.

Lion, L. S. 1978. Psychological effects of jogging: A preliminary study. *Perceptual and Motor Skills* 47:1215–18.

Little, J. C. 1969. The athlete's neurosis: A deprivation crisis. *Acta Psychiatrica Scandinavica* 45:187–97.

Lobstein, D. D.; Mosbacher, B. J.; and Ismail, A. H. 1983. Depression as a powerful discriminator between physically active and sedentary middle-aged men. *Journal of Psychosomatic Research* 27:69–76.

Luce, S. C.; Delquadri, J.; and Hall, R. V. 1980. Contingent exercise: A mild but powerful procedure for suppressing inappropriate verbal and aggressive behavior. *Journal of Applied Behavior Analysis* 13:583–94.

McCutcheon, L. E., and Hassani, K. H. 1981. Running away from illness. *Journal of Sport Behavior* 4:151–56.

Martin, J. E., and Dubbert, P. M. 1982. Exercise applications and promotion in behavioral medicine: Current status and future directions. *Journal of Consulting and Clinical Psychology* 50:1004–17.

Milvy, P., ed. 1977. The marathon: Physiological, medical, epidemiological, and psychological studies. *Annals of the New York Academy of Sciences,* vol. 301.

Morgan, R. L., and Hiebert, R. 1982. The changing-criterion design: Assessment of running behavior of a handicapped youth. *Psychological Reports* 50:1287–93.

Morgan, W. P. 1973. Influence of acute physical activity on state anxiety. *Proceedings, National College Physical Education Association for Men,* 76th annual meeting.

———. 1977. Involvement in vigorous physical activity with special reference to adherence. *Proceedings of the NCPEAM/NAPECW National Conference.*

———. 1979. Negative addiction in runners. *Physician and Sportsmedicine* 7(2):56–63, 67–70.

———. 1980. Psychological benefits of physical activity. In *Exercise, health and disease,* ed. F. J. Nagle and H. J. Montoye. Springfield, Ill.: Charles C Thomas.

Morgan, W. P., and Pollock, M. L. 1977. Psychologic characterization of the elite distance runner. *Annals of the New York Academy of Sciences* 301:382–403.

Muller, B., and Armstrong, H. E. 1975. A further note on the "running treatment" for anxiety. *Psychotherapy: Theory, Research, and Practice* 12:385–87.

Nash, J. E. 1979. Weekend racing as an eventful experience: Understanding the accomplishment of well-being. *Urban Life* 8:199–217.

Orwin, A. 1973. "The running treatment": A preliminary communication on a new use for an old treatment (physical activity) in the agoraphobic syndrome. *British Journal of Psychiatry* 122:175–79.

———. 1974. Treatment of a situational phobia: A case for running. *British Journal of Psychiatry* 125:95–98.

Pargman, D. 1980. The way of the runner: An examination of motives for running. In

*Psychology in sports: Methods and applications,* ed. R. M. Suinn. Minneapolis: Burgess.

Peele, S. 1981. *How much is too much: Healthy habits or destructive addictions.* Englewood Cliffs, N.J.: Prentice-Hall.

Pennebaker, J. W., and Lightner, J. M. 1980. Competition of internal and external information in an exercise setting. *Journal of Personality and Social Psychology* 39:165–74.

Perry, S. W., III, and Sacks, M. H. 1981. The psychodynamics of running. In *Psychology of running,* ed. M. H. Sacks and M. L. Sachs. Champaign, Ill.: Human Kinetics Publishers.

Prosser, G.; Carson, P.; Phillips, R.; Gelson, A.; Buch, N.; Tucker, H.; Neophytou, M.; Lloyd, M.; and Simpson, T. 1981. Morale in coronary patients following an exercise programme. *Journal of Psychosomatic Research* 25:587–93.

Ransford, C. P. 1982. A role for amines in the antidepressant effect of exercise: A review. *Medicine and Science in Sports and Exercise* 14:1–10.

Reilly, T. 1977. Pre-start moods of cross-country runners and their relationship to performance. *International Journal of Sport Psychology* 8:210–17.

Renfrow, N. E., and Bolton, B. 1979. Personality characteristics associated with aerobic exercise in adult males. *Journal of Personality Assessment* 43:261–66.

Rindskopf, K. D., and Gratch, S. E. 1983. Women and exercise: A therapeutic approach. *Women and Therapy* 1(4).

Robbins, J. M., and Joseph, P. 1980. Commitment to running: Implications for the family and work. *Sociological Symposium,* no. 30:87–108.

Roth, W. T. 1974. Some motivational aspects of exercise. *Journal of Sports Medicine and Physical Fitness* 14:40–47.

Sachs, M. L. 1981. Running therapy for the depressed client. *Topics in Clinical Nursing* 3(2):77–86.

———. 1982. Change agents in the psychology of running. In *Sports medicine, sports science: Bridging the gap,* ed. R. C. Cantu and W. J. Gillespie. Lexington, Mass.: Collamore Press.

Sachs, M. L., and Pargman, D. 1979. Running addiction: A depth interview examination. *Journal of Sport Behavior* 2:143–55.

Sacks, M. H. 1981. Running addiction: A clinical report. In *Psychology of running,* ed. M. H. Sacks and M. L. Sachs. Champaign, Ill.: Human Kinetics Publishers.

Sacks, M. H.; Milvy, P.; Perry, S. W., III; and Sherman, L. 1981. Mental status and psychological coping during a one hundred-mile race. In *Psychology of running,* ed. M. H. Sacks and M. L. Sachs. Champaign, Ill.: Human Kinetics Publishers.

Sacks, M. H., and Sachs, M. L., eds. 1981. *Psychology of running.* Champaign, Ill.: Human Kinetics Publishers.

Schwartz, G. E.; Davidson, R. J.; and Goleman, D. J. 1978. Patterning of cognitive and somatic processes in the self-regulation of anxiety: Effects of meditation versus exercise. *Psychosomatic Medicine* 40:321–28.

Sinyor, D.; Brown, T.; Rostant, L.; and Seraganian, P. 1982. The role of a physical fitness program in the treatment of alcoholism. *Journal of Studies on Alcohol* 43:380–86.

Solomon, E. G., and Bumpus, A. K. 1978. The running meditation response: An adjunct to psychotherapy. *American Journal of Psychotherapy* 32:583–92.

Sonstroem, R. J. 1982. Exercise and self-esteem: Recommendations for expository research. *Quest* 33(2):124–39.

Sours, J. A. 1981. Running, anorexia nervosa, and perfection. In *Psychology of running,* ed. M. H. Sacks and M. L. Sachs. Champaign, Ill.: Human Kinetics Publishers.

Spino, M. 1976. *Beyond jogging: The inner spaces of running.* New York: Berkeley.

Summers, J. J.; Sargent, G. I.; Levey, A. J.; and Murray, K. D. 1982. Middle-aged, non-elite marathon runners: A profile. *Perceptual and Motor Skills* 54:963–69.

Thompson, C. E., and Wankel, L. M. 1980. The effects of perceived choice upon frequency of exercise behavior. *Journal of Applied Social Psychology* 10(5):436–43.

Tokunaga, M.; Tatano, H.; Hashimoto, K.; and Kanezaki, R. 1980. A study on behavioral intention, attitude and belief as the factors predicting sport behavior. II. Comparison on attributes between joggers and nonjoggers. *Journal of Health Science* 2:91–101.

Tu, J., and Rothstein, A. L. 1979. Improvement of jogging performance through application of personality specific motivational techniques. *Research Quarterly* 50:97–103.

Turner, R. D.; Pooly, S.; and Sherman, A. R. 1976. A behavioral approach to individualized exercise programming. In *Counseling methods,* ed. J. D. Krumboltz, and C. E. Thoresen. New York: Holt, Rinehart and Winston.

Valliant, P. M. 1980. Injury and personality traits in noncompetitive runners. *Journal of Sports Medicine and Physical Fitness* 20:341–46.

Valliant, P. M.; Bennie, F. A. B.; and Valiant, J. J. 1981. Do marathoners differ from joggers in personality profile: A sports psychology approach. *Journal of Sports Medicine and Physical Fitness* 21:62–67.

Vernacchia, R. A. 1977. Humanistic research for the sport psychologist: The case profile approach. *Canadian Journal of Applied Sports Sciences* 2:105–8.

Wankel, L. M., and Thompson, C. 1977. Motivating people to be physically active: Self-persuasion vs. balanced decision making. *Journal of Applied Social Psychology* 7:332–40.

Wilson, V. E.; Berger, B. G.; and Bird, E. I. 1981. Effects of running and of an exercise class on anxiety. *Perceptual and Motor Skills* 53:472–74.

Wilson, V. E.; Morley, N. C.; and Bird, E. I. 1980. Mood profiles of marathon runners, joggers and non-exercisers. *Perceptual and Motor Skills* 50:117–18.

Yates, A.; Leehey, K.; and Shisslak, C. M. 1983. Running: An analogue of anorexia? *New England Journal of Medicine* 308 (3 February): 251–55.

Young, R. J. 1979. The effect of regular exercise on cognitive functioning and personality. *British Journal of Sports Medicine* 13:110–17.

Zarski, J. J.; West, J. D.; and Bubenzer, D. L. 1982. Social interest, running, and life
adjustment. *Personnel and Guidance Journal* 61(3):146–49.

Zimmerman, J. D., and Fulton, M. 1981. Aerobic fitness and emotional arousal: A
critical attempt at replication. *Psychological Reports* 48:911–18.

*Bonnie G. Berger*, Ed.D., is professor and director of the sport psychology laboratory at Brooklyn College of the City University of New York.

*Gary W. Buffone*, Ph.D., is a psychologist in private practice and a consulting psychologist at Riverside Hospital in Jacksonville, Florida.

*Richard A. Dienstbier*, Ph.D., is a professor of psychology at the University of Nebraska at Lincoln.

*E. Thomas Dowd*, Ph.D., is an associate professor of counseling psychology at the University of Nebraska at Lincoln.

*Roger R. Eischens*, M.S., is a running therapist with the Department of Psychiatry at the University of Wisconsin at Madison.

*John H. Greist*, M.D., is a professor of psychiatry at the University of Wisconsin at Madison.

*Frederick D. Harper*, Ph.D., is a professor of psychoeducational studies at Howard University.

*Thaddeus Kostrubala*, M.D., is program chief in the Humboldt County Community Mental Health Services, Eureka, California.

*David Pargman*, Ph.D., is a professor of movement science and physical education at Florida State University.

*Michael L. Sachs*, Ph.D., is a research project coordinator with the Department of Pediatrics, University of Maryland School of Medicine, Baltimore.

*Michael H. Sacks*, M.D., is an associate professor of psychiatry at Cornell University Medical College, New York City.

*W. Mark Shipman*, M.D., F.A.P.A., is an assistant clinical professor of psychiatry at the University of California at San Diego.

*Barry B. Shultz*, Ph.D., is an associate professor of physical education at the University of Utah.

*John M. Silva*, Ph.D., is an assistant professor of physical education at the University of North Carolina at Chapel Hill.

*Jaylene Summers*, Ph.D., is a psychotherapist in private practice in Kennebunkport, Maine.

*Henry Wolstat*, M.D., F.A.P.A., is a psychiatrist in private practice in Portsmouth, New Hampshire.

# Index